The Neurophysiological Foundations of Mental and Motor Imagery

The Neurophysiological Foundations of Mental and Motor Imagery

Edited by

Aymeric Guillot
Centre de recherche et d'innovation
sur le Sport, Equipe Performance Motrice,
Mentale et du Matériel (P3M)
Université Claude Bernard Lyon1
France

Christian Collet
Centre de recherche et d'innovation sur le Sport,
Equipe Performance Motrice,
Mentale et du Matériel (P3M)
Université Claude Bernard Lyon1
France

OXFORD
UNIVERSITY PRESS

OXFORD
UNIVERSITY PRESS

Great Clarendon Street, Oxford OX2 6DP

Oxford University Press is a department of the University of Oxford.
It furthers the University's objective of excellence in research, scholarship,
and education by publishing worldwide in

Oxford New York

Auckland Cape Town Dar es Salaam Hong Kong Karachi
Kuala Lumpur Madrid Melbourne Mexico City Nairobi
New Delhi Shanghai Taipei Toronto

With offices in

Argentina Austria Brazil Chile Czech Republic France Greece
Guatemala Hungary Italy Japan Poland Portugal Singapore
South Korea Switzerland Thailand Turkey Ukraine Vietnam

Oxford is a registered trade mark of Oxford University Press
in the UK and in certain other countries

Published in the United States
by Oxford University Press Inc., New York

British Library Cataloguing in Publication Data
Data available

Library of Congress Cataloging in Publication Data
Data available

Typeset in Minion by Glyph International, Banglore, India
Printed in Great Britain
on acid-free paper by the
MPG Books Group, Bodmin and King's Lynn

ISBN 978–0–19–954625–1

10 9 8 7 6 5 4 3 2 1

Oxford University Press makes no representation, express or implied, that the drug dosages in this book
are correct. Readers must therefore always check the product information and clinical procedures with the
most up-to-date published product information and data sheets provided by the manufacturers and the most
recent codes of conduct and safety regulations. The authors and the publishers do not accept responsibility
or legal liability for any errors in the text or for the misuse or misapplication of material in this work. Except
where otherwise stated, drug dosages and recommendations are for the non-pregnant adult who is not
breastfeeding.

Preface

Mental motor imagery is a fascinating phenomenon. Yet, contrary to visual imagery, which has been on the forefront of neurological and psychological research for decades, motor imagery seems to have been somewhat neglected until recently. Already at the end of the nineteenth century, Alfred Binet considered that what he called the 'motor type' of mental imagery was 'perhaps the most interesting of all, and certainly the one of which least is known' At that time, however, the dominant explanation for all types of mental imagery, including the motor one, was that they were of a sensory nature. William James in the chapter *Imagination* of his famous *Principles of Psychology* discussed the issue of whether motor imagery was a 'resuscitated feeling' arising in the body parts that had been influenced by prior movements. Forming the mental image of an object, for example, involved not only its visual features, but also cues acquired during the motor exploration of that object. To James, sensation and imagination were closely related phenomena.

It is not until the 1980s that the true motor nature of motor imagery was fully recognized. This move was a noted contribution of sport psychologists, who had understood the potential importance of motor imagery for training and rehearsing motor performance in athletes. The first systematic laboratory experiments, using the introspective method for exploring the content of motor images in normal subjects, clearly confirmed this view. The parameters of the imagined action, which could be extracted from these introspective reports, revealed its striking similarity with the same action when it was performed, up to the point where 'mental kinematics' of an action appeared to closely match its physical kinematics. This discovery was soon supported by neuroimaging studies showing a similar involvement of the motor system in the two modalities.

One of the major issues to be addressed in this book will be to explore the boundaries of the phenomenon of motor imagery. Is the term 'imagery', widely used among the people who study this phenomenon, still appropriate? An image refers to a conscious mental state which can be voluntarily controlled by the subject: any of us can quickly generate the bodily sensations of running or swimming, for example. In fact, it is now widely accepted that the phenomenon extends far beyond what can be consciously elicited. Firstly, the conscious content of an imagined action is paralleled by non-conscious neurophysiological changes, notably in the autonomic nervous system where they have been extensively studied by A. Guillot and C. Collet, the two co-editors of this book. Secondly, the notion of motor imagery should also include those many situations in everyday life where an action remains covert, but is non-consciously 'simulated' by the motor system. Examples of such situations are: evaluating the feasibility of an action, observing tools, hearing action verbs, observing somebody acting. Although not accompanied by conscious images, they all have in common to activate the motor system to the same extent as during classically understood motor imagery. The inclusion of these states of action simulation within the realm of motor imagery considerably extends the functional relevance of this phenomenon, for both motor behaviour and motor cognition.

Clearly defining the resemblances and dissimilarities of covert (simulated) and overt (executed) actions thus should be another important outcome of this book. This point is obviously critical when practical issues are considered. Following its use in elite sport practice, the potential impact of motor imagery on domains, like skill learning and motor rehabilitation, has raised considerable interest.

Not only do music performers and dancers consistently use mental rehearsal as part of their training, but mental rehearsal is now included in rehabilitation procedures for patients suffering from pathological motor impairments and associated troubles, like phantom pain, for example. Yet, we know that activation of the motor system during motor imagery is not identical to that during motor execution: the distribution of activity in the two modalities only partially overlaps, with cortical and cerebellar zones of activation specific for each of them; the activity within motor cortex is weaker during imagery than during execution. These differences might become critical for extending the practice of mental rehearsal to other domains, like brain/computer interfacing. Using cortical activity for moving a prosthetic arm, for example, should imply that the information picked up for signal processing is compatible with action execution. The fact that the activity generated by the motor cortex during the mental representation of an action is weaker, and also possibly coarser, than during execution of that action, is a potential difficulty for these techniques.

The two editors have succeeded in compiling contributions from the most representative research groups in this rapidly expanding field. The neural and physiological aspects of mental imagery are discussed in the first two sections. The first section, mostly based on the contribution of neuroimaging studies, is devoted to the cortical involvement during imagery in the perceptual and the motor domains; the second section deals with functional correlates of motor imagery, such as EEG changes or changes at the level of effectors like muscles and autonomic system, which are essential for identifying the content of these mental states. The other two sections are devoted to more practical applications of motor imagery. Not surprisingly, the section on the role of motor imagery in rehabilitation is the most important in terms of the number of contributions. This extensive coverage reflects the level of expectation and hope among clinicians for improving recovery after lesions of the central nervous system. Finally, the last section on motor imagery and learning processes is possibly the most open to future developments, for improving the efficiency of mental training in the acquisition of new skills.

Pr. M. Jeannerod (MD)
Past director of the Cognitive Sciences Institute (Lyon, France)
Member of the French Scientific Academy

Contents

Contributors

Amélie M. Achim
Centre de recherche Université Laval
Robert-Giffard, Québec,
Canada

Christian Collet
Centre de Recherche et d'innovation
sur le sport,
Equipe Performance Motrice,
Mentale et du Matériel (P3M),
Université Claude Bernard Lyon1,
UFR STAPS,
France

Jennifer Cumming
School of Sport and Exercise Sciences,
College of Life and Environmental Sciences,
University of Birmingham,
UK

Ursula Debarnot
Centre de Recherche et d'innovation
sur le sport,
Equipe Performance Motrice,
Mentale et du Matériel (P3M),
Université Claude Bernard Lyon1,
France

Ruth Dickstein
Department of Physical Therapy,
Faculty of Social Welfare and Health Sciences,
University of Haifa,
Israel

Chris H. Dijkerman
Experimental Psychology,
Helmholtz Institute,
Utrecht University,
The Netherlands

Julien Doyon
Department of Psychology
Functional Neuroimaging Unit,
University of Montreal Geriatric Institute,
Québec,
Canada

Martin G. Edwards
School of Sport and Exercise Sciences,
College of Life and Environmental Sciences,
University of Birmingham,
UK

Giorgio Ganis
Massachusetts General Hospital and
Harvard Medical School
Boston, MA,
USA

Aymeric Guillot
Centre de recherche et d'innovation
sur le sport, Equipe Performance Motrice,
Mentale et du Matériel (P3M),
Université Claude Bernard Lyon1,
UFR STAPS,
France

Paul S. Holmes
Research Institute for Health
and Social Change,
Manchester Metropolitan University,
Alsager,
UK

Luís Aureliano Imbiriba
Laboratory of Biomechanics,
School of Physical Education,
Federal University of Rio de Janeiro,
Rio de Janeiro,
Brazil

Nady Hoyek
Centre de Recherche et d'innovation
sur le sport,
Equipe Performance Motrice,
Mentale et du Matériel (P3M),
Université Claude Bernard Lyon1,
France

Magdalena Ietswaart
School of Psychology and Sport Sciences,
University of Northumbria,
UK

Philip L. Jackson
École de Psychologie, Laval University,
Center for Interdisciplinary Research in
Rehabilitation and Social Integration
and Centre de recherche Robert-Giffard,
Québec,
Canada

Sylvia B. Joffily
Laboratory of Cognition and Language,
State University of The North Fluminense
Darcy Ribeiro of Campos dos Goytacazes,
Rio de Janeiro,
Brazil

Marie Johnston
Health Psychology Research Group,
School of Psychology,
University of Aberdeen,
UK

Stephen M. Kosslyn
Psychology Department,
Harvard University,
Cambridge,
USA

Florent Lebon
Centre de Recherche et d'innovation
sur le sport,
Equipe Performance Motrice,
Mentale et du Matériel (P3M),
Université Claude Bernard Lyon1,
France

Martin Lotze
Functional Imaging Unit Centre of
Diagnostic Radiology and Neuroradiology,
University of Greifswald,
Germany

Magali Louis
Centre de Recherche et d'innovation
sur le sport,
Equipe Performance Motrice,
Mentale et du Matériel (P3M),
Université Claude Bernard Lyon1,
France

Tadhg MacIntyre
School of Sports Studies,
University of Ulster,
Newtownabbey,
UK

Francine Malouin
Department of Rehabilitation, Laval
University and Center for Interdisciplinary
Research in Rehabilitation and
Social Integration,
Québec,
Canada

Emmanuel Mellet
Ci-NAPS, UMR 6232,
CEA, CNRS,
Universités de Caen et Paris Descartes,
GIP Cyceron,
Boulevard Henri Becquerel,
France

Aidan Moran
School of Psychology
University College Dublin
Newman Building
Belfield,
Dublin
Ireland

Christa Neuper
Department of Psychology,
University of Graz,
Austria

Stephen J. Page
Departments of Rehabilitation Sciences,
Physical Medicine and Rehabilitation,
Neurology, and Neurosciences,
University of Cincinnati
Academic Medical Center,
Cincinnati, OH;
Director, Neuromotor Recovery and
Rehabilitation laboratory,
Drake Center,
Cincinnati, OH
USA

Laurent Petit
Ci-NAPS, UMR 6232,
Groupe d'Imagerie Neurofonctionnelle,
CEA, CNRS,
Universités de Caen et Paris Descartes
GIP Cyceron,
Boulevard Henri Becquerel,
France

Gert Pfurtscheller
Institute for Knowledge Discovery,
BCI Laboratory,
Graz University of Technology,
Krenngasse, Graz
Austria

Nicolas Poirel
Ci-NAPS, UMR 6232,
Groupe d'Imagerie Neurofonctionnelle,
CEA, CNRS,
Universités de Caen et Paris Descartes
GIP Cyceron,
Boulevard Henri Becquerel,
France

Carol L. Richards
Department of Rehabilitation,
Laval University and Center for
Interdisciplinary Research in Rehabilitation
and Social Integration,
Québec,
Canada

Erika Carvalho Rodrigues
Laboratory of Neurobiology II,
Institute of Biophysics Carlos Chagas Filho,
Federal University of Rio de Janeiro,
Rio de Janeiro,
Brazil

Rebecca G. Rogers
Midwifery Division,
Department of Obstetrics and Gynecology,
University of New Mexico,
Albuquerque,
USA

Robert E. Sapien
Department of Emergency Medicine,
University of New Mexico Health
Sciences Center,
University of New Mexico, Albuquerque,
USA

Cathy M. Stinear
Neurology Research Group,
Department of Medicine,
Faculty of Medical and Health Sciences,
University of Auckland, Auckland,
New Zealand

Ruth Tamir
Department of Physical Therapy,
Faculty of Social Welfare and Health Sciences,
University of Haifa, Mount Carmel, Haifa,
Israel

William L. Thompson
Department of Psychology,
Harvard University,
Cambridge, MA,
USA

Claudia D. Vargas
Laboratory of Neurobiology II,
Institute of Biophysics Carlos Chagas Filho,
Federal University of Rio de Janeiro,
Rio de Janeiro
Brazil

Laure Zago
Ci-NAPS, UMR 6232,
Groupe d'Imagerie Neurofonctionnelle,
CEA, CNRS,
Universités de Caen et Paris Descartes
GIP Cyceron,
Boulevard Henri Becquerel,
France

Karen Zentgraf
Bender Institute of Neuroimaging,
Giessen University, Germany and
Institute of Sports Science,
University of Bern,
Switzerland

Introduction

Mental imagery is probably, among others, one of the more sophisticated operations allowed by the human brain abilities. Forming mental images of things or events is a self-power that can prepare the individual to act properly in the environment. It is also the way to build your own world, to transform the existing world by letting your thoughts imagining what your will wants. Mental imagery has no limit because the human brain imagination has no limit.

Motor imagery is more often used when the human body is involved, hence requiring the individual to imagine the body as the generator of acting forces and not only the effects of these forces on the external world (Jeannerod 1994). Imagery experience is understood as evocation, copy, or reconstruction of actual perceptual experience from the past. At other times, each of us may anticipate possible or forthcoming events through imagery as a function of what they are awaiting for. Understanding the neural correlates of goal-directed action, whether executed or imagined, has been an important aim in the field of cognitive brain research since the advent of functional imaging studies. Since the earliest studies at the end of the eighties, providing evidence of the brain activity that accompanies the mental representation of movement, much progress has been made in this area of research. Practical implications have also emerged from these studies. For instance, the use of mental practice including motor imagery in the rehabilitation of patients with cerebral motor impairments is currently one of the most actual growing topics in the field of imagery research. Such data provide evidence for imagery as an original method in stroke rehabilitation, a reliable help in cerebral reconstruction by neural networks stimulation, and thus to functional recovery due to cerebral plasticity. Recent data also suggest that different types of imagery, for example visual or kinaesthetic, are mediated through separate neural systems, and, thus, can contribute differently to motor (re)learning and neurological rehabilitation. Despite these converging assumptions, several intensive debates have emerged, thus revealing unresolved issues. Now is the time to draw up a review of the scientific state in this field of research, both from theoretical and applied viewpoints.

This book is designed to consider four main aspects of mental/motor imagery. In the first part, we aim to gather articles related to the neural basis of mental and motor imagery, as well as papers focusing on the relationships between mental imagery and perception, on the one hand, and motor imagery and physical execution, on the other. The second part is devised to collect data referring to the evaluation of imagery accuracy, including both central and peripheral nervous system recordings. In the third part, we adopt a different viewpoint by examining in some detail the effectiveness of mental practice on motor recovery after stroke, while the last section is focused on the imagery-related effects on learning processes.

All chapters are written by internationally or nationally well-known experts in the imagery research area. The book includes 19 chapters and discusses theories, experimental research, and clinical applications. We express our deepest appreciation to all contributors for their fine work in spite of the short deadlines they had been given. We further cordially thank the staff of Oxford University Press, and particularly Martin Baum and Charlotte Green for their patience and guidance throughout the project. A special word of gratitude goes to Stephen Kosslyn for his help during the project initiation phase. Finally, we are very grateful to Marc Jeannerod, who is a worldwide authority on this research area and has been a pioneer in the motor imagery topic, and are honoured that he accepted writing the preface of this book. Below is a general overview of each section.

Section 1: Neural substrate of mental and motor imagery

In the first chapter, S.M. Kosslyn, G. Ganis, and W.L. Thompson review the main results of the neuroimaging experiments that have investigated the neural underpinning of mental imagery and its comparison with visual perception. Specifically, visual imagery, as well as auditory and motor imagery, are considered. They also focus on a new research area, the use of imagery in stimulating the social world.

The second chapter by N. Poirel, L. Zago, L. Petit, and E. Mellet summarizes the experiments that have contributed to document the functional and structural similarities between mental images and the perceptual events from which they were formed. Especially, the authors consider the neural substrate mediating mental navigation and mental exploration following different modes of perceptual learning. The first part of the chapter describes the core network of topographical representations, while the second part examines the importance of the nature of the information which is used to form the mental images.

The book will then focus on the individual ability to imagine the physical execution of an action, i.e. to consider the body as a generator of acting forces. Neuroimaging results are described by M. Lotze and K. Zentgraf in the third chapter by integrating a discussion on the structural equivalence between motor imagery and motor execution. This chapter shows that motor imagery and motor execution share many anatomical substrates but are not completely overlapping, especially when sensorial cues on which motor imagery is constructed are considered. The central question of the contribution of the primary motor cortex to motor imagery forms the heart of this section, as some conflicting results have rendered this question somewhat unresolved.

The fourth chapter by C. Stinear is devised to investigate whether motor imagery may facilitate corticospinal activity in the areas corresponding to the muscles involved in the imagined movement. Again, neuroimaging data provide evidence that the increase in brain activity is specific to the representation of the body part whose movement is imagined. Interestingly, this section demonstrates that the facilitation of corticospinal excitability during motor imagery is associated with specific reductions in intracortical inhibition.

Section 2: Neurophysiological correlates of motor imagery

In the first chapter of this section, C. Neuper and G. Pfurtscheller describe and illustrate the electroencephalographic changes following motor imagery practice. Specifically, the sensorimotor activation and deactivation through event-related (de)synchronization pattern recordings are considered. The authors demonstrate that measuring the neuronal activity with high temporal resolution brings researchers a reliable tool to study the time-course of short-lasting changes of neuronal activity in distinct time windows before, during and after motor imagery. Finally, they specifically examine the effectiveness of using multimodal techniques (e.g. combining functional magnetic resonance imagery and electroencephalography) to study the neuronal processes engaged in motor imagery.

In the second chapter, A. Guillot, F. Lebon and C. Collet consider a topic of research that has received inconsistent results, hence resulting in interesting, but opposite, insights into the nature of motor imagery. The first part of the chapter therefore reviews the papers highlighting the lack of muscular activity during motor imagery of an effortful movement, supporting the central explanation of motor imagery. In contrast, the second part provides evidence that motor imagery may be accompanied by a subliminal electromyographic activity, and that the nature of this muscular activity may differ as a function of muscle contraction and load constraints related to movement characteristics. The authors then discuss these inconsistent findings, with particular attention on the neural origin of these peripheral changes and the inhibition of the action during imagined movements.

The third chapter by C. Collet and A. Guillot is devised to review the experimental studies investigating motor imagery through the recording of the autonomic nervous system activity. This section further outlines the goals and methods of such peripheral recordings in studying mental processes. In addition, the authors discuss how the motor commands sent to the autonomic effectors are facilitated during motor imagery, whereas the direct voluntary commands transmitted through the pyramidal tract are, at least partially, inhibited.

In reference to recent experimental data, the last chapter of this section by A. Guillot, M. Louis, and C. Collet shows whether motor imagery accuracy and vividness may be estimated using a set of several indicators, psychological, behavioural and physiological recordings. This discussion will be hooked into other approaches of the previous chapter. More generally, the authors consider whether the different neurophysiological methods may be combined to evaluate the individual ability to form accurate mental images.

Section 3: Motor imagery in rehabilitation

In the first chapter of this section, H.C. Dijkerman, M. Ietswaart, and M. Johnston provide an overview on how motor imagery can be helpful in the rehabilitation of patients. Accordingly, they primarily focus on the behavioural and kinematic effects of imagery following neurologic disorders. The aim is to understand how to select groups of patients that could benefit from a therapeutic approach using motor imagery and why motor imagery may be helpful during the different stages of the rehabilitation process. How to integrate motor imagery into classical rehabilitation programmes, as well as data regarding the appropriate delivery and dosing of mental practice, are then considered, to ascertain the efficiency of this technique during the rehabilitation process.

The second chapter by S.J. Page focuses more extensively on the neuroimaging studies dealing with motor imagery and neurorehabilitation. The chapter is primarily focused on the functional relation of imagery to hemiparesis. The discussion further highlights the basic principles of plasticity, followed by the promise of motor imagery for hemiparesis recovery.

The aim of the third chapter is to provide evidence of the effectiveness of mental practice during motor recovery of gait and locomotor skills. Especially, F. Malouin, C.L. Richards, P. Jackson, and J. Doyon review the use of imagery during rehabilitation, as well as the specific findings that provide the rationale for the use of motor imagery as a tool for improving locomotor skills after stroke.

In this and in all subsequent chapters, one central purpose is to describe how to select groups of patients that could benefit from a therapeutic approach including motor imagery. In the chapter, R. Dickstein and R. Tamir consider that motor imagery is impaired in patients with Parkinson's disease. Specifically, they review literature to determine whether similar or distinct neural networks are recruited during motor imagery in patients with Parkinson's disease and healthy individuals. They also examine the effectiveness of using motor imagery during motor rehabilitation, as well as the effect of surgical treatments on motor imagery in patients with Parkinson's disease.

The next chapter by L.A. Imbiriba, S.B. Joffily, E.C. Rodrigues, and C.D. Vargas focuses on the use of mental and/or motor imagery in patients with early and late onset blindness. A review of literature indicates that blind people are able to form mental images, even though they do not use the same strategies than sighted people. Further, the authors discuss whether early and late blind subjects make use of distinct body representation during motor imagery. The question of how blind patients keep the ability to form mental image is of particular interest.

In the last chapter by G. Pfurtscheller and C. Neuper, the brain/computer used to drive robots from the brain activity during imagined actions is considered, as it opens new possibilities for helping patients with various forms of paralysis. In particular, the authors demonstrate that motor imagery is an efficient strategy to operate a brain–computer interface through the imagery-related encephalographic changes, classified in real time.

Section 4: Motor imagery in learning processes

The effects of motor imagery on performance and on motor skill learning are well-established. The chapter by A. Guillot, U. Debarnot, M. Louis, N. Hoyek, and C. Collet reviews the literature providing evidence that imagery may be used during the different stages of the motor learning process and that this technique may help to reach several different outcomes during the preparation phase preceding a competitive event.

The chapter by T. McIntyre and A. Moran investigates meta-imagery processes in elite sports performers. The nature and types of metacognition that have been postulated by the two researchers are first explored, before considering the metacognitive processes in athletes. Then, the section articulates some of the possible reasons for the neglect of meta-imagery and subsequently describes some preliminary investigations of meta-imagery processes in athletes. Finally, the authors consider the neglected role of meta-imagery processes in current theoretical models of imagery processes in athletes.

An original chapter by R.E. Sapien and R.G. Rogers will be devised to explore the potential role of mental and/or motor imagery during the acquisition of surgical skills, i.e. training and maturation of surgeons. Hence, this chapter will review data showing that acquisition and performance of emergency procedure can be improved by the use of imagery, and the authors will provide some guidelines for the implementation of imagery in surgical procedures.

The fourth chapter of this section by P.S. Holmes, J. Cumming, and M.G. Edwards then reviews literature evidencing that motor imagery and observation can modulate skill. First, the neuroscientific processes thought to be involved in physical movement skill acquisition and modulation are considered. Then, the chapter reviews the case for movement imagery and observation, supporting change within the neuronal system through similar processes.

Finally, the last chapter by P. Jackson and A.M. Achim aims at understanding in greater details the role of imagery in social behaviours. Especially, the relationship between imagery and empathy, i.e. imagining how another person feels and how one would feel in a similar situation, will be considered.

Although many other subsections could have been approached, for example developmental and ageing processes, pathological aspects of motor imagery such as in schizophrenic patients, this book offers a complete survey of present knowledge related to recent theoretical findings and practical applications. One of the next challenges would probably be to better understand the processes of the motor command inhibition during motor imagery. Experimental investigation in patients with spinal cord stroke is perhaps the way to take to solve this important issue in fundamental as well as in applied research.

A . Guillot and C. Collet
Université Claude Bernard Lyon 1,
France … a country that you can easily mentally imagine in the south-west of Europe!
15 May 2009

Section 1

The neural substrates of mental and motor imagery

Chapter 1

Multimodal images in the brain

Stephen M. Kosslyn, Giorgio Ganis,
and William L. Thompson

Multimodal images in the brain

Mental imagery is like perceiving, but in the absence of an immediate appropriate sensory stimulation. As such, imagery is often identified with specific phenomenology, such as the experience of 'seeing with the mind's eye', 'hearing with the mind's ear', and so on. However, the experience itself is not the image; and, in fact, it is not even clear that mental images must always be accompanied by a specific experience. Rather, mental images consist of internal representations of the same types as those that arise during the early phases of like-modality perception. Mental images are internal representations that are based on information stored in memory. In contrast, perception occurs when information is registered directly from the senses.

This conception of mental imagery leads us to characterize many sorts of imagery. First, each perceptual modality should, in principle, be accompanied by the ability to generate images in that modality. And, in fact, people commonly report visual, auditory, and kinaesthetic images (e.g., Kosslyn *et al.* 1990). Second, not all forms of imagery need give rise to distinct phenomenology. For example, spatial images may give rise to only the most impoverished sense of 'where things are'. Third, mental images need not be simply the recall of previously perceived objects or events; they also can be created by combining and modifying stored perceptual information in novel ways.

Mental imagery has played a central role in theories of mental function at least since the time of Plato. It has fallen in and out of fashion, in large part because it is inherently a private affair – by definition restricted to the confines of one's mind. (In this context, by 'mind' we mean brain function.) Thus, imagery has been difficult to study. In fact, in 1913 the founder of Behaviourism (the school of psychology that focused solely on observable stimuli, responses, and the consequences of responses), John B. Watson, denied that mental images even existed. Instead, he suggested, thinking consists of subtle movements of the vocal apparatus (Watson 1913).

Nevertheless, clever researchers developed empirical methods for studying imagery. Notably, Alan Pavio and his colleagues (see, for example, Paivio 1971) were able to show that the use of imagery dramatically improves memory. However, even in the face of such findings, some researchers were not convinced that imagery is a distinct form of thought. Indeed, Watson's position was echoed 60 years later by Zenon Pylyshyn, who championed the view that mental images are not 'images' at all, but rather rely on mental descriptions no different in kind from those that underlie language. According to Pylyshyn (1973), the pictorial aspects of imagery that are evident to conscious experience are entirely epiphenomenal, like the heat from a light bulb when you read (which plays no role in the reading process). That is, according to this descriptivist view, the fact that we experience visual images as akin to pictures in the mind's eye says nothing about the nature of the underlying mental representation.

The emergence of cognitive neuroscience has opened a new chapter in the study of mental imagery. An enormous amount has been learned about the neural underpinnings of visual perception, memory, emotion, and motor control. Much of this information has come from the study of animal models. Unlike language and reasoning, these more basic functions have many common features among higher mammals, including humans. In addition, neuroimaging technologies, especially positron emission tomography (PET) and functional magnetic resonance imaging (fMRI), have allowed theories of imagery to be tested objectively in humans. Researchers have taken advantage of these developments to show that mental imagery draws on much of the same neural machinery as perception in the same modality, and can engage mechanisms used in memory, emotion, and motor control.

In this chapter we draw on results from a variety of methods, including studies of the effects of selective brain damage on behaviour, neuroimaging, and studies examining the effects of transcranial magnetic stimulation (TMS). Each method has its strengths and weaknesses, but they are complementary. Thus, for example, neuroimaging provides only correlational data (when engaged in a particular task, a particular set of brain areas is activated) but can monitor the entire brain; TMS can be used to establish causal roles of distinct areas (e.g., by showing that performance in a task that draws on a specific brain area is impaired following TMS to that area), but must be targeted to a specific location. To the extent that the same conclusions are reached using different methods, these conclusions can be taken increasingly seriously.

We briefly review three main classes of research: evidence that imagery engages brain mechanisms that are used in perception and action; evidence that visual mental imagery engages even the earliest visual cortex (Areas 17 and 18); and evidence that imagery engages mechanisms that control physiological processes such as heart rate and breathing, having effects much like those that occur with the corresponding perceptual stimuli.

Mental imagery, perception, and action

We begin with visual imagery, which is by far the most intensively studied modality, and then turn to auditory and motor imagery.

Visual mental imagery

Well over 100 years ago, researchers described brain-damaged patients who had lost the ability to form visual mental images after they became blind (for review, see Farah 1984; however, see also Chatterjee and Southwood 1995). Methods from cognitive psychology have allowed researchers to characterize such deficits in imagery with increasing precision, typically by building on knowledge about perception. For example, some patients have perceptual deficits in only one of the two major cortical visual functions. One major visual pathway runs from the occipital lobe down to the inferior temporal lobes (the so-called 'object properties processing' pathway; see Ungerleider and Mishkin 1982). This pathway in turn can be broken down into two sub-pathways, which subserve shape and colour. Depending on the nature of brain damage, the animal or person cannot easily recognize shape or colour. The other major visual pathway runs from the occipital lobe to the posterior parietal lobes (the so-called 'spatial properties processing' pathway); when damaged, the animal or person cannot easily register location. As we summarize in the following, such detailed knowledge about perception has guided much research on imagery.

Imagery and perception

Typically, parallel deficits appear in mental imagery and perception: damage to the occipital-temporal pathway disrupts the ability to visualize shape (as used, for example, to recollect whether George Washington had a beard) and/or colour (as used, for example, to determine the colour of the inside of a cantaloupe), whereas damage to the occipital-parietal pathway disrupts the ability to visualize locations (as used, for example, to indicate the locations of furniture in a room when one's eyes are closed; see, for example, Levine *et al.* 1985). Indeed, very subtle deficits can occur in imagery that parallel the deficits found in perception. For example, some brain-damaged patients can no longer distinguish colours perceptually or in imagery (De Vreese 1991) and others can no longer distinguish faces perceptually or in imagery (Young *et al.* 1994).

However, although the deficits in imagery and perception often parallel each other, this is not always the case. In a seminal literature review and analysis, Farah (1984) showed that some patients have selective problems in generating visual mental images (i.e. producing them on the basis of information stored in long-term memory) even though they are able to recognize and identify comparable perceptual stimuli (for a review, see also Ganis *et al.* 2003). In addition, patients have been reported who could visualize but had impaired perception (e.g., Behrmann *et al.* 1992; Jankowiak *et al.* 1992). In short, the results from research with brain-damaged patients suggest that visual mental imagery and visual perception share many common mechanisms, but do not draw on identical processes. Although shape, location, and surface characteristics are represented and interpreted in comparable ways during both functions, the two differ in key ways: imagery, unlike perception, does not require low-level organizational processing; and perception, unlike imagery, does not require us to activate information in memory when the stimulus is not present (see Behrmann 2000).

The results of neuroimaging studies, that compare imagery and perception have dovetailed nicely with those from studies of brain-damaged patients (for a review, see Kosslyn and Thompson 2003). One study, for example, found that of all the brain areas activated during perception and imagery, approximately two-thirds were activated in common (Kosslyn *et al.* 1997). Another study reported that the amount of overlap is considerably greater, over 90 % (Ganis *et al.* 2004). But it is clear that imagery and perception do not activate identical neural systems. Presumably, lesions in the areas not activated in common produce the dissociations, where imagery or perception is disrupted independently; whereas lesions in the areas activated in common produce the more frequently reported parallel deficits in imagery and perception.

Structure of visual mental imagery

Finally, studies of deficits following brain damage have underscored the fact that 'imagery' – like all other cognitive functions – is not a single, undifferentiated ability. Rather, it is a collection of abilities, each of which can be disrupted independently. For example, some patients can make imagery judgements about the shape or colour of objects but have difficulty imagining an object rotating (e.g., when trying to decide whether the letter 'p' would be another letter when rotated 180°, or whether 'Z' would be another letter when rotated 90° clockwise). Other patients have the reverse pattern of deficits. Indeed, when participants perform different imagery tasks while their brain activity is monitored, different patterns of activation are observed while they process images in different ways. For example, when participants mentally rotate patterns, their parietal lobes (often bilaterally) and right frontal lobes typically are strongly activated (e.g., Cohen *et al.* 1996; Kosslyn *et al.* 1998; Richter *et al.* 2000; Jordan *et al.* 2001; Ng *et al.* 2001; for a review, see Zacks 2008). In contrast, if they are asked to visualize previously memorized patterns of stripes and judge which are longer, wider, and so on (all on the basis of their mental images, with eyes closed), these areas are not activated, but other areas in the occipital lobe and left association cortex are activated (Kosslyn *et al.* 1999; Thompson *et al.* 2001).

Depending on the precise task, different sets of processes are activated (O'Craven and Kanwisher 2000; Downing *et al.* 2006; Kanwisher and Yovel 2006). Indeed, brain activation during mental imagery may vary according to the type of object that is visualized. Using fMRI, O'Craven and Kanwisher (2000) found activation in the fusiform face area (FFA) when participants visualized faces. Conversely, when participants visualized indoor or outdoor scenes depicting a spatial layout, these researchers found activation in the parahippocampal place area (PPA). There was no hint of activation of the PPA during face imagery or of the FFA during place imagery. These results are similar to what was observed when participants actually perceived faces and places. The findings underscore that imagery and perception share very specific, specialized mechanisms.

Visual mental imagery and early visual cortex

A large portion of research on the neural bases of imagery focuses on whether early visual cortex is activated during imagery (for a review, see Kosslyn and Thompson 2003; Kosslyn *et al.* 2006.). Early visual cortex consists of Areas 17 and 18, the first two cortical areas to receive input from the eyes. Researchers have wanted to know whether visual imagery activates these early areas for three main reasons. First, these areas are known to be topographically organized; that is, they preserve (roughly) the local spatial geometry of the retina – and thus patterns of activation in them serve to depict shape. If these areas are activated during imagery, and such activation plays a functional role, this would be evidence that imagery relies on representations that depict information, not describe it. In other words, this would be evidence that mental imagery relies on actual images.

Second, such findings cannot be explained by appeal to 'tacit knowledge', which Pylyshyn (1981) used to explain away the findings from earlier behavioural experiments that attempted to demonstrate that imagery relies on depictive representations. According to this view, participants in imagery experiments may have unconsciously tried to imitate what they thought they would have done in the corresponding perceptual situation (such as by taking more time to scan farther distances across an imaged scene). But such tacit knowledge, stored as descriptions, would not explain why early visual cortex would be activated when participants had their eyes closed during imagery.

Third, if imagery can alter the activation of early visual cortex, this suggests that one's beliefs and expectations can (at least under some circumstances) modulate what one actually sees during perception. And this finding would have clear-cut implications for the reliability of eyewitness testimony and the veracity of visual memory, more generally.

More than 50 neuroimaging studies have examined activation in early visual cortex (for reviews, see Thompson and Kosslyn 2000; Kosslyn and Thompson 2003). The following studies seem to provide the strongest support for activation in early visual cortex during visual mental imagery. The participants had their eyes closed during all of the neuroimaging tasks, and thus activation of early visual cortex could not have been caused by seeing visual stimuli.

In one study (Kosslyn *et al.* 1995), participants were asked to visualize line drawings of objects at different sizes (as if they fit into different-sized boxes that were memorized before the PET scan). Not only was Area 17 activated, compared to a control condition in which identical auditory cues were provided but no imagery was used, but also the specific locus of activation depended on the size of the imaged object. Even though their eyes were closed, the mere fact of visualizing an object at a larger size shifted the activation to more anterior parts of the calcarine sulcus (the major anatomical landmark of Area 17) – just as is found in perception proper (e.g., Sereno *et al.* 1995). This result was replicated by Tootell *et al.* (1998) with fMRI and using a precise method to localize Area 17; there is no doubt that varying the size of objects in mental images shifts the locus of activation along Area 17 comparably to what occurs in perception.

In addition, Klein *et al.* (2000) used event-related fMRI to chart activation in Area 17 when visual mental images were formed. They found clear activation in every participant, with a clear-cut temporal pattern; activation began about 2 seconds after an auditory cue, and peaked around

4–6 seconds later, before dropping off during the next 8 seconds or so. But is such activation playing a functional role in imagery? In another study (Kosslyn *et al.* 1999), participants memorized four quadrants, each with black-and-white stripes (which varied in length, width, orientation, and separation), and later had to visualize them and make subtle shape comparisons, such as deciding which set had longer or wider stripes. PET scanning revealed that Area 17 was activated during this task. Moreover, when repetitive TMS was applied to Area 17 (in a separate group of participants) prior to the task, every participant subsequently required more time to make these judgements than when repetitive TMS was applied so that it did not affect Area 17. Indeed, the magnitude of the decrement in performance was the same when participants had their eyes closed and visualized the stripes as when they had their eyes open and made judgements based on visible stripes. This makes sense if Area 17 is critical in both the imagery and perceptual versions of the task. These findings are consistent with those of Farah *et al.* (1992) who found that after one occipital lobe was surgically removed from a patient (as part of a medical treatment), the apparent size of images decreased by approximately half – as expected if each occipital lobe represents the contra-lateral part of space.

In another PET study (Kosslyn *et al.* 1996), participants closed their eyes and visualized named letters of the alphabet, in upper case form. Four seconds after forming the image, they were asked to judge whether the letter had a specific characteristic (such as any curved lines); the response times and error rates were recorded at the same time that their brains were scanned. Not only were variations in the level of activation in Area 17 significantly correlated with the time participants required to make the judgements, but this correlation was present even after all other correlations between variations in regional cerebral blood flow and response time were statistically removed.

Finally, Slotnick *et al.* (2005) designed a study to examine whether mental imagery could evoke cortical activation with precise retinotopy. Participants took part in a standard retinotopic mapping procedure with three conditions: perception, imagery, and attention. In the perception condition, participants viewed two wedges with a checkerboard texture rotating around a central point. In the imagery condition, participants merely viewed the arcs (edges) of the wedge stimuli and filled in the rest of the figure using visual imagery. In the attention condition, participants also viewed the arcs of the wedge stimuli, but now they paid attention to where the stimulus wedges would have been, without having learned the appearance of the wedges; thus it was not possible for them to visualize the wedge stimuli. The perceptual retinotopic mapping activation was taken as the standard to which the imagery and attention conditions were compared. Statistical analyses revealed that imagery did activate retinotopic maps, and did so (at least for some participants) more strongly than attention alone. These results lend support to the view that mental imagery relies on the same early visual cortical areas as perception.

These results, taken together, indicate that: (1) Activation in early visual cortex is systematically related to spatial properties of the imaged object; (2) if Area 17 is impaired, via TMS or brain damage, so is the use of visual imagery; and (3) the activation in early visual cortex is not likely to be an artefact of activation in other areas, which is merely incidentally sent (via neural connections) to early visual cortex.

Given these positive results, why have many studies failed to find activation in early visual cortex? Kosslyn and Thompson (2003) report a meta-analysis that led to three conclusions: First, if a task requires participants to find a high-resolution detail in an image (such as by evaluating the shape of an animal's ears or comparing two similar sets of stripes), activation in early visual cortex is likely. Second, if a task requires a spatial judgement (which may be mediated by the parietal lobe), activation is less likely. Indeed, many of the studies that did not report activation in early visual cortex used spatial tasks (Mellet *et al.* 1995, 1996, 2000). Third, not surprisingly, the more sensitive the neuroimaging technique, the more likely the researchers were to detect activation in early visual cortex.

A second puzzle is why some brain-damaged patients continue to have some use of imagery, in spite of the fact that early visual cortex has been severely damaged (see, for example, Chatterjee and Southwood 1995). Probably the most straightforward account for this finding is that early visual cortex is not necessary for all forms of visual imagery. Indeed, Crick and Koch (1995) make a good case that the experience of visual perception does not arise from early visual cortex, but rather from later areas that receive input from the earlier ones. The same is probably true in imagery: if later areas are activated in the absence of the appropriate immediate sensory input, one may experience visual imagery. However, such later areas do not make fine spatial variations accessible to later processes, and hence one apparently needs to reconstruct the local geometry in earlier areas (which have much smaller receptive fields, and hence higher resolution) if one must extract fine-grained details from the imaged object (for a review of imagery abilities in brain-damaged patients, see Ganis *et al.* 2003).

Auditory imagery

Do the first three notes of the children's song 'Three blind mice' ascend or descend? Most people report that they 'hear' the song in the process of deciding (that the three notes ascend). Such phenomenology has been taken to signal the presence of modality-specific internal representations, which correspond to auditory images. Research on auditory imagery has been far less extensive than on visual imagery. Zatorre and Halpern (1993) studied brain-damaged patients to find out whether specific brain areas are critical for auditory imagery. They studied a group of patients who had had the left or right temporal lobe removed (for the treatment of otherwise intractable epilepsy) and compared them to similar control participants. In one condition, the participants heard a familiar song while also reading the lyrics, and judged which of two particular words had the higher pitch. In another condition, the participants saw the lyrics and made the same judgements, but did not actually hear the song – and thus had to rely on their mental imagery. The patients with right-temporal lesions were impaired in both conditions, compared to both other groups. These findings demonstrate that at least some of the neural structures that play a key role in pitch discrimination in perception also play a comparable role in imagery.

Most research on auditory imagery has focused on imagery for music (for a review, see Zatorre and Halpern 2005). Zatorre *et al.* (1996) asked whether auditory imagery draws on the same mechanisms used in auditory perception. The participants either listened to songs and judged the relative pitch of pairs of words, or imagined hearing songs and made the same judgements. No auditory stimulation was present during the baseline condition, which required the participants to judge the relative length of visually presented words. PET revealed that many of the same areas were in fact activated in common in auditory imagery and perception. Although activation was stronger during perception than imagery, it was located in comparable regions in the temporal lobes in both conditions. The activated areas included bilateral associative auditory cortex (BA 21/22, in spite of the fact that the left temporal lobe has often been identified with the perception of language and the right with music or environmental sounds), bilateral frontal cortex (BA 45/9 and 10/47), left parietal cortex (BA 40/7), and supplementary motor cortex (BA 6). The bilateral activation in associative auditory cortex may reflect the fact that these researchers used verbal melodies.

Indeed, in a subsequent study, Halpern and Zatorre (1999) asked musically trained participants to listen to the opening notes of familiar (non-verbal) melodies and then continue 'hearing the melody with the mind's ear'. Again using PET, they found activation in two regions of the right temporal lobe (the superior and inferior temporal cortex), which is consistent with their earlier study of brain-damaged patients; both of these areas are involved in storing and interpreting nonverbal sounds. Moreover, auditory imagery of a melody that required retrieval from memory also activated two right-hemisphere regions, in the frontal lobe and superior temporal gyrus (which is critical for auditory perception). Finally, the supplementary motor area (SMA) was also activated by auditory imagery, regardless of whether the melody was retrieved or simply rehearsed on-line. This is interesting because no overt behaviour was required. Halpern and Zatorre believe that stored movements are used in this sort of imagery – which makes sense for melodies, where one can subvocalize the tune as part of the process of retrieving the information.

Finally, Griffiths (2000) reports a novel study of patients who became deaf and then hallucinated hearing music. These patients were neither psychotic nor beset with an obvious neurological problem, such as epilepsy. Griffiths was able to perform PET while the patients had such hallucinations, and reports that the posterior temporal lobes, in auditory cortex, as well as several other areas (specifically, the right basal ganglia, the cerebellum and the inferior frontal cortices) were activated.

In short, auditory imagery appears to draw on most of the neural structures used in auditory perception. However, unlike visual imagery, there is little evidence that the first auditory cortical area to receive input from the ears, Area A1, is activated during auditory imagery (see Kleber *et al.* 2007).

Motor imagery

When people are asked to imagine walking to a specific goal placed in front of them and to indicate when they would have arrived, their estimates of transit time are remarkably similar to the actual time they subsequently require to walk that distance (Decety and Jeannerod 1995). In such tasks, people report that they imagine moving; and such imagery typically is referred to as 'motor imagery'. However, in our view the term 'motor imagery' may be slightly misleading. It is likely that participants do not activate the motor commands alone, but also activate representations of kinaesthetic feedback. To be sure, there is a difference between imagining moving one's own arm and imagining having somebody else move it for you in the same way. Nevertheless, both sorts of imagery involve kinaesthetic perceptual representations, along with representations of any motor commands that may accompany such perceptual feedback.

Many studies have now been carried out to investigate the neural bases of such motor imagery, and to distinguish motor imagery from purely visual mental imagery. Although visual imagery may often accompany motor imagery, researchers have documented that motor imagery relies on distinct mechanisms. Specifically, many researchers have shown that cortex used in movement control also plays a role in motor imagery. Indeed, in a classic study, Georgopoulos *et al.* (1989) recorded activity in individual neurons in the motor strip of monkeys while the animals were planning to move a lever along a specific arc. They found that these neurons fired in a systematic sequence, depending on their orientation tuning. Specifically, at first, only neurons tuned for orientations near the starting position of the lever fired, followed by those tuned for orientations slightly farther along the trajectory, and so on. All of this occurred before the animal actually began moving. These findings do not, however, show that mental imagery of movement occurs in the motor strip itself; it is possible that the computation takes place elsewhere in the brain (e.g., the posterior parietal lobes), and that the results of such computation are simply being executed in the motor strip.

Indeed, a host of neuroimaging studies on 'mental rotation' have now been reported, all of which have shown that multiple brain areas are activated during mental rotation. For example, Richter *et al.* (2000) measured brain activation with fMRI while participants mentally rotated the three-dimensional multi-armed angular stimuli invented by Shepard and Metzler (1971) (which look as if they had been constructed by gluing small cubes together to form the arms). Participants were shown pairs of such shapes in which one member was rotated relative to the other; the participants were asked to report whether the figures in each pair were the same or mirror-reversed. Richter *et al.* report that the superior parietal lobules (in both hemispheres) were activated during this task, as well as premotor cortex (in both hemispheres), supplementary motor cortex, and also the left primary motor cortex.

Other neuroimaging studies have provided strong support for the role of motor processes in mental transformations. For example, Parsons *et al.* (1995) showed participants a picture of a hand, which could be rotated to various degrees; the pictures were presented in the left visual field (so the image was registered first by the right hemisphere) or in the right visual field (so the image was registered first by the left hemisphere). The participants were to decide whether each picture was a left or right hand. Parsons *et al.* expected motor cortices to be activated in this task if participants imagined rotating their own hand into congruence with the stimulus. And, in fact, not only was supplementary motor cortex activated bilaterally, but also prefrontal and insular premotor areas were activated in the hemisphere contralateral to the stimulus handedness – suggesting that participants did in fact imagine the appropriate movements. Many other regions, including areas in the frontal and parietal lobes, and basal ganglia and cerebellum, were active, as was Area 17.

Is motor imagery used only to rotate parts of one's body? Some researchers (Jeannerod 1994; Jeannerod and Decety 1995; Decety 1996) have suggested that people often transform images by imagining what they would see if the objects were manipulated in a specific way. One PET study (Kosslyn *et al.* 1998) directly compared rotation of hands versus inanimate objects, again using the three-dimensional multi-armed angular stimuli invented by Shepard and Metzler (1971). The participants compared pairs of drawings and decided whether they were identical or mirror images (using the task and stimuli from the original Shepard and Metzler study). In the experimental condition, the figures were presented at different relative orientations, and one had to be 'mentally rotated' into congruence with the other; in the baseline condition, the figures were presented at the same orientation, and thus no mental rotation was necessary. The comparison of the two conditions revealed the areas that were activated specifically by mental rotation. The corresponding design was used for drawings of hands, but now the participants decided whether the two hands in a pair were both left or both right, or whether one was a left hand and one a right hand.

In this study, several motor areas were activated when participants mentally rotated hands, including primary motor cortex (Area M1), premotor cortex, and the posterior parietal lobe. None of the frontal motor areas were activated when the Shepard-Metzler figures were mentally rotated. However, Cohen *et al.* (1996) used fMRI to study mental rotation of exactly the same inanimate objects and found that premotor cortex was activated in this task, but only in half the participants.

The fact that only some participants had activation in a motor area during mental rotation of inanimate objects suggests that there may be two strategies for performing such rotations. One strategy involves imagining what you would see if you manipulated an object; the other involves imagining what you would see if someone else (or an external force, such as a motor) manipulated an object. To test this idea, Kosslyn *et al.* (2001) asked participants to perform the same mental rotation task used by Cohen *et al.* (1996), but with a twist: Immediately prior to the task, the participants saw a wooden model of that type of stimulus (one not actually used in the task) either being rotated by an electric motor or they themselves physically turned the stimulus. They were told that during the task they should imagine the stimuli being rotated just as they had seen the model rotate at the outset. In this experiment, Area M1 was activated when participants mentally rotated stimuli after having themselves physically rotated the stimulus (and then imagined themselves doing so), and not when they saw the electric motor rotating the stimulus at the outset.

Similarly, Wraga *et al.* (2003) examined activation when participants mentally rotated images of inanimate objects. They found that activation in motor regions of the brain was greater when participants had just completed mental rotation of body parts (hands) than when they had just completed another session of rotating inanimate objects. In this study, the participants were never instructed to use a motor strategy, but this method of accomplishing the mental rotation task apparently transferred from having just rotated images of hands.

These results showed that imagining oneself manipulating an object is one way in which mental transformation of objects, in general (not just body parts), can take place – and also show that humans can voluntarily adopt this strategy or use a strategy in which they imagine what they would see if an external force transformed an object.

Finally, one can ask whether primary motor cortex plays a functional role in allowing participants to manipulate objects in images. It is possible that the actual computation is taking place in another area that incidentally sends activation to primary motor cortex. To test this hypothesis, Ganis *et al.* (2000) disrupted function in the left primary motor cortex (M1) by administering TMS while participants mentally rotated pictures of hands and feet (with the to-be-rotated stimulus appearing in the right visual field). The TMS was time-locked so that it disrupted neural processing only a specific amount of time after the stimulus appeared. Participants required more time to perform this task if a single magnetic pulse was delivered to the motor strip (roughly over the 'hand area') 650 ms after the stimuli were presented (but not at the other temporal delays tested); moreover, rotation of hands was impaired more than rotation of feet, as expected if this area is specialized for controlling the hand per se. Within the limits of the spatial resolution afforded by the TMS technique, these results suggest that activation in this area reflects processing used to perform the task. As in the case of TMS stimulation of area 17, we cannot be entirely sure, however, that M1 is the primary site of processing because the information could be computed elsewhere in the brain. However, the finding that primary motor cortex is involved in the mental rotation of hands has been replicated by Tomasino *et al.* (2005), using similar materials and paradigms.

In short, mental imagery can engage the motor system. This finding may help to explain why 'mental practice' can improve actual performance (Maring 1990; Driskell *et al.* 1994; Weiss *et al.* 1994; MacIntyre *et al.* 2002; Guillot and Collet 2008; Guillot *et al.* in this volume; MacIntyre and Moran in this volume). In this case, to imagine making movements may not only exercise the relevant brain areas, but also may build associations among processes implemented in different areas – which in turn facilitate complex performance.

Simulating the social world

The great Behaviourist B. F. Skinner (1977, p. 6) wrote, 'There is no evidence of the mental construction of images to be looked at or maps to be followed. The body responds to the world, at the point of contact; making copies would be a waste of time'. We hope that the reader is convinced that the first part of this claim is incorrect; images are in fact internal representations. We now briefly consider the second part, whether having such representations is a 'waste of time'. We focus on a relatively new area, the use of imagery in simulating social interactions.

Mirror neurons and 'mental simulations'

Mental imagery has many possible uses, ranging from helping one to memorize new information to visual problem solving. Among such functions, researchers have suggested that images can function as 'mental simulations' of a possible real-world event. Why take the trouble of lugging furniture around your living room if you can get a sense of how an arrangement will look simply by visualizing it?

One important role of such simulations is in anticipating the consequence of someone's performing an action – or of your performing it. Such simulations apparently depend not simply on the neural machinery used to recognize objects or to situate them in space. In addition, an important role may be played by a subpopulation of neurons in the frontal lobe (area F5 of the monkey brain, which is part of premotor cortex). These neurons respond selectively not only when the animal performs specific actions with the hand and/or mouth, but also when the animal merely observes the same actions being performed by another monkey (or human; Rizzolatti *et al.* 1998). Because of this property, such neurons have been labelled 'mirror neurons'.

Neuroimaging and TMS studies have shown that human premotor cortex is activated when humans observe other people's actions (e.g., Fadiga *et al.* 1995; Grafton *et al.* 1996; Rizzolatti *et al.* 1996; Hari *et al.* 1998; Gangitano *et al.* 2001), which is consistent with the existence of mirror neurons in the human brain. The likely homologue of Area F5 in humans is Broca's area (typically characterized as being involved in speech production), which has prompted some authors to theorize that the mirror neurons in humans may have a crucial role not only in imitation, but also in language acquisition. Mirror neurons may also play a role in motor imagery, consistent with the idea that people often transform images by imagining what they would see if the objects were manipulated in a specific way.

Imagery and emotion

One reason that simulating other people may be useful is that those simulations allow us to anticipate emotional responses. In fact, many findings indicate that imagery of emotional events activates the autonomic nervous system and (as also evident in single-cell recordings in humans) the amygdala. That is, visualizing an object has much of the same effects on the body as actually seeing the object. For example, Lang *et al.* (1993) showed that skin conductance increases, as do heart rate and breathing rate, when participants view pictures of threatening objects. And the same result occurs when they merely visualize the objects. Indeed, Kosslyn *et al.* (1996) found that mental images of aversive stimuli activate the anterior insula, the major cortical site of feedback from the autonomic nervous system. In addition, Kreiman *et al.* (2000) recorded from single cells in the human brain (hippocampus, amygdala, enthorinal cortex, and parahippocampal gyrus) while participants were shown pictures or formed mental images of those same pictures. Some of the cells that responded selectively when participants viewed specific visual stimuli (e.g., faces) also responded selectively when those same stimuli were visualized. Of particular interest, this pattern was seen in the amygdala, which is known to play a key role in certain emotions, especially fear and anger (LeDoux 1995, 1996)**.** Thus, imagery can engage neural structures that are also engaged in perception, and these in turn can affect events in the body itself.

Conclusions

Mental imagery is not a single function. Rather, like all other cognitive activities, mental imagery arises from the joint action of numerous systems. Moreover, there are different types of imagery, and each type can be used in the service of performing many types of tasks. Researchers agree that most of the processes underlying like-modality perception are also used in mental imagery, and imagery in many ways can 'stand in' for a perceptual stimulus or situation. Imagery can not only engage the motor system, but also affect the body much as can actual perceptual experience.

Nevertheless, many questions remain. For example: Why do people differ so much in their imagery abilities? Does genetics affect some aspects of imagery more than others? How does semantic content in images engage specific mechanisms? How do different types of imagery interact? And, the perennial favourite question, What is the relationship between information processing during imagery and conscious experience? Unlike 25 years ago, questions such as these can now begin to be answered.

Acknowledgements

Preparation of this chapter was made possible through funding from National Institutes of Health (NIH) grant R01 MH060734 to Stephen M. Kosslyn. Any opinions, findings, and conclusions or recommendations expressed in this material are those of the authors and do not necessarily reflect the views of NIH. Portions of this chapter are adapted from an earlier work by the same authors: Kosslyn, S. M., Ganis, G., and Thompson, W. L. (2001) Neural foundations of imagery. *Nature Reviews Neuroscience*, **2**, 635–42.

References

Behrmann, M. (2000). The mind's eye mapped onto the brain's matter. *Current Directions in Psychological Science*, **9**(2), 50–4.

Behrmann, M., Winocur, G., and Moscovitch, M. (1992). Dissociation between mental imagery and object recognition in a brain-damaged patient. *Nature*, **359**, 636–37.

Chatterjee, A. and Southwood, M.H. (1995). Cortical blindness and visual imagery. *Neurology*, **45**(12), 2189–95.

Cohen, M.S., Kosslyn, S.M., Breiter, H.C., *et al.* (1996). Changes in cortical activity during mental rotation: a mapping study using functional MRI. *Brain*, **119**, 89–100.

Crick, F. and Koch, C. (1995). Are we aware of neural activity in primary visual cortex? *Nature*, **375**(6527), 121–3.

Decety, J. (1996). Neural representation for action. *Reviews in the Neurosciences.* **7**(4), 285–97.

Decety, J. and Jeannerod, M. (1995). Mentally simulated movements in virtual reality: does Fitts's law hold in motor imagery? *Behavioral Brain Research*, **72**(1–2), 127–34.

De Vreese, L.P. (1991). Two systems for colour-naming defects: verbal disconnection vs colour imagery disorder. *Neuropsychologia*, **29**(1), 1–18.

Downing, P.E., Chan, A.W., Peelen, M.V., Dodds, C.M., and Kanwisher, N. (2006). Domain specificity in visual cortex. *Cerebral Cortex*, **16**(10), 1453–61.

Driskell, J., Copper, C., and Moran, A. (1994). Does mental practice enhance performance? *Journal of Applied Psychology*, **79**(4), 481–92.

Fadiga, L., Fogassi, L., Pavesi, G., and Rizzolatti, G. (1995). Motor facilitation during action observation: a magnetic stimulation study. *Journal of Neurophysiology*, **73**(6), 2608–11.

Farah, M.J. (1984). The neurological basis of mental imagery: a componential analysis. *Cognition*, **18**, 245–72.

Farah, M.J., Soso, M.J., and Dasheiff, R.M. (1992). Visual angle of the mind's eye before and after unilateral occipital lobectomy. *Journal of Experimental Psychology: Human Perception and Performance*, **18**(1), 241–6.

Gangitano, M., Mottaghy, F.M., and Pascual-Leone, A. (2001). Phase-specific modulation of cortical motor output during movement observation. *NeuroReport*, **12**(7), 1489–92.

Ganis, G., Keenan, J.P., Kosslyn, S.M., and Pascual-Leone, A. (2000). Transcranial magnetic stimulation of primary motor cortex affects mental rotation. *Cerebral Cortex,* **10**, 175–80.

Ganis, G., Thompson, W.L., and Kosslyn, S.M. (2004). Brain areas underlying visual mental imagery and visual perception: an fMRI study. *Cognitive Brain Research*, **20**, 226–41.

Ganis, G., Thompson, W.L., Mast, F.W., and Kosslyn, S.M. (2003). Visual imagery in cerebral visual dysfunction. *Neurologic Clinics of North America*, **21**, 631–46.

Georgopoulos, A.P., Lurito, J.T., Petrides, M., Schwartz, A.B., and Massey. J.T. (1989). Mental rotation of the neuronal population vector. *Science, 243*, 234–6.

Grafton, S.T., Arbib, M.A., Fadiga, L., and Rizzolatti, G. (1996). Localization of grasp representations in humans by positron emission tomography: 2. Observation compared with imagination. *Experimental Brain Research,* **112**(1), 103–11.

Griffiths, T.D. (2000). Musical hallucinosis in acquired deafness. Phenomenology and brain substrate. *Brain, 123*(Pt 10), 2065–76.

Guillot, A. and Collet, C. (2008). Construction of the motor imagery integrative model in sport: a review and theoretical investigation of motor imagery use. *International Review of Sport and Exercise Psychology,* **1**, 31–44.

Guillot, A. *et al.* (2009). Motor imagery in sports sciences: an overview, in A. Guillot and C. Collet (eds), *The Neural Foundations of Mental and Motor Imagery*. Oxford, UK: Oxford University Press.

Halpern, A.R. and Zatorre, R.J. (1999). When that tune runs through your head: a PET investigation of auditory imagery for familiar melodies. *Cerebral Cortex,* **9**, 697–704.

Hari, R., Forss, N., Avikainen, S. Kirveskari, E., Selenius, S., and Rizzolatti, G. (1998). Activation of human primary motor cortex during action observation: a neuromagnetic study. *Proceedings of the National Academy of Sciences of the United States of America,* **95**(25), 15061–5.

Jankowiak, J., Kinsbourne, M., Shalev, R.S., and Bachman, D.L. (1992). Preserved visual imagery and categorization in a case of associative visual agnosia. *Journal of Cognitive Neuroscience,* **4**(2), 119–31.

Jeannerod, M. (1994). The representing brain: neural correlates of motor intention and imagery. *Behavioral and Brain Sciences,* **17**(2), 187–245.

Jeannerod, M. and Decety, J. (1995). Mental motor imagery: a window into the representational stages of action. *Current Opinion in Neurobiology,* **5**(6), 727–32.

Jordan, K., Heinze, H.J., Lutz, K., Kanowski, M., and Jancke, L. (2001). Cortical activations during the mental rotation of different visual objects. *Neuroimage,* **13**(1), 143–52.

Kanwisher, N. and Yovel, G. (2006). The fusiform face area: a cortical region specialized for the perception of faces. *Philosophical Transactions of the Royal Society B: Biological Sciences,* **361**(1476), 2109–28.

Kleber, B., Birbaumer, N., Veit, R., Trevorrow, T., and Lotze, M. (2007). Overt and imagined singing of an Italian aria. *NeuroImage,* **36**(3), 889–900.

Klein, I., Paradis, A.-L., Poline, J.-B., Kosslyn, S.M., and Le Bihan, D. (2000). Transient activity in human calcarine cortex during visual imagery. *Journal of Cognitive Neuroscience,* **12**(6), 15–23.

Kosslyn, S.M., Segar, C., Pani, J., and Hillger, L.A. (1990). When is imagery used in everyday life? A diary study. *Journal of Mental Imagery,* **14**, 131–52.

Kosslyn, S.M., Shin, L.M., Thompson, W.L., *et al.* (1996). Neural effects of visualizing and perceiving aversive stimuli: a PET investigation. *NeuroReport,* **7**, 1569–76.

Kosslyn, S.M., Pascual-Leone, A., Felician, O., *et al.* (1999). The role of area 17 in visual imagery: convergent evidence from PET and rTMS. *Science,* **284**, 167–70.

Kosslyn, S.M., DiGirolamo, G., Thompson, W.L., and Alpert, N.M. (1998). Mental rotation of objects versus hands: neural mechanisms revealed by positron emission tomography. *Psychophysiology,* **35**, 151–61.

Kosslyn, S.M. and Thompson, W.L. (2003). When is early visual cortex activated during visual mental imagery? *Psychological Bulletin,* **129**, 723–46.

Kosslyn, S.M., Thompson, W.L., and Alpert, N.M. (1997). Neural systems shared by visual imagery and visual perception: a positron emission tomography study. *NeuroImage,* **6**, 320–34.

Kosslyn, S.M., Thompson, W.L., and Ganis, G. (2006). *The Case for Mental Imagery*. New York: Oxford University Press.

Kosslyn, S.M., Thompson, W.L., Kim, I.J., and Alpert, N.M. (1995). Topographical representations of mental images in primary visual cortex. *Nature,* **378**, 496–8.

Kosslyn, S.M., Thompson, W.L., Kim, I.J., Rauch, S.L., and Alpert, N.M. (1996). Individual differences in cerebral blood flow in area 17 predict the time to evaluate visualized letters. *Journal of Cognitive Neuroscience,* **8**, 78–82.

Kosslyn, S.M., Thompson, W.L., Wraga, M., and Alpert, N.M. (2001). Imagining rotation by endogenous and exogenous forces: distinct neural mechanisms for different strategies. *NeuroReport,* **12**, 2519–25.

Kreiman, G., Koch, C., and Fried, I. Imagery neurons in the human brain. (2000). *Nature,* **408**(6810), 357–61.

Lang, P.J., Greenwald, M.K., Bradley, M.M., and Hamm, A. O. (1993). Looking at pictures: affective, facial, visceral, and behavioral reactions. *Psychophysiology,* **30**(3), 261–73.

LeDoux, J.E. (1995). Emotion: Clues from the brain. *Annual Review of Psychology,* **46**, 209–35.

LeDoux, J.E. (1996). *The Emotional Brain:The Mysterious Underpinnings of Emotional Life.* New York: Simon and Schuster.

Levine, D.N., Warach, J., and Farah, M.J. (1985). Two visual systems in mental imagery: dissociation of 'what' and 'where' in imagery disorders due to bilateral posterior cerebral lesions. *Neurology,* **35**, 1010–8.

MacIntyre, T. and Moran, A. (2009). Meta-imagery processes among elite sport performers, in A. Guillot and C. Collet (eds), *The Neural Foundations of Mental and Motor Imagery.* Oxford, UK: Oxford University Press.

MacIntyre, T., Moran, A., and Jennings, D.J. (2002). Are mental imagery abilities related to Canoe-Slalom performance? *Perceptual and Motor Skills,* **94**, 1245–50.

Maring, J.R. (1990). Effects of mental practice on rate of skill acquisition. *Physical Therapy,* **70**(3), 165–72.

Mellet, E., Tzourio, N., Crivello, F., Joliot, M., Denis, M., and Mazoyer, B. (1996). Functional anatomy of spatial mental imagery generated from verbal instructions. *Journal of Neuroscience,* **16**(20), 6504–12.

Mellet, E., Bricogne, S., Tzourio-Mazoyer, N., *et al.* (2000). Neural correlates of topographic mental exploration: the impact of route *versus* survey perspective learning. *NeuroImage,* **12**, 588–600.

Mellet, E., Tzourio N., Denis, M., and Mazoyer, B. (1995). A positron emission tomography study of visual and mental spatial exploration. *Journal of Cognitive Neuroscience,* **4**, 433–45.

Ng, V.W., Bullmore, E.T., de Zubicaray, G.I., Cooper, A., Suckling, J., and Williams, S. C. (2001). Identifying rate-limiting nodes in large-scale cortical networks for visuospatial processing: an iIllustration using fMRI. *Journal of Cognitive Neuroscience,* **13**(4), 537–45.

O'Craven, K.M. and Kanwisher, N. (2000). Mental imagery of faces and places activates corresponding stimulus-specific brain regions. *Journal of Cognitive Neuroscience,* **12**(6), 1013–23.

Paivio, A. (1971). *Imagery and Verbal Processes.* New York: Holt, Rinehart and Winston.

Parsons, L.M., Fox, P.T., Downs, J.H., *et al.* (1995). Use of implicit motor imagery for visual shape discrimination as revealed by PET. *Nature,* **375**, 54–8.

Pylyshyn, Z.W. (1973). What the mind's eye tells the mind's brain: a critique of mental imagery. *Psychological Bulletin,* **80**, 1–24.

Pylyshyn, Z.W. (1981). Psychological explanations and knowledge-dependent processes. *Cognition,* **10**(1–3), 267–74.

Richter, W., Somorjai, R., Summers, R., *et al.* (2000). Motor area activity during mental rotation studied by time resolved single-trial fMRI. *Journal of Cognitive Neurosicence,* **12**(2), 310–20.

Rizzolatti, G., Fadiga, L., Matelli, M., *et al.* (1996). Localization of grasp representations in humans by PET: 1. Observation versus execution. *Experimental Brain Research,* **111**(2), 246–52.

Rizzolatti, G., Luppino, G., and Matelli, M. (1998). The organization of the cortical motor system: new concepts. *Electroencephalography and Clinical Neurophysiology,* **106**(4), 283–96.

Sereno, M.I., Dale, A.M., Reppas, J.B., *et al.* (1995). Borders of multiple visual areas in humans revealed by functional magnetic resonance imaging. *Science,* **268**(5212), 889–93.

Shepard, R.N. and Metzler, J. (1971). Mental rotation of three-dimensional objects. *Science,* **171**, 701–3.

Skinner, B.F. (1977). Why I am not a cognitive psychologist. *Behaviorism,* **5**, 1–10.

Slotnick, S.D., Thompson, W.L., and Kosslyn, S.M. (2005). Visual mental imagery induces retinotopically organized activation of early visual areas. *Cerebral Cortex,* **15,** 1570–83.

Thompson, W.L. and Kosslyn, S.M. (2000). Neural systems activated during visual mental imagery. A review and meta-analyses, in A. W. Toga and J. C. Mazziotta (eds), *Brain Mapping II: The Systems,* pp. 535–60. San Diego: Academic Press.

Thompson, W.L. Kosslyn, S.M., Sukel, K.E., and Alpert, N. M. (2001). Mental imagery of high- and low-resolution gratings activates Area 17. *NeuroImage,* **14,** 454–64.

Tomasino, B., Borroni, P., Isaja, A., and Rumiati, R. I. (2005). The role of the primary motor cortex in mental rotation: a TMS study. *Cognitive Neuropsychology,* **22,** 348–63.

Tootell, R.B.H., Hadjikani, N.K., Mendola, J.D., Marrett, S., and Dale, A.M. (1998). From retinotopy to recognition: fMRI in human visual cortex. *Trends in Cognitive Sciences,* **2,** 174–83.

Ungerleider, L.G. and Mishkin, M. (1982). Two cortical visual systems, in D.J. Ingle and R.J.W. Mansfield (eds), *Analysis of Visual Behavior,* pp. 549–86. Cambridge, MA: MIT Press.

Watson, J.B. (1913). Psychology as the behaviorist views it. *Psychological Review,* **20,** 158–77.

Weiss, T., Hansen, E., Rost, R., and Beyer, L. (1994). Mental practice of motor skills used in poststroke rehabilitation has own effects on central nervous activation. *International Journal of Neuroscience,* **78**(3–4),157–66.

Wraga, M.J., Thompson, W.L., Alpert, N.M., and Kosslyn, S.M. (2003). Implicit transfer of motor strategies in mental rotation. *Brain and Cognition,* **52,** 135–43.

Young, A.W., Humphreys, G.W., Riddoch, M.J., Hellawell, D.J., and de Haan, E.H. (1994). Recognition impairments and face imagery. *Neuropsychologia,* **32**(6), 693–702.

Zacks, J. (2008). Neuroimaging studies of mental rotation: a meta-analysis and review. *Journal of Cognitive Neuroscience,* **20**(1), 1–19.

Zatorre, R.J. and Halpern, A.R. (1993). Effect of unilateral temporal-lobe excision on perception and imagery of songs. *Neuropsychologia,* **31**(3), 221–32.

Zatorre, R.J. and Halpern, A.R. (2005). Mental concerts: musical imagery and auditory cortex. *Neuron,* **47,** 9–12.

Zatorre, R.J., Halpern, A.R., Perry, D.W., Meyer, E., and Evans, A.C. (1996). Hearing in the mind's ear: A PET investigation of musical imagery and perception. *Journal of Cognitive Neuroscience,* **8,** 29–46.

Chapter 2

Neural bases of topographical representation in humans: Contribution of neuroimaging studies

Nicolas Poirel, Laure Zago, Laurent Petit, and Emmanuel Mellet

Introduction

The human mind is able to internalize motor and sensory events and to evoke them mentally, giving rise to mental imagery activity. Topographical representation is a type of mental image that accounts for numerous and essential activities in humans. We are reasonably good at reaching or moving to a specific location, and are also able to navigate and reach a goal along novel routes. As such, our brains store locations that can be continually updated to reflect our new current spatial position. Remembering specific locations, and how to get there, requires reference to our knowledge of an environment, mainly embodied in our brain by means of topographical representations. While the psychological properties of mental images of an environment have been widely studied, neuroimaging techniques provide new insights into the neural bases of this type of spatial cognition.

The first part of this chapter is devoted to the psychological definition of the topographical representation. The next section focuses on the description of the neural network of topographical representations as revealed by neuroimaging studies. The final section shows that this neural network can be modulated, based on the way the environment is learned.

Definition of topographical representation

Topographical representation refers to spatial mental imagery limited to the internal representation of environments such as rooms, landscape, and towns. Included in these representations are the geometry and the arrangement of the landmarks and the objects of the environment. This topographical mental image allows the representation of a previous perceived environment to be activated, and gives one the possibility to mentally move from one point to another, despite the absence of visual perception input. A cornerstone experiment demonstrating the materiality of such images came from Kosslyn's work (Kosslyn *et al.* 1978). In this experiment, subjects had to memorize a map of an imaginary island in which many landmarks were present (a tree, a hut, a pit, and others). Subjects were then asked to generate a mental map of the island and to travel mentally from one landmark to another. This experiment revealed a strong correlation between the time needed to move mentally from one landmark to another and the actual distance between the landmarks. These results showed, for the first time, a structural similarity between a real scene and the mental representation of that scene.

To build such spatial representations, one can acquire information in different ways, e.g., by actually navigating the environment (information is then acquired via an egocentric or 'route' perspective) or by learning maps (information is acquired in an allocentric or 'survey' perspective).

In the route perspective, the localization of objects is defined relative to the location of the subject in the scene. Accordingly, the terms 'right', 'left', 'top', 'bottom', 'in front of', and 'behind' are usually used to describe an object's location. This representation is then constructed linearly (temporally and spatially), in a 'step by step' manner, by coding the different landmarks from a starting point to a final point. This perspective is natural and constitutes what is likely the first basic reference for humans. However, this kind of representation suffers from a lack of flexibility, because of the requirement to memorize a constrained sequence of objects in succession as presented in the mental scene. As a result, each sequence depends inescapably on the precedent; the landmarks are linked together both temporally and spatially. The route perspective is, thus, mostly based on action. However, if some crucial landmarks are missing, forgotten, or cannot be accessed because a usual road is blocked, the topographical representation becomes useless to find one's way.

In the survey perspective, the topographical representation is built from an allocentric perspective, in a two-dimensional view. Unlike the route representation, the localization of objects in a survey representation does not depend on the location of the subject. The localization of an object is specified in relation to the whole space or to the other objects present in the environment. The terms 'north', 'south', 'east', and 'west' are used to localize objects and places. Survey perspective provides direct access to the global configuration of a scene, contrary to the route perspective in which the subject has only fractionated local views of the environment. This representation is, then, very flexible, and it is very easy to find a new itinerary on this mental map when an obstacle is present on a usual road. This flexibility is highly sensible to individual characteristics, such as visuospatial abilities or gender (Astur *et al.* 2004). For instance, females rely predominantly on landmark information while males more readily use both landmark and geometric information (Sandstrom *et al.* 1998).

Topographical representations and the brain

In this section, we will focus on the results obtained by the neuroimaging methods. The two main techniques are positron emission tomography (PET) and functional magnetic resonance imaging (fMRI) (Raichle and Mintun, 2006). Both are aimed at measuring the variation of regional cerebral blood flow (rCBF). Indeed, fluctuations of rCBF are correlated to neuronal activity. Using the classical subtraction paradigm, it is thus possible to infer which regions are more activated in a given condition than in a reference situation. To provide an estimation of CBF, PET requires the injection of a labelled tracer (usually H_2O^{15}-labelled water). The fMRI signal depends on the ratio between oxygenated and deoxygenated blood, which varies according to the CBF. This last technique does not require participants to be injected. Neuroimaging techniques provide considerable new insights regarding the nature and the organization of the brain regions involved in topographical memory. Briefly, cerebral regions involved in the processing of mental images of environments can be arranged in two categories. Parietal and frontal regions, constituting a parieto-frontal network, play a general role in spatial cognition (see Figure 2.1). The hippocampus and the parahippocampus, in the medial part of the temporal lobe, and posterior cingulate cortex, in the retrosplenial region, appear more specific to topographical processing.

The parieto-frontal network

As suggested above, this network is not specific to topographical imagery. In fact, the proposition is that this parieto-frontal network constitutes the smallest set of regions necessary to deal with spatial representation, including spatial working memory and spatial mental imagery (Mellet *et al.* 2000a).

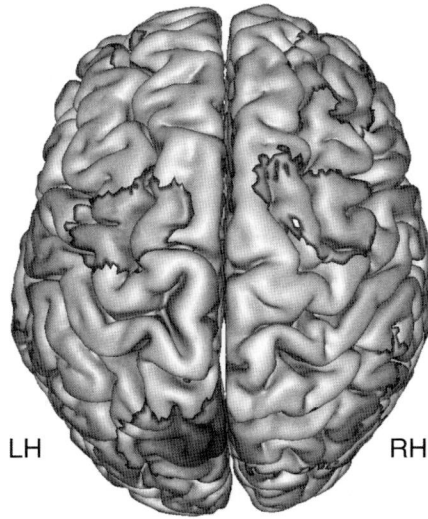

Fig. 2.1 3-D rendering of areas activated during a mental navigation task in environments learned from different modalities (actual navigation learning, map learning, and text learning, see Mellet *et al.*, 2000a, 2002). This conjunction analysis revealed the basic parieto-frontal network involved as soon as subjects use a spatial mental representation ($P_{uncorr} < 0.001$, LH: left hemisphere, RH: right hemisphere). See colour plate section.

The intraparietal sulcus is a structure commonly involved during visuospatial attention (Corbetta 1998; Beauchamp *et al.* 2001), spatial working memory (Petit *et al.* 1996; Smith *et al.* 1996), and spatial mental imagery (Mellet *et al.* 1995, 1996, 2000a). The second component of the network is constituted by a bilateral region located in the depth of the superior frontal sulcus, near its intersection with the pre-central sulcus. This region is reported to be activated in spatial working memory studies (Jonides *et al.* 1993; Petit *et al.* 1996) and in spatial mental imagery studies (Mellet *et al.* 1996), when visual input is no longer present and spatial information must be held on-line (Courtney *et al.* 1998; Zago *et al.* 2008). It should be noted that this region is anatomically distinct from the Frontal Eye Field (Courtney *et al.* 1998; Mellet *et al.* 2000a).

The third component, common to the two mental exploration tasks, corresponds to the pre-Supplementary Motor Area (SMA). This region has been functionally distinguished from the SMA in that it is involved in complex motor tasks, as opposed to the SMA proper located posteriorly, which is involved in simpler motor tasks (Picard and Strick 1996). It has been proposed that pre-SMA is tightly linked to working memory, being involved in the preparation for selecting a motor response based on information held on-line (Petit *et al.* 1998). In agreement with its role in spatial cognition, this parieto-frontal network has been repeatedly found activated in various topographical tasks. This network was evidenced during the coding and learning of topographic information (Aguirre *et al.* 1996; Shelton and Gabrieli 2002; Blanch *et al.* 2004; Wolbers *et al.* 2004; Wolbers and Buchel 2005). The parieto-frontal network is also involved when participants have to remember the location of places and during wayfinding—a navigational task in which subjects have to find their way between two locations (Hartley *et al.* 2003; Iaria *et al.* 2003; Jordan *et al.* 2004; Rosenbaum *et al.* 2004). It was also evidenced during purely mental tasks, such as mental exploration of learned environments (Mellet *et al.* 2000b, 2002; Ino *et al.* 2002).

The role of parietal structures (from the intraparietal sulcus to the superior and inferior parietal lobes and the precuneus) in the processing of egocentric perspective was emphasized in previous research. Their activation is reported in learning routes and environments from an ego-centric perspective (Blanch *et al.* 2004; Wolbers *et al.* 2004; Wolbers and Buchel 2005). In addition, the activity of the posterior part of inferior parietal regions increased linearly with the behavioural measures of route expertise (Wolbers *et al.* 2004). However, the involvement of parietal structures is not confined to the egocentric perspective (Shelton and Gabrieli 2002; Blanch *et al.* 2004). In fact, it is proposed that these structures play a role in the translation of a survey representation into a route perspective (Ino *et al.* 2002).

In addition to the parietal regions, the frontal lobe plays a crucial role during visuospatial navigation and during the learning of routes and environments (Shelton and Gabrieli 2002). It is suggested that frontal activations reflected the spatial working memory involvement needed for the memorization of the temporo-spatial sequence of environmental features (Wolbers *et al.* 2004). This hypothesis is strengthened by the work of Pine, who found a positive correlation between the activity of the frontal lobe and a navigation score during a wayfinding task (Pine *et al.* 2002).

While the involvement of the parieto-frontal network in topographical processing is well established, the precise role of the hippocampus and the parahippocampus, which represent other fundamental structures involved in topographical representation, is still under debate.

The hippocampus: a controversial role

The discovery of the so-called 'place cells' in the hippocampus of rats has been the cornerstone of the putative role of this region in topographical cognition (O'Keefe and Dostrovsky 1971). These neurons increased their activity selectively when the animal reached a given spatial position in its environment. Morris and collaborators showed that a lesion to the hippocampus could produce deficits regarding topographic learning in the rat (Morris *et al.* 1982). These results are consistent with the view that the hippocampus represents the structure responsible for the elaboration of a cognitive map of the environment, which, in turn, allows an allocentric view of the space (O'Keefe and Nadel 1978). Using single neuron recordings in epileptic patients, Ekstrom and collaborators discovered 'place cells' in the human hippocampus. These neurons responded selectively according to the given space position of the subject, whatever his orientation (Burgess and O'Keefe 2003; Ekstrom *et al.* 2003). This suggested that, as in rodents, the human hippocampus is engaged in the maintenance of a cognitive map of the environment. However, some diverging results make this result less clear (Aguirre and D'Esposito 1999). Some neuroimaging studies report an activation of the hippocampus during a task in which subjects have to use topographical representations (Maguire *et al.* 1998a; Hartley *et al.* 2003; Wolbers *et al.* 2004), whereas other studies found no activation in this area (Aguirre *et al.* 1996, 1998; Blanch *et al.* 2004; Rosenbaum *et al.* 2004). Several factors could explain these discrepancies.

Extent of learning

Wolbers asked participants to repeatedly encode a complex environment from an egocentric perspective, while they were to infer the spatial layout of the environment. Left hippocampal activation was most prominent during the initial learning phase, and decayed when performances approached ceiling level (Wolbers and Buchel 2005). This suggests that during navigational learning, the hippocampus is required to incorporate new information into an emerging memory representation. The decreased activation in the hippocampus, in relation to task expertise, is a possible explanation for the lack of activation of this structure in some fMRI studies. Moreover, Barrash suggested that the right hippocampus played a role in the consolidation of the topographical information in long-term memory (Barrash *et al.* 2000). After the consolidation period, the hippocampus would not be necessary for recalling topographical information. In addition,

Rosenbaum proposed that this structure could be involved only in the spatial memory of recent events, but not in the case of recalling spatial information encoded a long time ago (Rosenbaum *et al.* 2004).

Individual spatial abilities

Maguire *et al.* evidenced a positive relationship between performance in a wayfinding task and the amount of activation in the hippocampus (Maguire *et al.* 1998a). This assumption was confirmed by some other works. Pine *et al.* showed that during a wayfinding memory task in an allocentric perspective, the level of activation of the left posterior part of the hippocampus positively correlated with the performances to the test (Pine *et al.* 2002). Hartley *et al.* also reported that good navigators exhibited increased activity in the hippocampus while bad navigators presented a decrease of activity in this structure (Hartley *et al.* 2003). In this case, it seems that the hippocampus is specifically implicated when the task is successfully performed. Inter-individual variability in performance could thus explain, at least in part, the discrepancies between studies.

Gender

A behavioural study demonstrated that women and men rely on distinct strategies to process spatial information (Sandstrom *et al.* 1998). Women use predominantly landmark cues whereas men use both landmarks and geometric cues. To elucidate whether this behavioural difference has some consequences at the brain's organization level, Grön *et al.* compare the fMRI results in women and men while they navigated a virtual maze (Grön *et al.* 2000). The authors showed that the left hippocampus was more activated in men whereas women recruited right parietal and right pre-frontal regions. The male-specific hippocampal activity may reflect a more efficient strategy (accordingly, their performances were better). Note, however, that this result has not been found in another work that used both route and survey perspectives in a learning task and which evidenced no difference between women and men, whatever the perspective (Blanch *et al.* 2004).

The parahippocampal gyrus: spatial scenes and landmarks

Unlike the hippocampus, activation in the parahippocampus has been found in almost all works studying navigation in humans. This region, strongly connected to the hippocampus, has been shown to be specifically involved in the perception and mental imagery of spatial scenes and places, such as rooms and landscapes. It has been termed the parahippocampal place area (Epstein and Kanwisher 1998; Epstein *et al.* 1999; O'Craven and Kanwisher 2000). The parahippocampal gyrus has also been involved in the encoding of objects during navigation (Aguirre *et al.* 1996; Maguire *et al.* 1998b). Recent research provided new insights into this latter aspect (Janzen and Van Turennout 2004). In the first phase of this study, participants viewed a route in a virtual environment (VE) with objects placed at locations relevant for navigation (an intersection for example) or, at simple turn, useless for navigation. The authors then monitored brain activity in fMRI while the participants were asked to recognize both types of objects in isolation. The results of the participants showed that parahippocampal responses increased for objects previously placed at locations with a navigational relevance (Janzen and Van Turennout 2004). Interestingly, this increase was independent from attentional demand and also occurred even when subjects viewed objects they had forgotten. The navigational information thus appears automatically activated, in the absence of any spatial cues.

The issue of how parahippocampus and hippocampus work together to provide a coherent topographical representation is still not clear. One reason for this is that the hippocampus has been inconsistently found activated in neuroimaging studies (see Figure 2.1) and might not be indispensable in path integration (Shrager *et al.* 2008). Another reason is that the type of represen-tation processed by the parahippocampus is not entirely settled. It has been suggested that the early representation is largely viewpoint-specific (Epstein *et al.* 2003). However, this representa-tion could evolve over time and become viewpoint-invariant, thus being closer to a cognitive map (Epstein *et al.* 2005).

Impact of learning modalities on the neural bases of topographical representation

A feature of topographical representations is that they can be built from numerous modalities. The final part of this chapter emphasizes that, besides the core network involved in topographical representations, some regions might be additionally involved, depending on the modality from which this representation is built. As previously mentioned, the most natural way to memorize an environment is to walk within this environment. From here, one builds a representation in a route perspective where the position of landmarks is specified in relation to the body. It is also possible to learn from a map. In this case, the representation is elaborated in a survey perspective. The landmarks are then specified independently of one's position. A third possibility is to men-tally build a spatial image of the environment from a verbal or written description. Finally, it is possible to memorize an environment by using a virtual reality device. In fact, the growing use of video games and realistic simulation devices made VEs that are new and powerful materials with which to build topographical representations. In this framework, the central question of this final section is: Do these different modalities lead to a unique representation in the brain, or is there some difference at the cortical level that could be related to the way the representation of the environment has been built?

Effect of perspective: can we distinguish in the brain an environment learnt by navigation from an environment learnt by map reading?

Some studies have found an effect of the learning perspective on the properties of the topograph-ic representation built from either text descriptions (Schneider and Taylor 1999) or visual experi-ence (Thorndyke and Hayes-Roth 1982; Taylor *et al.* 1999). For example, route distance estimations are more accurate than Euclidean distance (straight-line) estimations when informa-tion has been initially acquired by actual navigation, while the reverse pattern is observed when the spatial information has been encoded through survey learning (Thorndyke and Hayes-Roth 1982). In the same vein, survey-learning subjects make more errors when judging orientation (e.g., are asked to indicate the direction of a landmark using a compass wheel) than navigation-learning subjects. The structure of the topographic representation seems, therefore, in part, con-strained by the route or survey perspective in which spatial information is acquired. It is thus natural to investigate whether such behavioural differences could be reflected at the brain level. A neuroimaging study including two groups of participants tackled this question (Mellet *et al.* 2000a). In order to ensure optimal homogeneity of the sample of the subjects, all participants were selected as high-visuospatial imagers. They scored beyond the 75th percentile of a popula-tion of 100 male subjects on the basis of the Minnesota Paper Form Board and on the Mental Rotation Test. The first group learned the environment by means of an actual walk within this environment. During this walk, the subjects encountered landmarks (such as a gas station, a stat-ue, etc.), and were instructed to memorize the position of the landmarks. The second group learned the same environment on a map with coloured dots standing in for the landmarks. In both groups, the task in the PET camera was the same: with eyes closed, the participants were to move mentally between two landmarks, delivered through earphones, and press a key when they reached the second landmark. In addition to the CBF, the reaction times were collected. When the relationship between the reaction time and the distance was examined, the same relationship as evidenced by Kosslyn thirty years ago was discovered (Kosslyn *et al.* 1978); this relationship was true regardless of the type of learning. This strengthened the fact that the isomorphism between spatial mental images and the configurations they represent is a general property of topographic representations, and does not depend on which way the survey or route perspective was acquired.

With respect to these behavioural similarities, a fronto-parietal network, as well as the right hippocampus, was activated during the mental tasks, as compared to a rest condition, whatever the type of learning. As such, this study demonstrated that the core network of topographical representations was activated, whatever the route or survey perspective of learning.

Interestingly, the contrast of the two mental exploration tasks revealed a major difference confined to the parahippocampal gyrus that was specific to the route perspective learning. As discussed earlier, this region plays a key role in the processing of natural landmarks. Learning the route by walking included encountering the actual landmarks (unlike the survey perspective learning landmarks, which were represented by coloured dots). At first glance, it seems that retrieval of topographical representation is poorly affected by the perspective in which it has been learned. Shelton and Gabrieli (2002) contrasted the two perspectives with fMRI during the learning phase rather than the retrieval stage. The results suggested that the differences between the two perspectives could be more prominent during encoding. In particular, survey encoding recruited a subset of areas recruited by route encoding, but it did so with greater activation in some areas (inferior temporal cortex and posterior superior parietal cortex). By contrast, route encoding recruited regions that were not activated by survey encoding (medial temporal lobe structures, anterior superior parietal cortex, and postcentral gyrus).

Mental images are not restricted to the reactivation of visual memories. In fact, the importance of mental imagery in human cognition comes, in part, from the interaction between mental imagery and language. Humans have the ability to translate symbolic information into an analogical format, to build a mental image from a verbal description, and vice-versa. Interestingly, mental images built from a verbal description or built from visual memorization not only share properties at the behavioural level (Denis and Cocude 1992; Denis 2008) but also activate common neural networks (Mellet *et al.* 1996, 2000b). This observation elicits the second question.

Can we distinguish in the brain an environment learnt visually (map reading) from an environment learnt verbally (reading a text which describes a map)?

Researchers suggest that the representation built from a verbal description shares some structural properties with the mental image of the environment built from visual perception. It is now widely accepted that the topographic representation built from a text not only includes the spatial relations that have been explicitly described in the text, but also, as for topographic representation built from perception, allows people to deduce a number of non-stated relations (Perrig and Kintsch 1985; Taylor and Tversky 1992a,b). Empirical support is provided by studies showing that when people perform mental scanning across spatial configurations containing several landmarks, a positive correlation between scanned distances and scanning times is obtained in both cases. This is true whether the images were built from the visual perception of a map or the processing of a verbal description of that map, where the relative distances between landmarks could be inferred (Denis and Cocude 1992; Denis and Kosslyn 1999; Denis 2008). The existence of features common to representations built from visual and verbal inputs raises the hypothesis that both types of representation could share some neural components. However, the topographic knowledge obtained through verbal information differs in several aspects from that acquired through visual experience. In particular, metric information, which is naturally included in the topographic representation built visually, may be absent or incomplete in a text description. Thus, the structural isomorphism between a physical environment and its mental counterpart may not be achieved when mental scanning (or some other form of mental processing) is performed on an environment that has been verbally described. Consequently, the neural components involved in the storage and the retrieval of topographic knowledge that is acquired from these two modalities may not be identical.

A PET study tested this hypothesis using neuroimaging (Mellet *et al.* 2002). Two groups of subjects participated in this study. In the first group, the participants had to visually memorize a map during the learning phase as described in the study presented above. The second group had to read a text describing an environment until they were able to build a spatial image of this environment, including the landmarks described in the text in survey perspective. Importantly, no metric information was included in the text. In both groups, the task in the PET camera was the same: with eyes closed, participants had to mentally imagine the environment and to move from one landmark to another, the name of landmarks being delivered through earphones. They pressed a key when they reached the second landmark. Thus, map learners heard, for example, 'red dot, yellow dot' and travelled mentally between the two dots. The text learners heard 'white hills-fairy road' and did the same task between the two landmarks. In addition to the CBF, the reaction times were collected. After the PET session, the subjects were invited to draw maps of the environments that they had built from the texts. They produced accurate maps, suggesting that they were able to translate the verbal information included in the text in a spatial representation. Moreover, the map they drew was used to assess the relation between the time the subject spent to mentally travel between landmarks and the normalized distance between the landmarks. Most subjects (four out of six) exhibited a significant positive correlation between distance and mental scanning time, although they had no metric constraint to build their maps. This meant that these subjects incorporated their own metric in their representation and kept it constant throughout the task. However, some subjects did not show such correlation, suggesting that the spatial representations they built and scanned were less stable with a less consistent metric.

Turning to the PET results, the authors reported a fronto-parietal network, very similar to the one described earlier, involved in the task, whatever the visual or verbal modality of learning. This is in line with its very general role in the processing of spatial representation. When the two groups were compared, the hippocampus was more activated in map learners than in text learners to the point that the hippocampus was actually deactivated in most of text learners. Thus, while the fronto-parietal network remains the core set of region for visuospatial processing, the hippocampal activity was modulated by the way the topographical representation was built. In particular, this result suggested that the medial temporal lobe plays a more limited role than previously assumed. According to the results, this structure is crucial only when the information from which the topographic representation is built is visual, or when accurate metric information is provided.

The most striking results were discovered when looking at the regions more activated in text readers than in map readers. Activation of Broca's area (left inferior frontal gyrus) and of Wernicke's area (the posterior part of the left superior temporal gyrus) was evidenced. These activations are likely related to the verbal nature of the original input. These results suggested that Broca's and Wernicke's areas could be activated even when the task did not explicitly include any language components. These activations demonstrated that areas belonging to the language network (Vigneau *et al.*, 2006), and presumably active during the construction and the encoding of the representation (i.e., the mental map), were also implicated during the retrieval of this representation. These activations could reflect that there is a representation of the text encoded in the brain from which the analogue 'picture-like' representation used during the mental scanning task is derived. Moreover, these results were in line with the neuroimaging findings, suggesting that some of the brain regions active during the encoding of specific piece of information were reactivated during this information retrieval (Nyberg *et al.* 2000; Wheeler *et al.* 2000). In addition to these language areas, the authors reported a parietal activation extending downward to a region that straddles the angular gyrus and the middle occipital gyrus. The angular gyrus belongs to the heteromodal cortex, and seems to be involved in processes that combine symbolic and analogue representations. For example, the left angular gyrus is engaged in reading tasks that combine visuospatial and linguistic processing. It is also involved in calculation which merge symbols (figures and number) and analogue representations of magnitude (Dehaene 1992; Chochon *et al.* 1999; Zago *et al.* 2001). In the present study, the specific implication of the angular gyrus in the mental scanning, after learning by reading condition, may reflect that the symbolic information has been transformed in analogue 'map-like' information used during mental scanning.

We can conclude from this study that, although the brain has converted verbal information into a visuospatial format, an effect of the learning modality remains present in the cortical representation of the learned environment. Would this effect still be present when the difference between the two learning modalities is much closer? Virtual reality was used to address this issue and to answer the following question.

Does the brain keep a trace of learning modality when it only differs in the real or virtual nature of the environment explored?

Even though the use of realistic simulation devices grows in a variety of domains, including neuroimaging studies, the question of whether VEs are represented differently from real environment (RE) within the brain is still unknown. In contrast to what has been observed, with learning by visual map or descriptive text, spatial knowledge acquired by moving in VE (in a route perspective) is broadly similar to that gained from walking within an RE, at least when the VE used is highly realistic (immersive VE) and has a simple spatial configuration (Ruddle *et al.* 1997; Richardson *et al.* 1999; Lessels and Ruddle 2005).

However, even if immersive VE provides a realistic display, a crucial difference with the real world exists: exploring and learning a VE usually involves simulated locomotion through a joystick. It thus requires the conversion of visual information, arising from the visual display, into motor manipulation of the joystick to control one's trajectory within the virtual space. If, as suggested above, the learning modality shapes the cortical representation of an environment, then the use of a tool dedicated to navigation should have consequences at the cortical level. In particular, the process related to the complex use of a tool for learning should leave a cortical fingerprint. This was tested by an experiment wherein participants freely navigated using a joystick within an immersive virtual indoor environment containing ten landmarks (Mellet *et al. in press*). A control group explored the real version of a strictly identical environment by actual walking. The day after the learning phase, all subjects were scanned with fMRI while performing a topographical memory task where they had to mentally compare bird-flight distances between pairs of landmarks in the previously learned environment. At the behavioural level, there was no difference between virtual and real learners. In particular, there was no difference in time spent to learn the environment outside the camera and during scanning; response times and error rates were identical in both groups. Also, after the scanning session, both groups were able to draw accurate maps confirming that they could easily produce a survey representation of the environment. These behavioural similarities are in line with previous work, which evidenced broadly similar topographical knowledge between RE and VE, at least when simple and immersive VEs were used, as is the case in this experiment (Ruddle *et al.* 1997; Richardson *et al.* 1999; Lessels and Ruddle 2005). Obviously, a network common to both groups, which included the fronto-parietal network and the parahippocampus bilaterally, was activated. As discussed previously, this latter region is a key area for landmarks processing. An accurate positioning of landmarks is essential to perform the mental task, whatever the way the environment was learned. More interestingly, despite similar behavioural results, some regions were more activated in virtual learners than in real ones. In particular, this was the case for three regions: the left inferior frontal gyrus (IFG), the left inferior parietal lobule (IPL), and the left posterior part of the middle temporal gyrus (MTG). Strikingly, this network is repeatedly implicated in semantic knowledge of actions and tools (Johnson-Frey 2004; Noppeney *et al.* 2005) and is similar to the network described in action tool representation (Kellenbach *et al.* 2003). More specifically, the left IFG appears to play a key role in conceptual knowledge of tool use (Goldenberg *et al.* 2007). This region interacts with the left IPL in hand–object interactive movement and more generally when visuomotor coordination is required (Culham and Valyear 2006). Finally, the posterior MTG is activated during retrieval of information about tools and when making semantic decision about action (Chao *et al.* 1999; Noppeney *et al.* 2005). Critically, these regions are involved in the execution or the motor imagery of hand movements with a joystick (Stephan *et al.* 1995). It is worth noting that the cortical signature of the virtual nature of the learned environment spared medial temporal regions. This is likely related to the absence of difference in performance between virtual and real learners. As a conclusion to this last study, these results strongly suggest that, compared to real learners, virtual learners exhibited more activation in a strongly left, lateralized set of regions involved in the representations of hand–object interaction and high-level representation of action. This is likely related to the use of a joystick that allowed a simulated walk within the VE. Thus, a neural fingerprint of learning by virtual reality related to the use of a tool to navigate during the learning phase was detected. However, this conclusion remains somewhat speculative. To confirm that the cortical difference evidenced was indeed related to the use of a tool, we designed an additional experiment where subjects learned actively or passively either the RE or its virtual replication. A joystick in the virtual version or actual locomotion in the RE allowed participants to explore actively. For virtual learners, the experimenter used the joystick according to their indications while real learners were driven in a wheeling chair by the experimenter to allow passive exploration. If the differences observed in the first study were actually related to the use of the joystick, then they should no longer be detected when virtual passive learners are compared to real passive learners. In general, this study should also provide new insights on the neural substrate of the motor component included in topographic learning. The data analysis is currently in progress.

The first part of this chapter described the core network of topographical representations. It included a fronto-parietal network generally involved in spatial cognition, and the hippocampus and the parahippocampus in the medial part of the temporal lobe, regions more specific to the topographical nature of the spatial representation. Some aspects of the role of the hippocampus remain to be clarified. The identification of the factors that could modulate its involvement, such as gender and skill, gave rise to an abundance of literature over the last few years. On the other hand, the role of the parahippocampus in spatial scenes perception and landmarks identification is well established. The second part of the chapter suggested that the visual, verbal, real, or virtual nature modality of the initial information is used to build the representation matters for the brain. The modality left a neural fingerprint that is revealed when the spatial representation is used. This supports the view developed by Barsalou that knowledge is not amodal but rather grounded in sensorimotor systems (Barsalou *et al.* 2003).

References

Aguirre, G.K. and D'Esposito, M. (1999). Topographical disorientation: a synthesis and taxonomy. *Brain*, **122**, 1613–28.

Aguirre, G.K., Dettre, J.A., Alsop, D.C., and D'Esposito, M. (1996). The parahippocampus subserves topographical learning in man. *Cerebral Cortex*, **6**, 823–9.

Aguirre, G.K., Zarahn, E., and D'Esposito, M. (1998). Neural components of topographical representation. *Proceedings of the National Academy of Sciences of the United States of America*, **95**, 839–46.

Astur, R.S., Tropp, J., Sava, S., Constable, R.T., and Markus, E.J. (2004). Sex differences and correlations in a virtual Morris water task, a virtual radial arm maze, and mental rotation. *Behavioural Brain Research*, **151**, 103–15.

Barrash, J., Damasio, H., Adolphs, R., and Tranel, D. (2000). The neuroanatomical correlates of route learning impairment. *Neuropsychologia*, **38**, 820–36.

Barsalou, L.W., Kyle, S.W., Barbey, A.K., and Wilson, C.D. (2003). Grounding conceptual knowledge in modality-specific systems. *Trends in Cognitive Sciences*, **7**, 84–91.

Beauchamp, M.S., Petit, L., Ellmore, T.M., Ingeholm, J., and Haxby, J.V. (2001). A parametric fMRI study of overt and covert shifts of visuospatial attention. *NeuroImage*, **14**, 310–21.

Blanch, R.J., Brennan, D., Condon, B., Santosh, C., and Hadley, D. (2004). Are there gender-specific neural substrates of route learning from different perspectives? *Cerebral Cortex*, **14**, 1207–13.

Burgess, N. and O'Keefe, J. (2003). Neural representations in human spatial memory. *Trends in Cognitive Sciences*, **7**, 517–9.

Chao, L.L., Haxby, J.V., and Martin, A. (1999). Attribute-based neural substrates in temporal cortex for perceiving and knowing about objects. *Nature Neuroscience*, **2**, 913–9.

Chochon, F., Cohen, L., Vandemoortele, P.F., and Dehaene, S. (1999). Differential contributions of the left and right inferior parietal lobules to number processing. *Journal of Cognitive Neuroscience*, **11**, 617–30.

Corbetta, M. (1998). Frontoparietal cortical networks for directing attention and the eye visual locations: identical, independent, or overlapping neural systems? *Proceedings of the National Academy of Sciences of the United States of America*, **95**, 831–8.

Courtney, S.M., Petit, L., Maisog, J.M., Ungerleider, L.G., and Haxby, J.V. (1998). An area specialized for spatial working memory in human frontal cortex. *Science*, **279**, 1347–51.

Culham, J.C. and Valyear, K.F. (2006). Human parietal cortex in action. *Current Opinion in Neurobiology*, **16**, 205–12.

Dehaene, S. (1992). Varieties of numerical abilities. *Cognition*, **44**, 1–42.

Denis, M. (2008). Assessing the symbolic distance effect in mental images constructed from verbal descriptions: a study of individual differences in the mental comparison of distances. *Acta Psychologica (Amsterdam)*, **127**, 197–210.

Denis, M. and Cocude, M. (1992). Structural properties of visual images constructed from poorly or well-structured verbal descriptions. *Memory and Cognition*, **20**, 497–506.

Denis, M. and Kosslyn, S.M. (1999). Scanning visual mental images: a window on the mind. *Current Psychology of Cognition*, **18**, 409–65.

Ekstrom, A.D., Kahana, M.J., Caplan, J.B., *et al.* (2003). Cellular networks underlying human spatial navigation. *Nature*, **425**, 184–8.

Epstein, R., Graham, K.S., and Downing, P.E. (2003). Viewpoint-specific scene representations in human parahippocampal cortex. *Neuron*, **37**, 865–76.

Epstein, R., Harris, A., Stanley, D., and Kanwisher, N. (1999). The parahippocampal place area: recognition, navigation, or encoding. *Neuron*, **23**, 115–25.

Epstein, R. and Kanwisher, N. (1998). A cortical representation of the local visual environment. *Nature*, **392**, 598–601.

Epstein, R.A., Higgins, J.S., and Thompson-Schill, S.L. (2005). Learning places from views: variation in scene processing as a function of experience and navigational ability. *Journal of Cognitive Neuroscience*, **17**, 73–83.

Goldenberg, G., Hermsdorfer, J., Glindemann, R., Rorden, C., and Karnath, H.O. (2007). Pantomime of tool use depends on integrity of left inferior frontal cortex. *Cerebral Cortex*, **17**, 2769–76.

Grön, G., Wunderlich, A.P., Spitzer, M., Tomczak, R., and Riepe, M.W. (2000). Brain activation during human navigation: gender-different neural networks as substrate of performance. *Nature Neuroscience*, **3**, 404–8.

Hartley, T., Maguire, E.A., Spiers, H.J., and Burgess, N. (2003). The well-worn route and the path less traveled: distinct neural bases of route following and wayfinding in humans. *Neuron*, **37**, 877–88.

Iaria, G., Petrides, M., Dagher, A., Pike, B., and Bohbot, V.D. (2003). Cognitive strategies dependent on the hippocampus and caudate nucleus in human navigation: variability and change with practice. *The Journal of Neuroscience*, **23**, 5945–52.

Ino, T., Inoue, Y., Kage, M., Hirose, S., Kimura, T., and Fukuyama, H. (2002). Mental navigation in humans is processed in the anterior bank of the parieto-occipital sulcus. *Neuroscience Letters*, **322**, 182–6.

Janzen, G. and Van Turennout, M. (2004). Selective neural representation of objects relevant for navigation. *Nature Neuroscience*, **7**, 673–7.

Johnson-Frey, S.H. (2004). The neural bases of complex tool use in humans. *Trends in Cognitive Sciences*, **8**, 71–8.

Jonides, J., Smith, E.E., Koeppe, R.A., Awh, E., Minoshima, S., and Mintun, M.A. (1993). Spatial working memory in humans as revealed by PET. *Nature*, **363**, 623–4.

Jordan, K., Schadow, J., Wuestenberg, T., Heinze, H.J., and Jancke, L. (2004). Different cortical activations for subjects using allocentric or egocentric strategies in a virtual navigation task. *Neuroreport*, **15**, 135–40.

Kellenbach, M.L., Brett, M., and Patterson, K. (2003). Actions speak louder than functions: the importance of manipulability and action in tool representation. *Journal of Cognitive Neuroscience*, **15**, 30–46.

Kosslyn, S.M., Ball, T.M., and Reiser, B.J. (1978). Visual images preserve metric spatial information: evidence from studies of image scanning. *Journal of Experimental Psychology: Human Perception and Performance*, **4**, 47–60.

Lessels, S. and Ruddle, R.A. (2005). Movements around real and virtual cluttered environments. *Presence*, **14**, 580–96.

Maguire, E.A., Burgess, N., Donnett, J.G., Frackowiak, R.S.J., Frith, C.D., and O'Keefe, J. (1998a). Knowing where and getting there: a human navigation network. *Science*, **280**, 921–4.

Maguire, E.A., Frith, C.D., Burgess, N., Donnett, J.G., and O'Keefe, J. (1998b). Knowing where things are: parahippocampal involvement in encoding object locations in virtual large-scale space. *Journal of Cognitive Neuroscience*, **10**, 61–76.

Mellet, E., Bricogne, S., Crivello, F., Mazoyer, B., Denis, M., and Tzourio-Mazoyer, N. (2002). Neural basis of mental scanning of a topographic representation built from a text. *Cerebral Cortex*, **12**, 1322–30.

Mellet, E., Briscogne, S., Tzourio-mazoyer, N. *et al.* (2000a). Neural correlates of topographic mental exploration: the impact of route versus survey perspective learning. *NeuroImage*, **12**, 588–600.

Mellet, E., Kosslyn, S.M., Mazoyer, N., Bricogne, S., Denis, M., and Mazoyer, B. (2000b). Functional anatomy of high resolution mental imagery. *Journal of Cognitive Neuroscience*, **12**, 98–109.

Mellet, E., Laou, L., Petit, L., Zago, L., Mazoyer, B., and Tzourio-Mazoyer, N. (In press) Impact of the virtual reality on the neural representation of an environment. *Human Brain Mapping*.

Mellet, E., Tzourio, N., Crivello, F., Joliot, M., Denis, M., and Mazoyer, B. (1996). Functional anatomy of spatial mental imagery generated from verbal instruction. *The Journal of Neuroscience*, **16**, 6504–12.

Mellet, E., Tzourio, N., Denis, M., and Mazoyer, B. (1995). A positron emission tomography study of visual and mental spatial exploration. *Journal of Cognitive Neuroscience*, **7**, 433–45.

Morris, R.G.M., Garrud, P., Rawlins, J.N., and O'Keefe, J. (1982). Place navigation impaired in rats with hippocampal lesions. *Nature*, **297**, 681–3.

Noppeney, U., Josephs, O., Kiebel, S., Friston, K.J., and Price, C.J. (2005). Action selectivity in parietal and temporal cortex. *Cognitive Brain Research*, **25**, 641–9.

Nyberg, L., Habib, R., McIntosh, A.R., and Tulving, E. (2000). Reactivation of encoding-related brain activity during memory retrieval. *Proceedings of the National Academy of Science U.S.A.*, **97**, 11120–4.

O'Craven, K.M. and Kanwisher, N. (2000). Mental imagery of faces and places activates corresponding stimulus-specific brain regions. *Journal of Cognitive Neuroscience*, **12**, 1013–23.

O'Keefe, J. and Dostrovsky, J. (1971). The hippocampus as a cognitive map: preliminary evidence from unit activity in the freely moving rat. *Brain Research*, **34**, 171–5.

O'Keefe, J. and Nadel, L. (1978) *The hippocampus as a cognitive map*. Oxford: Clarendon.

Perrig, W. and Kintsch, W. (1985). Propositional and situational representations of text. *Journal of Memory and Language*, **24**, 503–18.

Petit, L., Courtney, S.M., Ungerleider, L.G., and Haxby, J.V. (1998). Sustained activity in the medial wall during working memory delays. *The Journal of Neuroscience*, **18**, 9429–37.

Petit, L., Orssaud, C., Tzourio, N., Crivello, F., Berthoz, A., and Mazoyer, B. (1996). Functional anatomy of a sequence of prelearned saccades in man. *The Journal of Neuroscience*, **16**, 3714–26.

Picard, N. and Strick, P.L. (1996). Motor area of the medial wall: a review of their location and functional activation. *Cerebral Cortex*, **6**, 342–53.

Pine, D.S., Grun, J., Maguire, E.A., *et al.* (2002). Neurodevelopmental aspects of spatial navigation: a virtual reality fMRI study. *NeuroImage*, **15**, 396–406.

Raichle, M.E. and Mintun, M.A. (2006). Brain work and brain imaging. *Annual Review of Neuroscience*, **29**, 449–76.

Richardson, A.E., Montello, D.R., and Hegarty, M. (1999). Spatial knowledge acquisition from maps and from navigation in real and virtual environments. *Memory and Cognition*, **27**, 741–50.

Rosenbaum, R.S., Ziegler, M., Winocur, G., Grady, C.L., and Moscovitch, M. (2004). 'I have often walked down this street before': fMRI studies on the hippocampus and other structures during mental navigation of an old environment. *Hippocampus*, **14**, 826–35.

Ruddle, R.A., Payne, S.J., and Jones, D.M. (1997). Navigating buildings in 'desk-top' virtual environments: experimental investigations using extended navigational experience. *Journal of Experimental Psychology: Applied*, **3**, 143–59.

Sandstrom, N.J., Kaufman, J., and Huettel, S.A. (1998). Males and females use different distal cues in a virtual environment navigation task. *Cognitive Brain Research*, **6**, 351–60.

Schneider, L.F. and Taylor, H.A. (1999). How do you get there from here? Mental representations of route description. *Applied Cognitive Psychology*, **13**, 415–41.

Shelton, A.L. and Gabrieli, J.D. (2002). Neural correlates of encoding space from route and survey perspectives. *Journal of Neuroscience*, **22**, 2711–7.

Shrager, Y., Kirwan, C.B., and Squire, L.R. (2008). Neural basis of the cognitive map: path integration does not require hippocampus or entorhinal cortex. *Proceedings of the National Academy of Science U.S.A.*, **105**, 12034–8.

Smith, E.E., Jonides, J., and Koeppe, R.A. (1996). Dissociating verbal and spatial working memory using PET. *Cerebral Cortex*, **6**, 11–20.

Stephan, K.M., Fink, G.R., Passingham, R.E., *et al.* (1995). Functional anatomy of the mental representation of upper extremity movements in healthy subjects. *Journal of Neurophysiology*, **73**, 373–86.

Taylor, H.A., Naylor, S.J., and Chechile, N.A. (1999). Goal-specific influences on the representation of spatial perspective. *Memory and Cognition*, **27**, 309–19.

Taylor, H.A. and Tversky, B. (1992a). Descriptions and depictions of environments. *Memory and Cognition*, **20**, 483–96.

Taylor, H.A. and Tversky, B. (1992b). Spatial mental models derived from survey and route description descriptions. *Journal of Memory and Language*, **31**, 261–92.

Thorndyke P.W. and Hayes-Roth, B. (1982). Differences in spatial knowledge acquired from maps and navigation. *Cognitive Psychology*, **14**, 560–89.

Vigneau, M., Beaucousin, V., Hervé, P.Y., *et al.* (2006). Meta-analyzing left hemisphere language areas: phonology, semantics, and sentence processing. *NeuroImage*, **30**, 1414–32.

Wheeler, M.E., Petersen, S.E., and Buckner, R.L. (2000). Memory's echo: vivid remembering reactivates sensory-specific cortex. *Proceedings of the National Academy of Science U.S.A.*, **97**, 11125–9.

Wolbers, T. and Buchel, C. (2005). Dissociable retrosplenial and hippocampal contributions to successful formation of survey representations. *The Journal of Neuroscience*, **25**, 3333–40.

Wolbers, T., Weiller, C., and Buchel, C. (2004). Neural foundations of emerging route knowledge in complex spatial environments. *Cognitive Brain Research*, **21**, 401–11.

Zago, L., Pesenti, M., Mellet, E., Crivello, F., Mazoyer, B., and Tzourio-Mazoyer, N. (2001). Neural correlates of simple and complex mental calculation. *NeuroImage*, **13**, 314–27.

Zago, L., Petit, L., Turbelin, M.R., Andersson, F., Vigneau, M., and Tzourio-Mazoyer, N. (2008). How verbal and spatial manipulation networks contribute to calculation: an fMRI study. *Neuropsychologia*, **46**, 2403–14.

Chapter 3

Contribution of the primary motor c to motor imagery

Martin Lotze and Karen Zentgraf

The functional equivalence between motor imagery and motor execution

According to Jeannerod (1994, 1995), motor imagery (in this chapter, we shall use the abbreviation IM for motor imagery to avoid confusion with M1, the primary motor cortex) represents the process of accessing the intention to perform a movement that may be carried out also unconsciously during movement preparation. IM and motor preparation therefore share common mechanisms and can be viewed as functionally equivalent processes. As a result, it is not surprising that movement execution (ME) and IM reveal a high overlap of active brain regions. This has been demonstrated convincingly by imaging studies in the last 15 years (Lotze and Halsband 2006; Munzer et al. 2009, for overviews). As we have already learned about these overlapping networks in the Chapter 2, we shall now focus on the contribution of the primary motor cortex to IM.

The involvement of the contralateral primary motor cortex (cM1) in IM reflects a fundamental shift in our understanding of the functional organization of the motor system. If cM1 were to be related purely to execution, no activity would be expected during IM; and if it were to be found, it should be due to undetected execution during IM. On the other hand, if M1 were active during IM, even when any ME is avoided, this would drastically modify our understanding of the function of M1 during movement preparation and execution. We already have good reasons to change our concept of the primary motor cortex, because neurons in M1 code not only for mere ME but also for differences in movement complexity (Lotze et al. 2000), and play an important role in motor learning – as demonstrated by the training-associated changes in M1 recruitment that accompany improvements in performance (Karni et al. 1995; Lotze et al. 2003).

The relation between motor execution and imagination

James (1890) and Jacobson (1930) both maintained that the mental image of a movement is always followed by discharges of its target muscles. In contrast, recent scientific approaches to IM try to exclude any motor execution. By inhibiting the execution of a movement, it becomes possible to gain conscious access to motor preparation (Jeannerod 1994). Early work on imagery clearly demonstrates the relation between a movement-related mental image and peripheral processes. During imagined weight lifting, the forearm muscles show a linear increase of amplitude in EMG recordings as a function of increasing weight (Shaw 1940). Since the autonomous nervous system cannot be modulated directly on a voluntary basis, the immediately observed changes of heart rate during imagined foot movements along with the increases in CO_2 pressure and in respiration frequency (Decety et al. 1991, 1993; Wuyam et al. 1995) are probably caused by cerebral processes that are part of motor programming. Guillot et al. (2008) underline the connection between IM and its consequences for bodily processes. They used skin conductance responses (SCR) during imagined and executed movements to separate good from bad motor imagers. Good imagers show a task-related increase in SCR during IM and a decrease during rest. Therefore, it is essential to take vividness of IM into consideration when talking about mental accuracy. This issue is extensively elaborated in Chapter 8 of this book and the importance for measuring physiological and psychological parameters to control the imagery performance of subjects has been stressed in detail previously (Guillot and Collet 2005a).

Decety (1996a, 1996b) also proposed that during imagined activities, a significant portion of the observed increase in autonomic response is of central origin. They suggested that in IM, the mind deludes the body into believing that some movements are being executed. Additionally, subjective ratings of the mental effort to imagine a task correlate with the amount of force needed for task execution.

Another argument for a common basis of ME and IM is provided by studies using a mental chronometry paradigm. Executed and imagined writing of the same letters, regardless of which hand is used, or executed and imagined walking of the same distances show the same durations (Decety and Michel 1989; Bakker *et al.* 2008). If the task is more difficult, for example, when carrying a heavy load, participants tend to overestimate the duration of IM. Visual imagery of walking on a thin line, for instance, does not reveal any delayed duration in contrast to imagery of walking on a broad comfortable path. However, there is a significant delay in kinaesthetic imagination for the thin line walk when compared with the broad path (Bakker *et al.* 2008). In addition, Fitts' law (Fitts 1954), which states that more difficult movements take more time to be executed than easier ones, also holds for imagined movements (Decety and Jeannerod 1995; Maruff *et al.* 1999). Hence, the validity of Fitts' law can be used to distinguish between participants who are able to imagine a task kinaesthetically and those who cannot.

Further investigations on the durations of imagined movements have, however, also revealed differences compared with executed movements. In a review of the durations of mentally simulated movements, Guillot and Collet (2005b) concluded that when athletes simulate only dynamic phases of movement or perform IM just before competing, environmental and time constraints lead to an underestimation of actual duration. Conversely, complex attention-demanding movements take longer to imagine. In line with previous assumptions, the process of imagination is not fully dependent on the ability to execute a movement, but depends rather on central processing mechanisms. Compared with healthy controls, patients with lesions of the motor cortex and patients with Parkinson's disease (Dominey *et al.* 1995) show decreased movement velocity during ME and IM. Patients with incomplete spinal lesions show only prolonged duration of ME but the same durations of IM (Decety and Boisson 1990). Most interestingly, activation in M1 is even enhanced after complete peripheral deafferentation due to spinal cord injury or peripheral nerve lesion (Lotze *et al.* 2001, 2006; Alkadhi *et al.* 2005). This finding indicates that M1 can be accessed by IM even after years of deafferentation and deefferentation.

Differences between IM and ME

The lack of execution of the task

Scientific approaches to imagery differ from those in applied fields. For athletes and musicians, a perfect avoidance of ME during IM is not necessarily important, and some tension or even movement of the target muscles during IM is tolerable. Some athletes even report that bringing their body into a position similar to the motor task and moving slightly helps them to generate a vivid motor image. However, in order to distinguish clearly between IM and ME, from a scientific viewpoint, it is essential to avoid any motor activity during IM. This would mean that cortical neuronal assemblies involved only in ME (if there are some) should not be involved in IM. We shall deal with issues in controlling avoidance of motor execution during IM in the methodological section of this chapter. In addition, Chapters 4 and 6 of this book carefully consider inhibitory mechanisms for motor commands in IM.

The lack of somatosensory feedback

Interacting with the environment is always associated with sensory input from changes in body position and dynamics (proprioceptive) as well as from objects in the external world transmitted by different sensory modalities (exteroceptive). The motor system is particularly dependent on feedback from somatosensory inputs. Anatomically, the somatosensory system is tightly connected to the primary motor cortex via U fibres. If there is no interaction with an external object, this special type of somatosensory input is lacking. Because the sensorimotor guidance of movement is coordinated predominantly by the ipsilateral anterior hemisphere of the cerebellum (Gao *et al.* 1996), it is not astonishing that some studies on IM, which had implemented a careful normalization of cerebellar anatomy, demonstrated that IM involves different structures within the cerebellar hemisphere than ME does (Lotze *et al.* 1999).

In the visual or auditory modality, the recruitment of primary areas during imagination has been shown to correlate highly with the vividness of imagery (Cui *et al.* 2007; Kraemer *et al.* 2005). In contrast, there are no explicit reports on vivid somatosensory imagery tasks. Some studies, however, demonstrated somatosensory activation during vivid IM (Stippich *et al.* 2002; Lorey *et al.* 2009) – even after deafferentation (Lotze *et al.* 2001).

Methodological issues

What is the primary motor cortex?

It is important to bear in mind that the assignment of cortical areas to M1 is based on different levels. Some authors use assignments to anatomical levels; others, functional; and others, cytoarchitectural. Roughly speaking, many studies have approximated M1 to the precentral gyrus. However, this becomes increasingly inaccurate for the more ventral parts of the precentral gyrus. In an early functional magnetic resonance imaging (fMRI) experiment, this issue was addressed by using individual anatomical masks to separate activation in the precentral gyrus, and compared the number of activated voxels in this area with those in a reference area during ME and IM (Lotze *et al.* 1999).

Transcranial magnetic stimulation (TMS) studies define M1 functionally as the area below the scalp in which maximal motor-evoked potentials of a target muscle can be elicited. Cytoarchitectural probability maps are now available as masks for the Montreal Neurological Institute (MNI) brain and the Talairach space to identify M1 (Eickhoff *et al.* 2005). Nonetheless, spatial impreciseness due to the normalization process necessary for the overlay of these masks is still an issue when applying this method.

There is also a further subdivision of Brodmann's area BA4: The dorsal bank of M1 is subdivided into an anterior area (BA 4a) closely connected to premotor areas and a more posterior area (BA 4p). Both areas contain different finger representations (Geyer *et al.* 1996). Whereas Area 4a is thought to relate predominantly to motor-executive aspects, BA 4p is modulated by attention during ME (Binkofski *et al.* 2002). In a very recent paper, Sharma *et al.* (2008) elegantly demonstrated how informative it is to use probability maps to highlight the involvement of M1 in IM. The authors found an involvement of both BA 4a and 4p in IM of a finger-to-thumb opposition task. Area 4p activation, however, was more robust and similar to executed movement (see Figure 3.1).

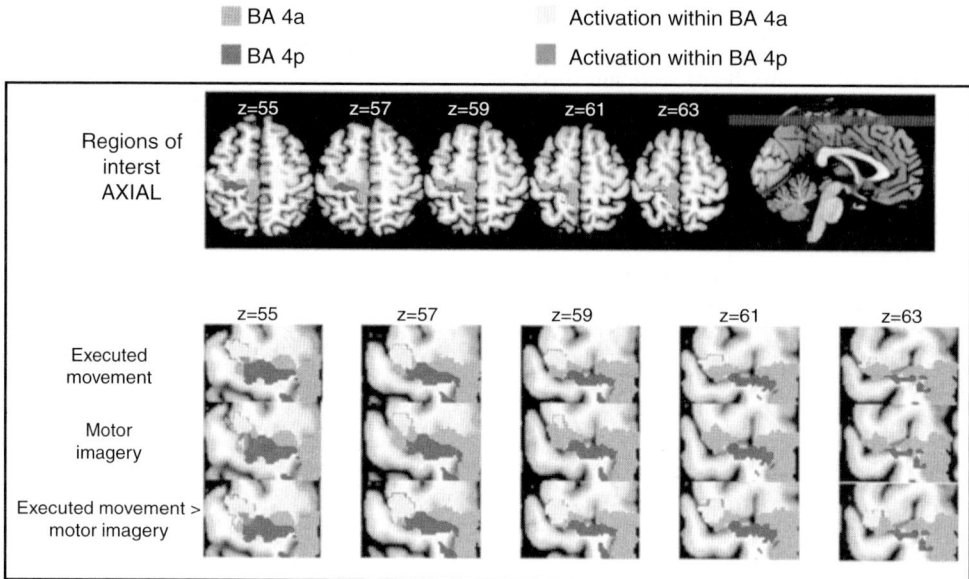

Fig. 3.1 Contribution of primary motor cortex during a finger opposition sequence. Activation clusters are shown in cytoarchitectural masks (indicated in green and blue) of highest probability for Brodmann's area 4a (yellow) and 4p (pink). The figure is printed with permission from Sharma, Carpenter, and Baron, NeuroImage 2008. See colour plate section.

Results on primary motor cortex activation during imagery

A direct comparison of ME minus IM during simple movements revealed significant differences in the cM1 (Stephan *et al.* 1995) and in the ipsilateral anterior cerebellar hemisphere (Nair *et al.* 2003). Similar differences were found during executed and imagined left-hand playing of a violin sonata (Lotze *et al.* 2003). One way to avoid the problem of false attribution of areas to neighbouring anatomical structures due to normalization (which is definitely more than 1 cm in imaging studies) is to use the precentral gyrus as an individual anatomical mask. Early fMRI studies applying this method described approximately 50% blood-oxygenation-level-dependent (BOLD) magnitude during IM compared with ME (Porro *et al.* 1996; Lotze *et al.* 1999). This 50% reduced activation magnitude might well lead to the impression that there is no M1 activation during imagery tasks when conservative thresholds are applied (e.g., family-wise error correction for false positive responses in the whole brain volume, random-effects statistics).

One way of verifying that a structure is not involved in a task is to compare its activation with a region *definitely* not involved. If activation in M1 is statistically increased in comparison with such a reference region, activation in M1 will most probably be associated with task performance. Unfortunately, imaging studies with PET and fMRI offer only correlative data. Therefore, it is impossible to decide definitely whether M1 is necessary for IM on the basis of this method. However, causal relationships can be revealed by TMS application, which produces a temporary functional lesion in the region of interest (Lotze *et al.* 2006).

Several fMRI studies did not reveal significant activation in M1 during IM (Binkofski *et al.* 2000; Gerardin *et al.* 2000; Boecker *et al.* 2002; Naito *et al.* 2002). However, none of these studies employed appropriate behavioural measures. In addition, the statistical power for detecting a decreased M1 contribution to IM was too low. In fact, direct cellular recordings in primates during IM of a prehensile task suggest that M1 is involved directly in encoding directional information (Georgopoulos *et al.* 1986). Therefore, more complex motor tasks are more likely to induce M1 activation during IM. This assumption is in line with the findings of Dechent and Frahm (2003), who reported an initial activation in M1 in five out of six participants that decreased over longer imagery periods. Additionally, Kristeva and colleagues (2003), using imagery of playing a violin, demonstrated in an EEG study that muscle activation can be detected during the initial phase of imagery. Nonetheless, it cannot be ruled out completely that the initial M1 activation observed in the Dechent and Frahm study was associated with short electromyographic (EMG) activity in the target muscles, as this was not controlled for.

Sharma *et al.* (2008) postulated that since spatial encoding of a movement precedes execution, it is plausible that methods with higher temporal resolution will show a contribution of M1 in IM. By using TMS, it has been possible to describe excitability changes over M1 during IM. A TMS study by Fadiga and colleagues (1999) demonstrated that IM results in increased excitability of only the muscle groups involved in the IM task but not of those muscles that are not involved. Corticospinal activity during imagined actions *per se* is described in Chapter 4 of this book. Some authors even described a somatotopic representation of the movements imagined in the sensorimotor cortex (Stippich *et al.* 2002; Ehrsson *et al.* 2003; Szameitat *et al.* 2007; Orr *et al.* 2008). Unfortunately, all these studies lack objective control of avoidance of actual execution during the IM task.

It is interesting to note that damage to the precentral gyrus after stroke does not result in decreased personal ratings of IM vividness (Sirigu *et al.* 1995). Therefore, during IM, the precentral gyrus seems to be activated in the same neuronal assemblies that are associated with ME, but the intactness of these neurons is not essential for a personal feeling of vividness of IM. It might be interesting to correlate vividness ratings with functional imaging maps during IM to discover areas associated with the personally felt intensity of IM vividness. Although many studies demonstrated that kinaesthetic imagery is associated with M1 activation, most of these failed to detect any significant lateralization within M1 to the contralateral hemisphere (see, also, Guillot *et al.* 2009). For ME, it has been shown several times that the simpler the executed movement, the clearer the lateralization (e.g., Lotze *et al.* 2000). The same might be true for IM: Whereas kinaesthetic imagery of complex movements did not show relevant lateralization (Guillot *et al.* 2009), it has been described for IM of simple hand movements (Michelon *et al.* 2006; Pfurtscheller *et al.* 1999).

The issue of motor execution control during scanning

Several fMRI studies reported cM1 activation during IM (Leonardo *et al.* 1995; Sabbah *et al.* 1995; Porro *et al.* 1996, 2000; Roth *et al.* 1996; Lotze *et al.* 1999; Gerardin *et al.* 2000; Stippich *et al.* 2002; Nair *et al.* 2003; Ehrsson *et al.* 2003; Kuhtz-Buschbeck *et al.* 2003; Szameitat *et al.* 2007; Guillot *et al.* 2008, 2009; Munzert *et al.* 2008; Orr *et al.* 2008). However, most of these studies were unable to control for possible muscle discharges during scanning. Some fMRI studies used EMG monitoring during IM prior to scanning, and demonstrated that this was negligible compared with EMG amplitudes during ME (Leonardo *et al.* 1995; Roth *et al.* 1996; Lotze *et al.* 1999; Gerardin *et al.* 2000; Lafleur *et al.* 2002). However, when elicited by different muscle contraction types, this residual activity has been shown to be specific to the content of the imagined contraction (see Guillot *et al.* 2007). Only very recent studies have been able to control for avoidance of ME by using an artefact reduction of EMG during fMRI scanning (Bakker *et al.* 2008). One criticism of these studies is that marginal EMG activity might nonetheless not be detected after artefact reduction of EMG signals. Systems capable of dealing with these artefacts (if the electrodes are not moved in the magnetic field) have now become available (see Sehm *et al.* 2008).

Another possibility might be to monitor movement parameters themselves. This can be accomplished by video camera capture of the respective limb followed by a standardized evaluation of the data. A more elegant method is to detect movements by sensors affixed to the to-be-imagined limb. This can be achieved with a virtual reality glove equipped with optic fibre sensors. In a very recent paper, Sharma *et al.* (2008) used such an MRI-compatible glove. Although single muscle contractions might not be detected, even very small movements of hand and fingers can be identified.

When using methods such as magnetoencephalography (MEG), positron emission tomography (PET) or TMS, electromyographic activities during IM of target muscles can be controlled easily during data acquisition. When using MEG, two research groups have reported a contribution of cM1 in IM (Lang *et al.* 1996; Schnitzler *et al.* 1997). The use of dense-array electroencephalography (EEG) has made it possible to describe movement-associated mu and beta rhythm over the primary sensorimotor area (Pfurtscheller and Neuper 1997). By using TMS during IM, increased excitability was observed over the contralateral motor cortex somatotopically related to muscles involved in this specific imagery task (Fadiga *et al.* 1999; Pascual-Leone *et al.* 1995).

PET measurements allow for a control of muscle activation with EMG without fMRI-typical artefacts (Stephan *et al.* 1995; Naito *et al.* 1999). However, most PET studies did not show significant activation in cM1 during IM (e.g., Roland *et al.* 1980; Decety *et al.* 1994; Stephan *et al.* 1995). There may be two reasons for these discrepant results, and both are methodologically grounded. The first is the factor 'time'. It has been shown that cM1 activation during IM is shorter and smaller in magnitude than during ME (Kristeva *et al.* 2003). Therefore, it is easier to detect by electrophysiological measurements but not by methods with poor temporal resolution (such as PET). The other factor is the 'significance and size of activation loci'. Activation magnitude and representation size decrease during IM, so the methods with low spatial resolution will fail to detect activation in M1.

One highly interesting PET study described significant activation in the contralateral BA 4a using an illusory arm extension after vibration on the biceps tendon (Naito *et al.* 1999). However, this is a quite different task than IM, and since the vibration task involves BA 3a and 2 of the primary somatosensory cortex, it might automatically induce activation in the tightly anatomically and functionally associated motor neurons.

The importance of training, imagery abilities, and instructions

Imagery may not be imagery: which tasks are 'motor imagery' tasks?

The previous section presented an overview of the conflicting results on M1 activation during IM. The recruitment of M1 during IM seems to depend on the specific instructions given for the imagery task, the training regimen for imagery, the experience of the participants with imagery tasks, their IM ability, and the level of motor expertise in the task to be imagined. Also, the use of different methods to evaluate the content and the ability of IM is needed (see Guillot *et al.* 2008, 2009). The following section will elaborate on these issues in greater detail.

Instructions for imagery tasks possibly relate to brain activation

When reviewing the literature on IM, one problem faced is that many studies fail to provide detailed reports on the instructions given to participants when asked to imagine. As imagery defies direct control by the experimenter (i.e., quantification of imagery content is not possible, but see Heremans *et al.* 2008 for an approach in goal-directed movements), it is essential to constrain the imagery process by appropriate instructions. Additionally, it should be considered that instructional differences might lead to changes in motor cortical activation due to varying the participants' attentional focus on different aspects of motor control.

Solodkin *et al.* (2004) showed that visual and kinaesthetic imagery are based on differential neural substrates, because only IM, with its focus on kinaesthetic imagery contents but not visual imagery, involves M1. This finding was corroborated in a later fMRI study (Guillot *et al.* 2009), in which both tasks were given to the same group of participants.

Most authors agree that movement-related kinaesthetic sensations play a major role in the IM context. Instructions focusing on kinaesthetic contents of imagery ask participants, for instance, to concentrate on how their limbs feel during movement. In many studies, participants are also requested to imagine themselves moving in order to facilitate kinaesthetic sensations. When instructions for imagery are poorly reported in a study, it remains unclear which perspective participants have adopted during imagery. On a phenomenal level, there are several possibilities. For example, actions can be imagined as if oneself were acting, that is, adopting a first-person perspective (1PP). When expert ski runners mentally prepare for their race, they mostly adopt 1PP, focusing on kinaesthetic aspects during imagined skiing. In terms of somatosensory inputs, 1PP is referred to being within the acting body and experiencing oneself as the cause of the actions (being the 'agent'). In terms of visual inputs, 1PP resembles wearing a helmet camera, and the ski runners would 'see' their own body parts from a familiar viewpoint. This suggests that during IM, visual contents might be part of the imagery process, but the focus is on the kinaesthetic aspects. In contrast, third-person-perspective (3PP) imagery implies that other acting humans are the content of imagination, meaning they are agents of the actions. Here, the focus is clearly on the visual side. To complete the picture, another possibility is that participants adopt a 3PP, but imagine themselves acting. From a theoretical point of view (see Vogeley and Fink 2003), it is worth bearing this in mind, because perspective then does not determine agency, that is, one can imagine oneself from a 3PP, but still experience oneself as the agent of an action ('I see myself doing the dishes').

Other general differences in IM study procedures

It is striking that IM studies differ significantly with respect to the sources that guide imagery. Some studies employ designs with ME phases so that participants engage in IM after execution (e.g., Filimon *et al.* 2007). Other studies use observation of the to-be-imagined actions before imagery (e.g., Munzert *et al.* 2008) or even present visual stimuli during imagery (Iseki *et al.* 2008). Additionally, some studies get participants to perform imagery training phases (Hanakawa *et al.* 2003; Ehrsson *et al.* 2003), whereas others select participants who report experience in mental rehearsal (Lotze *et al.* 2003). Guillot *et al.* (2008) used different imagery ability measurements and autonomic measures before scanning to divide groups in good and bad imagers. They demonstrated that imagery ability is a major modulating factor of neural activation in IM. A relevant issue already brought up in a previous section of this chapter is the control of ME during IM. Some studies trained participants to avoid EMG responses of target muscles with EMG feedback (Lotze *et al.* 1999). By using this procedure, ME and muscle contractions can be reduced stepwise, and participants can attain high imagery vividness scores because of these training phases. The procedure also ensures that only participants able to perform IM vividly and without overt movement are fMRI-scanned.

More methodological influences in IM studies related to M1 activation

Kuhtz-Buschbeck *et al.* (2003) combined fMRI and TMS measurements in complex versus simple imagined movements and demonstrated that M1 is increasingly involved in more complex movements. This may support the hypothesis that the M1 contribution to IM is intensity- as well as threshold-dependent. A very recent fMRI study on IM clearly demonstrated that IM of complex finger movements involves M1 (Sharma *et al.* 2008). Jackson *et al.* (2001) summarized that 'contrary to the conditions in which a motor task can be learned implicitly with physical practice, mental practice with IM requires that subjects have all the necessary declarative knowledge about the different components of the task before practicing. However, as with physical practice, the rehearsing of the task with IM can also give access to the non-conscious processes involved in learning the skilled behaviour'. Jackson concluded, 'internally driven images which promote the kinaesthetic feeling of movements would best activate the different non-conscious processes involved during motor task training'.

A great variety of different types of actions involving different body parts have been used to elucidate the neural substrates of imagery in fMRI studies. These include singing (Kleber *et al.* 2007); walking (Iseki *et al.* 2008); gymnastic movements (Munzert *et al.* 2008); finger tapping (Hanakawa *et al.*, 2008); moving fingers, toes, and tongue (Ehrsson *et al.* 2003); object-related reaching (Filimon *et al.* 2007); flexion of the foot (Alkadhi *et al.* 2005; Cramer *et al.* 2007); or tango steps (Sacco *et al.* 2006). Some studies use familiar objects that participants need to act upon (Ruby and Decety 2001); others employ non-object movements (Naito *et al.* 2002).

Even though all the above-mentioned actions seem to differ widely, they are nonetheless alike in terms of how imagery is instructed explicitly, and in that participants can control them voluntarily. In many studies, participants even self-trigger their imagination, indicating the start and end of their imagination by button presses. This makes it possible to use mental chronometry as an indirect manipulation check (see Bruzzo *et al.* 2008, for a behavioural study and Sharma *et al.* 2008 for an fMRI study). It should be noted, however, that the term 'motor imagery' is also used for studies employing tasks in which the use of imagery is suggested only implicitly for instance, when action-related words are read (Tomasino *et al.* 2007), when body parts need to be rotated (Sharma *et al.* 2008), or when participants simulate manual rotation of objects in order to decide whether two objects are identical (Lamm *et al.* 2007). In implicit imagery paradigms, participants are not instructed explicitly to imagine these actions; they are asked to solve a task that implies motor simulation processes. Some participants in such studies might indeed use a simulation strategy, that is, use their own motor representations to solve the task, whereas others may not, and controlling the participant's compliance is a methodological issue here as well. The contribution of M1 in these studies (see, also, De Lange *et al.* 2006) could not be shown. In a recent study, Guillot *et al.* (2008) selected only those 13 members of a pre-investigated group of 50 healthy participants for the imagery task, who were able to achieve an imagery score more than one standard deviation higher than the group average. Other chapters in this book deal with the appropriate scores on imagery capabilities.

Latest studies combine many measures: scores in imagery, behavioural measures such as imagery duration in relation to execution duration, and physiological variables such as autonomic responses during IM and ME (Guillot *et al.* 2008, 2009). This will certainly help to understand what participants are actually doing when instructed to imagine a motor task.

Motor experience and its influence on IM

As the behavioural literature provides some hints that the use of the imagery mode is influenced by motor expertise (Hardy and Callow 1999), it is also plausible to argue that motor-system activation during IM may depend on refined motor representations. The latter should be 'stored' in an expert-specific format, because extensive practice requires the motor system to relate sensory signals and motor commands permanently. Which motor-related areas are essential for this aspect is still a matter of debate. The question whether this specifically depends on altered M1 activation in IM has not been comprehensively resolved. Kleber *et al.* (2007) did not find M1 activation in professional singers during imagery of singing and Guillot *et al.* (2008) only detected cM1 activation in poor imagers but not in good imagers during IM of a finger sequence task with their left hand (see, also, Lotze *et al.* 2003 for a similar result in musicians).

From a computational view in motor control, two highly influential models on motor control provide a framework for how this might be accomplished (Wolpert *et al.* 2003). The inverse model generates an appropriate motor command and the forward model maps the efference copy to the anticipated outcome of the action. It builds a template against which the incoming information (reafferences) can be compared. Normally, there is little discrepancy between the anticipated outcome and the real sensory feedback on moving. However, at times, greater discrepancies require a rapid adjustment of the motor command and, on this basis, of the anticipated consequences of actions as well. Whereas in the past, computational models have been used mainly as simulator tools to investigate small-range motor actions (such as reaching and grasping movements), they have now also been adapted for social interaction and other processes that might require hidden states of action (such as IM, see also Jeannerod 2001). In IM, the sensory feedback that normally occurs during ME might also be anticipated. Prediction, therefore, should also play a prominent role in IM. Behavioural studies have initially shown that kinaesthetic signals play a significant role in IM, because incompatible postural signals affect implicit and explicit imagery (Parsons 1994; Sirigu and Duhamel 2001; Funk *et al.* 2005; Ionta *et al.* 2007). In imaging studies, it could also be demonstrated that imagined and actual body positions influence activity in neural structures during own-body simulation processes (De Lange *et al.* 2006). These results suggest that the plastic and dynamic representation of spatial and biomechanical properties of the body, derived from highly redundant multiple sensory inputs as a result of physical practice, are involved in imagery. Therefore, modulation of neural activity by kinaesthetic feedback suggests that it may be particularly important when motor experts engage in IM.

Motor therapy and IM training

Mental practice improves performance in athletes (Driskell *et al.* 1994). Roure *et al.* (1999) showed a positive correlation between ratings of the quality of imagery using changes in autonomic measures such as heart rate, skin temperature as well as skin conductance and improvement in performance on volleyball. Chapters 15 and 18 in this book deal with this issue.

In a study using musical performance training, a period of 5 days of ME training and IM training combined with ME training resulted in an increase of cM1 map size of the long finger flexors and extensors as assessed with TMS (Pascual-Leone *et al.* 1995). Participants with ME training only displayed greatest increase in performance, but IM also resulted in a training effect. Most interestingly, the IM group demonstrated the same training effect after one additional ME training session as the ME-only group, pointing to the importance of *combining* IM and ME in musical performance training.

Some rehabilitation centres have been gathering experience for many years in IM training for stroke patients (e.g., Weiss *et al.* 1994; Miltner *et al.* 1999). However, they all select specially suited patients for this intervention: predominantly chronic stroke patients with low neuropsychological impairment and high imagery scores. In a comparison of conventional physiotherapy and physiotherapy combined with imagery training of movements of the hand in subacute to chronic stroke patients, Page and colleagues (2001) demonstrated a greater improvement of hand function after additional mental practice.

Since activation in the contralateral primary motor hand area is the best predictor for motor outcome of the hand function after lesion of the brain (Lotze and Cohen 2006), early access of M1

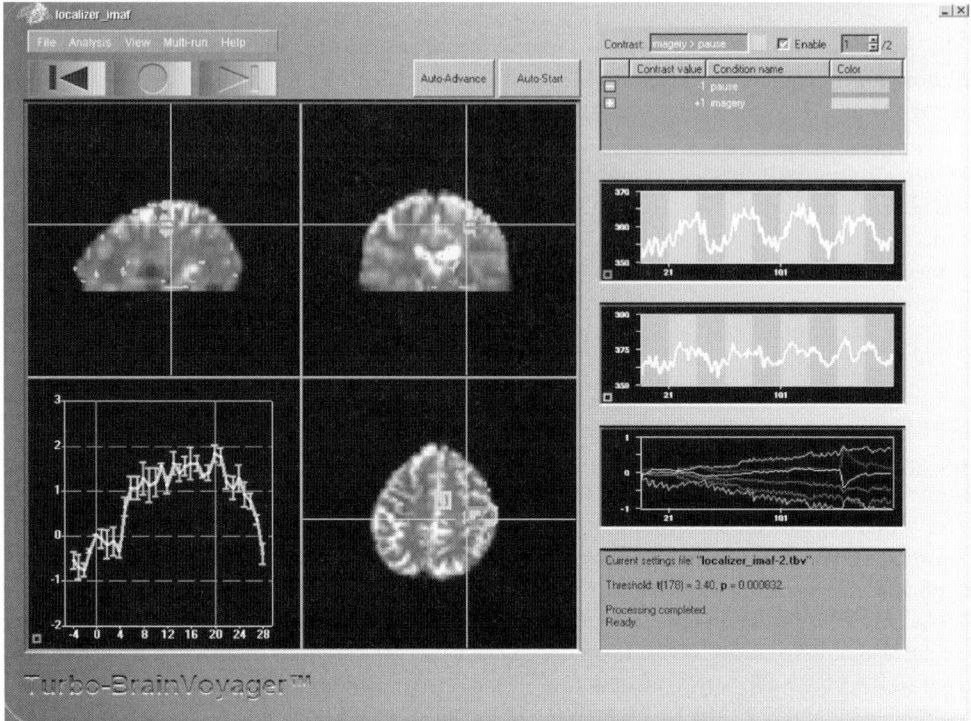

Fig. 3.2 Blood-oxygenation level-dependent (BOLD)-feedback training session of a patient suffering from motor impairment of the left hand due to a stroke in the internal capsule 3.5 years before fMRI. This is a screen shot of a Turbo Brain Voyager session of a left-hand imagery training session. Online visual inspection of the hand in the scanner was used to exclude execution. Left: The red rectangle in the three echo planar images indicates the Region-of-Interest (ROI) for M1c; the green, the reference area in the medial SMA. The bottom left panel shows the averaged BOLD plot of activation (%) over time (28 s) for one block. On the right, the top graph shows the BOLD time course for the ROI (cM1); the middle one, that for the reference area (SMA). The bottom graph indicates movement of the head in mm and rotations in degrees (each for 3 directions). This participant showed considerable problems with imagery intensity during training without fMRI (vividness score: 2 from a maximum of 6), but he was perfectly able to increase BOLD magnitude by fMRI visual feedback with an average temporal delay of 5 s. See colour plate section.

through IM training could be crucial, especially for patients who cannot execute movements due to complete plegia of the hand muscles. We tested an fMRI-based feedback training of M1 activation using imagery techniques (see Figure 3.2). Together with BOLD-feedback, activation in M1 without ME could be accomplished easily as demonstrated here. However, it is not clear whether increased access to M1 as established by feedback really does transfer to motor functioning in these patients. Recent research has demonstrated the value of both IM (Butler and Page 2006) and motor observation training for motor function improvement after stroke (Ertelt *et al.* 2007), and this technically less demanding method might be a useful complementary therapy approach for these patients.

Conclusions

1 Activation of the primary motor cortex is differentially influenced by instructions for IM, imagery ability, and motor expertise.

2 Imagery tasks need to be trained and described and controlled carefully to provide reliable results.

3 Methodological problems in describing M1 activity have to be solved by applying recent technical advances in data evaluation.

Consequences of the conclusions driven by this review:

1 The primary motor cortex (M1) does not just have an execution function for the motor system.

2 Imagery techniques can be used to either train the concept of movement and to (re)gain access to new assemblies of M1 in cases of cortical lesions and motor impairment.

References

Alkadhi, H., Brugger, P., Boendermaker, S.H., *et al.* (2005). What disconnection tells about motor imagery: evidence from paraplegic patients. *Cerebral Cortex*, **15**, 131–40.

Bakker, M., De Lange, F., Helmich, R.C., Scheeringa, R., Bloem, B.R., and Toni, I. (2008). Cerebral correlates of motor imagery of normal and precision gait. *NeuroImage*, **41**, 998–1010.

Binkofski, F., Amuts, K., Stephan, K.M., *et al.* (2000). Broca's region subserves imagery of motion: a combined cytoarchitectonic and fMRI study. *Human Brain Mapping*, **11**, 273–85.

Binkofski, F., Fink, G.R., Geyer, S., *et al.* (2002). Neural activity in human primary motor cortex areas 4a and 4p is modulated differentially by attention to action. *Journal of Neurophysiology*, **88**, 514–9.

Boecker, H., Ceballos-Baumann, A.O., Partenstein, P., et al. (2002). A H215O positron emission study on mental imagery of movement sequences – The effect of modulating sequence length and direction. *NeuroImage*, **17**, 999–1009.

Bruzzo, A., Gesierich, B., and Wohlschläger, A. (2008). Simulating biological and non-biological motion. *Brain and Cognition*, **66**, 145–9.

Butler, A. and Page, S. (2006). Mental practice with motor imagery: evidence for motor recovery and cortical reorganization after stroke. *Archives of Physical Medicine and Rehabilitation*, **87**, 2–11.

Cramer, S.C., Orr, E.L., Cohen, M.J., and Lacourse, M.G. (2007). Effects of motor imagery training after chronic, complete spinal cord injury. *Experimental Brain Research*, **177**, 233–42.

Cui, X., Jeter, C.B., Yang, D., Montague, P.R., and Eagleman, D.M. (2007). Vividness of mental imagery: individual variability can be measured objectively. *Vision Research*, **47**, 474–8.

De Lange, F.P., Helmich, R.C., and Toni, I. (2006). Posture influences motor imagery: an fMRI study. *NeuroImage*, **33**, 609–17.

Decety, J. (1996a). Do imagined and executed actions share the same neural substrate? *Cognitive Brain Research*, **3**, 87–93.

Decety, J. (1996b). The neurophysiological basis of motor imagery. *Behavioural Brain Research*, **77**, 45–52.

Decety, J. and Boisson, D. (1990). Effect of brain and spinal cord injuries on motor imagery. *European Archives of Psychiatry and Clinical Neuroscience*, **240**, 39–43.

Decety, J. and Jeannerod, M. (1996). Mentally simulated movements in virtual reality: does Fitt's law hold in motor imagery? *Behavioural Brain Research*, **72**, 127–34.

Decety, J., Jeannerod, M., Durozard, D., and Baverel, G. (1993). Central activation of autonomic effectors during mental simulation of motor actions in man. *Journal of Physiology*, **461**, 549–63.

Decety, J., Jeannerod, M., Germain, M., and Pastene, J. (1991). Vegetative response during imagined movement is proportional to mental effort. *Behavioural Brain Research*, **42**, 1–5.

Decety, J. and Michel, F. (1989). Comparative analysis of actual and mental movement times in two graphic tasks. *Brain and Cognition*, **11**, 87–97.

Dechent, P. and Frahm, J. (2003). Functional somatotopy of finger representations in human primary motor cortex. *Human Brain Mapping*, **18**, 272–83.

Dominey, P., Decety, J., Broussolle, E., Chazot, G., and Jeannerod, M. (1995). Motor imagery of a lateralized sequential task is asymmetrically slowed in hemi-Parkinson's patients. *Neuropsychologia*, **33**, 727–41.

Driskell, J. E., Copper, C., and Moran, A. (1994). Does mental practice enhance performance? *Journal of Applied Psychology*, **79**, 481–92.

Ehrsson, H.H., Geyer, S., and Naito, E. (2003). Imagery of voluntary movement of fingers, toes, and tongue activates corresponding body-part-specific motor representations. *Journal of Neurophysiology*, **90**, 3304–16.

Eickhoff, S.B., Stephan, K.E., Mohlberg, H., *et al.* (2005). A new toolbox for combining probabilistic cytoarchitectonic maps and functional imaging data. *NeuroImage*, **25**, 1325–35.

Ertelt, D., Small, S., Solodkin, *et al.* (2007). Action observation has a positive impact on rehabilitation of motor deficits after stroke. *NeuroImage*, **36**, Supplement 2, T164–T173.

Fadiga, L., Buccino, G., Craighero, L., Fogassi, L., Gallese, V., and Pavesi, G. (1999). Corticospinal excitability is specifically modulated by motor imagery: a magnetic stimulation study. *Neuropsychologia, **37**, 147–58.

Filimon, F., Nelson, J.D., Hagler, D.J., and Sereno, M.I. (2007). Human cortical representations for reaching: mirror neurons for execution, observation, and imagery. *NeuroImage*, **37**, 1315–28.

Fitts, P.M. (1954). The information capacity of the human motor system in controlling the amplitude of movement. *Journal of Experimental Psychology*, **47**, 381–91.

Funk, M., Brugger, P., and Wilkening, F. (2005). Motor processes in children's imagery: the case of mental rotation of hands. *Developmental Science*, **8**, 402–8.

Gao, J.-H., Parsons, L.M., Bower, J., Xiong, J., Li, J., and Fox, P.T. (1996). Cerebellum implicated in sensory acquisition and discrimination rather than motor control. *Science*, **272**, 545–7.

Georgopoulos, A.P., Schwartz, A.B., and Kettner, R.E. (1986). Neuronal population coding of movement direction. *Science*, **233**, 1416–9.

Gerardin, E., Sirigu, A., Lehericy, S., *et al.* (2000). Partially overlapping neural networks for real and imagined hand movements. *Cerebral Cortex, **10**, 1093–104.

Geyer, S., Ledberg, A., Schleicher, A., *et al.* (1996). Two different areas within the primary motor cortex of man. *Nature, **382**, 805–7.

Guillot, A. and Collet, C. (2005a). Contribution from neurophysiological and psychological methods to the study of motor imagery. *Brain Research Reviews*, **50**, 387–97.

Guillot, A. and Collet, C. (2005b). Duration of mentally simulated movement: a review. *Journal of Motor Behavior*, **37**, 10–20.

Guillot, A., Collet, C., Nguyen, V.A., Malouin, F., Richards, C., and Doyon, J. (2008). Functional neuroanatomical networks associated with expertise in motor imagery. *NeuroImage*, **41**, 1471–83.

Guillot, A., Collet, C., Nguyen, V.A., Malouin, F., Richards, C., and Doyon J. (2009). Brain activity during visual vs. kinaesthetic imagery: an fMRI study. *Human Brain Mapping*, **30**, 2157–72.

Guillot, A., Lebon, F., Rouffet, D., Champely, S., Doyon, J., and Collet, C. (2007). Muscular responses during motor imagery as a function of muscle contraction types. *International Journal of Psychophysiology*, **66**, 18–27.

Hanakawa, T., Immisch, I., Toma, K., Dimyan, M.A., van Gelderen, P., and Hallett, M. (2003). Functional properties of brain areas associated with motor execution and imagery. *Journal of Neurophysiology*, **89**, 989–1002.

Hanakawa, T., Dimyan, M.A., and Hallett, M. (2008). Motor planning, imagery, and execution in the distributed motor network: a time-course study with functional MRI. *Cerebral Cortex*, **18**, 2775–88.

Hardy, L. and Callow, N. (1999). Efficacy of external and internal visual imagery perspectives for the enhancement of performance on tasks in which form is important. *Journal of Sport and Exercise Psychology*, **21**, 95–112.

Heremans, E., Helsen, W.F., and Feys, P. (2008). The eyes as a mirror of our thoughts: quantification of motor imagery of goal-directed movements through eye movement registration. *Behavioural Brain Research*, **187**, 351–60.

Ionta, S., Fourkas, A.D., Fiorio, M., and Aglioti, S.S. (2007). The influence of hands posture on mental rotation of hands and feet. *Experimental Brain Research*, **183**, 1–7.

Iseki, K., Hanakawa, T., Shinozaki, J., Nankaku, M., and Fukuyama, H. (2008). Neural mechanisms involved in mental imagery and observation of gait. *NeuroImage*, **41**, 1021–31.

Jackson, P., Lafleur, M.F., Malouin, F., Richards, C., and Doyon, J. (2001). Potential role of mental practice using motor imagery in neurologic rehabilitation. *Archives of Physical Medicine and Rehabilitation*, **82**, 1133–41.

Jacobson, E. (1930). Electrical measurements of neuromuscular states during mental activities. Imagination of movement involving skeletal muscles. *American Journal of Physiology*, **91**, 547–608.

James, W. (1890). *The Principles of Psychology: Imagination,* pp. 44–75. NY, US: Henry Holt and Company.

Jeannerod, M. (1994). Object-oriented action. *Advances in Psychology*, **105**, 3–15.

Jeannerod, M. (1995). Mental imagery in the motor context. *Neuropsychologia*, **33**, 1419–32.

Jeannerod, M. (2001). Neural simulation of action: a unifying mechanism for motor cognition. *NeuroImage*, **14**, S103–S109.

Karni, A., Meyer, G., Jezzard, P., Adams, M.M., Turner, R., and Ungerleider, L.G. (1995). Functional MRI evidence for adult motor cortex plasticity during motor skill learning. *Nature*, **377**, 155–8.

Kleber, B., Birbaumer, N., Veit, R., Trevorrow, T., and Lotze, M. (2007). Overt and imagined singing of an Italian aria. *NeuroImage*, **36**, 889–900.

Kraemer, D.J.M., Macrae, C.N., Green, A.E., and Kelley, W.M. (2005). Musical imagery: sound of silence activates auditory cortex. *Nature,* **434**, 158.

Kristeva, R., Chakarov, V., Schulte-Mönting, J., and Spreer, J. (2003). Activation of cortical areas in music execution and imagining: a high-resolution EEG study. *NeuroImage*, **20**, 1872–83.

Kuhtz-Buschbeck, J.P., Mahnkopf, C., Holzknecht, C., Siebner, H., Ulmer, S., and Jansen, O. (2003). Effector-independent representations of simple and complex imagined finger movements: a combined fMRI and TMS study. *European Journal of Neuroscience,* **18**, 3375–87.

Lafleur, M.F., Jackson, P.L., Malouin, F., Richards, C.L., Evans, A.C., and Doyon, J. (2002). Motor learning produces parallel dynamic functional changes during the execution and imagination of sequential foot movements. *NeuroImage,* **16**, 142–57.

Lamm, C., Windischberger, C., Moser, E., and Bauer, H. (2007). The functional role of dorso-lateral premotor cortex during mental rotation: an event-related fMRI study separating cognitive processing steps using a novel task paradigm. *NeuroImage*, **36**, 1374–86.

Lang, W., Cheyne, D., Höllinger, P., Gerschlager, W., and Lindinger, G. (1996). Electric and magnetic fields of the brain accompanying internal simulation of movement. *Cognitive Brain Research*, **3**, 125–9.

Leonardo, M., Fieldman, J., Sadato, N., *et al.* (1995). A functional magnetic resonance imaging study of cortical regions associated with motor task execution and motor ideation in humans. *Human Brain Mapping*, **3**, 83–92.

Lorey, B., Bischoff, M., Pilgramm, S., Stark, R., Munzert, J., and Zentgraf, K. (2009). The embodied nature of motor imagery: the influence of posture and perspective. *Experimental Brain Research,* **194**, 233–43.

Lotze, M. and Cohen, L.G. (2006). Volition and Imagery in Neurorehabilitation. *Cognitive and Behavioural Neurology*, **19**, 135–40.

Lotze, M. and Halsband, U. (2006). Motor imagery. *Journal of Physiology-Paris*, **99**, 386–95.

Lotze. M., Markert. J., Sauseng. P., Hoppe. J., Plewnia. C., Gerloff. C. (2006). The role of multiple contralesional motor areas for complex hand movements after internal capsular lesion. *Journal of Neuroscience*, **26**, 6096–102.

Lotze, M., Scheler, G., Tan, H.-R.M., Braun, C., and Birbaumer, N. (2003). The musician's brain: functional imaging of amateurs and professionals during performance and imagery. *NeuroImage*, **20**, 1817–29.

Lotze, M., Erb, M., Flor, H., Huelsmann, E., Godde, B., and Grodd, W. (2000). FMRI evaluation of somatotopic representation in human primary motor cortex. *NeuroImage*, **11**, 473–81.

Lotze, M., Flor, H., Grodd, W., Larbig, W., and Birbaumer, N. (2001). Phantom movements and pain. An fMRI study in upper limb amputees. *Brain*, **124**, 2268–77.

Lotze, M., Montoya, P., Erb, M., Hülsmann, E., Flor, H., Klose, U., Birbaumer, N., and Grodd, W. (1999). Activation of cortical and cerebellar motor areas during executed and imagined hand movements: an fMRI study. *Journal of Cognitive Neuroscience*, **11**, 491–501.

Maruff, P., Wilson, P.H., De Fazio, J., Cerritelli, B., Hedt, A., and Currie, J. (1999). Asymmetries between dominant and non-dominant hands in real and imagined motor task performance. *Neuropsychologia*, **37**, 379–84.

Michelon, P., Vettel. J.M., and Zacks, J.M. (2006). Lateral somatotopic organization during imagined and prepared movements. *Journal of Neurophysiology*, **95**, 811–22.

Miltner, W.H.R., Bauder, H., Sommer, M., Dettmers, C., and Taub, E. (1999). Effects of constrained-induced movement therapy on patients with chronic motor deficits after stroke. *Stroke*, **30**, 586–92.

Munzert, J., Lorey, B., and Zentgraf, K. (2009). Cognitive motor processes: The role of motor imagery in the study of motor representations. *Brain Research Reviews*, **60**, 306–26.

Munzert, J., Zentgraf, K., Stark, R., and Vaitl, D. (2008). Neural activation in cognitive motor processes: comparing motor imagery and observation of gymnastic movements. *Experimental Brain Research*, **188**, 437–44.

Nair, D.G., Purcott, K.L., Fuchs, A., Steinberg, F., and Kelso, J.A.S. (2003). Cortical and cerebellar activity of the human brain during imagined and executed unimanual and bimanual action sequences: a functional MRI study. *Cognitive Brain Research*, **15**, 250–60.

Naito, E., Ehrsson, H.H., Geyer, S., Zilles, K., and Roland, P.E. (1999). Illusory arm movements activate cortical motor areas: a positron emission tomography study. *The Journal of Neuroscience*, **19**, 6134–44.

Naito, E., Kochiyama, T., Kitada, R., *et al.* (2002). Internally simulated movement sensations during motor imagery activate cortical motor areas and the cerebellum. *The Journal of Neuroscience*, **22**, 3683–91.

Orr, E., Lacourse, M.G., Cohen, M.J., and Cramer, S.C. (2008). Cortical activation during executed, imagined, and observed foot movements. *Neuroreport*, **19**, 625–30.

Page, S.J., Levine, P., Sisto, S.A., and Johnston, M.V. (2001). Mental practice combined with physical practice for upper-limb motor deficit in subacute stroke. *Physical Therapy*, **81**, 1455–62.

Parsons, L.M. (1994). Temporal and kinematic properties of motor behavior reflected in mentally simulated action. *Journal of Experimental Psychology*, **20**, 709–30.

Pascual-Leone, A., Dang, N., Cohen, L.G., Brasil-Neto, J.P, Cammarota, A., and Hallett, M. (1995). Modulation of muscle responses evoked by transcranial magnetic stimulation during the acquisition of new fine motor skills. *Journal of Neurophysiology*, **74**, 1037–43.

Pfurtscheller, G. and Neuper, C. (1997). Motor imagery activates primary sensorimotor area in humans. *Neuroscience Letters*, **239**, 65–8.

Pfurtscheller, G., Neuper, C., Ramoser, H., and Müller-Gerking, J. (1999). Visually guided motor imagery activates sensorimotor areas in humans. *Neuroscience Letters*, **269**, 253–156.

Porro, C.A., Cettolo, V., Francescato, M.P., and Baraldi, P. (2000). Ipsilateral involvement of primary motor cortex during motor imagery. *European Journal of Neuroscience*, **12**, 3059–63.

Porro, C.A., Francescato, M.P., Cettolo, V., Baraldi, P., and Diamond, M.E. (1996). Primary motor cortex activity during motor performance and motor imagery: an fMRI study. *NeuroImage*, **3**, S214.

Roland, P.E., Larsen, B., Lassen, N.A., Skinhoj, E. (1980). Supplementary motor area and other cortical areas in organisation of voluntary movements in man. *Journal of Neurophysiology*, **43**, 118–36.

Roth, M., Decety, J., Raybaudi, M., *et al.* (1996). Possible involvement of primary motor cortex in mentally simulated movement: a functional magnetic resonance imaging study. *Neuroreport*, **7**, 1280–84.

Roure, R., Collet, C., Deschaumes-Molinaro, C., Delhomme, G., Dittmar, A., and Vernet-Maury, E. (1999). Imagery quality estimated by autonomic response is correlated to sporting performance enhancement. *Physiology and Behavior*, **66**, 63–72.

Ruby, P. and Decety, J. (2001). Effect of subjective perspective taking during simulation of action: a PET investigation of agency. *Nature Neuroscience*, **4**, 546–50.

Sabbah, P., Simond, G., Levrier, O., *et al.* (1995). Functional magnetic resonance imaging at 1.5T during sensory motor and cognitive tasks. *European Neurology*, **35**, 131–5.

Sacco, K., Cauda, F., Cerliani, L., Mate, D., Duca, S., and Geminiani, G.C. (2006). Motor imagery of walking following training in locomotor attention. The effect of "the tango lesson". *NeuroImage*, **32**, 1441–49.

Schnitzler, A., Salenius, S., Salmelin, R., Jousmäki, V., and Hari, R. (1997). Involvement of primary motor cortex in motor imagery: a neuromagnetic study. *NeuroImage*, **6**, 201–8.

Sehm, B., Perez, M., Xu, B., Hidler, J., and Cohen, L.G. (In press). Functional neuroanatomy of mirroring during a unimanual force generation task. *Cerebral Cortex*, doi:10.1093/cercor/bhp075.

Sharma, N., Jones, P.S., Carpenter, T.A., and Baron, J.-C. (2008). Mapping the involvement of BA 4a and 4p during motor imagery. *NeuroImage*, **41**, 92–9.

Shaw, W.A. (1940). The relation of muscular action potentials to imaginal weight lifting. *Archives of Psychology (Columbia University)*, **247**, 50.

Sirigu, A. and Duhamel, J.R. (2001). Motor and visual imagery as two complementary but neurally dissociable mental processes. *Journal of Cognitive Neuroscience*, **13**, 910–9.

Sirigu, A., Duhamel, J.-R., Cohen, L., Pillon, B., Dubois, B., and Agid, Y. (1995). The mental representation of hand movements after parietal cortex damage. *Science*, **273**, 1564–2568.

Solodkin, A., Hlustik, P., Chen, E.E., and Small, S.L. (2004). Fine modulation in network activation during motor execution and motor imagery. *Cerebral Cortex*, **14**, 1246–55.

Stephan, K.M., Fink, G.R., Passingham, R.E., *et al.* (1995). Functional anatomy of the mental representation of upper extremity movements in healthy subjects. *Journal of Neurophysiology*, **73**, 373–86.

Stippich, C., Ochmann, H., and Sartor, K. (2002). Somatotopic mapping of the human primary sensorimotor cortex during motor imagery and motor execution by functional magnetic resonance imaging. *Neuroscience Letters*, **331**, 50–4.

Szameitat, A.J., Shen, S., and Sterr, A. (2007). Motor imagery of complex everyday movements. An fMRI study. *NeuroImage*, **34**, 702–13.

Tomasino, B., Werner, C.J., Weiss, P.H., and Fink, G.R. (2007). Stimulus properties matter more than perspective: an fMRI study of mental imagery and silent reading of action phrases. *NeuroImage*, **36**, T128–T141.

Vogeley, K. and Fink, G.R. (2003). Neural correlates of the first-person-perspective. *Trends in Cognitive Sciences*, **7**, 38–42.

Weiss, T., Hansen, E., Rost, R., *et al.* (1994). Mental practice of motor skills used in poststroke rehabilitation has own effects on central nervous activation. *International Journal of Neuroscience*, **78**, 157–66.

Wolpert, D.M., Goodbody, S.J., and Husain, M. (1998). Maintaining internal representations: the role of the superior parietal lobe. *Nature Neuroscience*, **1**, 529–33.

Wuyam, B., Moosavi, S.H., Decety, J., Adams, L., Lansing, R.W., and Guz, A. (1995). Imagination of dynamic exercise produced ventilatory responses which were more apparent in competitive sportsmen. *Journal of Physiology*, **482**, 713–24.

Chapter 4

Corticospinal facilitation during motor imagery

Cathy M. Stinear

Introduction

There is debate regarding the role of primary motor cortex (M1) in motor imagery. Functional neuroimaging studies have produced conflicting data, and have been discussed in detail in Chapter 3 of this book. The purpose of this chapter is to review the evidence for modulation of corticospinal excitability during motor imagery.

Pyramidal neurons within M1 form part of the corticospinal pathway, transmitting descending voluntary drive to motor neurons in the spinal cord. The excitability of the corticospinal pathway can be measured with transcranial magnetic stimulation (TMS), a painless, non-invasive technique. TMS activates pyramidal neurons trans-synaptically (Day *et al.* 1989; Rothwell 1991), producing a descending volley that can summate at the alpha motor neuron pool, and elicit a motor evoked potential (MEP) in the relevant musculature that can be recorded using electromyography. The amplitude of this MEP reflects the excitability of both the pyramidal and alpha motor neuron pools, collectively referred to as the corticomotor pathway. During motor imagery, facilitation of corticomotor excitability can be measured in the absence of detectable outflow in this pathway. This chapter reviews the evidence that this facilitation is at least partly due to alterations in the balance of excitatory and inhibitory input to pyramidal neurons.

However, MEPs are facilitated by even minimal levels of muscle activation. If participants inadvertently activate the muscles of interest during imagery, the resulting facilitation of MEPs can be wrongly attributed to the motor imagery process. Furthermore, electromyography (EMG) activity in the contralateral limb can also facilitate MEPs in the muscles of interest, even if they remain at rest (Liang *et al.* 2008). For these reasons, background EMG activity in the muscles of interest and contralateral homologous muscles must be closely monitored, and trials with non-resting levels of EMG activity discarded from analysis. In this review, all studies have monitored background EMG activity, though only a few report the actual levels of this activity, with a statistical analysis demonstrating no systematic changes that could confound results (Hashimoto and Rothwell 1999; Stinear and Byblow 2003a, 2004; Pelgrims *et al.* 2005; Stinear *et al.* 2006a, b, 2007; Cowley *et al.* 2008).

The following sections of this chapter provide an overview of the evidence for corticospinal facilitation during motor imagery. Motor imagery is usually explicit, in that it involves the deliberate use of imagery to mentally simulate the performance of a particular movement or sequence of movements. This is in contrast to implicit imagery, which is used 'unconsciously' during cognitive tasks such as mental rotation, and determining the appropriateness of potential hand–object interactions. The final sections of this chapter consider the site and mechanisms of corticospinal facilitation by motor imagery, and the possible continuum between imagined and executed movements.

Modulation of corticospinal excitability during explicit motor imagery

The facilitation of corticospinal excitability during explicitly imagined movement is similar to that observed during actual movement. The facilitation is graded, muscle-specific, and temporally modulated, and seems more effective when kinaesthetic imagery strategies are employed, as described in the following sections.

Muscle and movement specificity

When participants imagine a sustained isometric contraction of a muscle, the threshold for evoking a MEP in this muscle is lower (Kasai *et al.* 1997; Yahagi and Kasai 1998; Facchini *et al.* 2002), MEPs can be elicited from more scalp sites (Filippi *et al.* 2001; Marconi *et al.* 2007), and MEP amplitude is facilitated (Yahagi and Kasai 1999; Facchini *et al.* 2002) relative to rest, indicating an increase in corticospinal excitability.

The muscle specificity of this increase in excitability was first explored by Kasai *et al.* (1997), who found that imagined isometric wrist flexion facilitated MEPs in wrist flexors, and to a lesser extent in wrist extensors. This may parallel the co-contraction of wrist flexors and extensors commonly observed during isometric wrist flexion (Kasai *et al.* 1997). Motor imagery of thumb abduction facilitates the MEPs recorded from abductor pollicis brevis (APB), but not those recorded from first dorsal interosseous (FDI) (Facchini *et al.* 2002) or abductor digiti minimi (ADM, Figure 4.1A) (Stinear and Byblow 2003a, 2004; Stinear *et al.* 2006a). Similarly, MEPs recorded from FDI and ADM are specifically facilitated during imagined abduction of the index finger and little finger, respectively, while MEPs recorded from other muscles of the hand, forearm, and arm are unaffected (Rossini *et al.* 1999; Quartarone *et al.* 2005). Others have also shown that during actual and imagined thumb opposition, MEPs in the prime mover (opponens pollicis, OP) and a synergist (FDI) are facilitated (Marconi *et al.* 2007). At the same time, MEPs recorded from another intrinsic hand muscle (ADM) and the wrist extensors are unaffected, despite the large overlap in the cortical representations of these four muscles (Marconi *et al.* 2007). In the lower limb, MEPs are facilitated in the knee extensors (quadriceps), but not flexors (biceps femoris) during imagined knee extension (Tremblay *et al.* 2001).

In addition to this muscle specificity, the degree of MEP facilitation during imagery is graded according to the extent of muscle activation during actual movement. For example, FDI is most active during index finger flexion, then abduction, and extension. The degree of FDI MEP facilitation is greatest during imagined index finger flexion, then abduction, and then extension (Yahagi and Kasai 1998). In a later study it was shown that FDI is more active during index finger abduction when the forearm is pronated than when it is in a neutral position (Liang *et al.* 2007). This effect of posture was also observed during imagined index finger abduction, in that FDI MEPs were facilitated to a greater extent with the forearm in a prone position, than in a neutral position. Furthermore, the wrist extensors were activated synergistically with FDI activation when in the neutral forearm position, but not in the prone position. This was paralleled by facilitation of extensor MEPs during imagined index finger abduction with the forearm in a neutral position, but not a prone position (Liang *et al.* 2007). These studies indicate that the degree of MEP facilitation in a given muscle during an imagined movement reflects the extent to which the muscle is recruited during actual performance of that movement.

The individuation of actual and imagined finger movements has also been explored. TMS can be used to evoke a muscle twitch, and the force of this twitch measured as an indication of corticospinal excitability. When participants actually flex their index finger, small flexion forces are

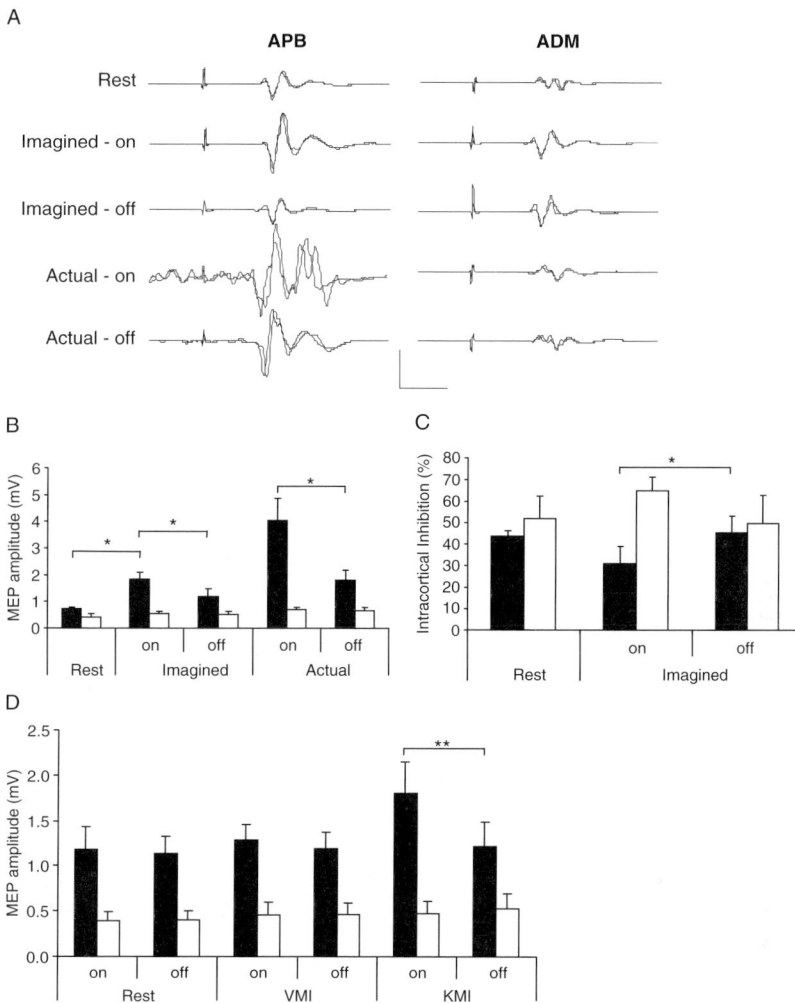

Fig. 4.1 A. EMG traces from right abductor pollicis brevis (APB) and abductor digiti minimi (ADM) while at rest, and during the 'on' and 'off' phases of imagined and actual thumb abduction. Imagined and actual task performance was paced with a 1 Hz auditory metronome. Two traces are overlaid for each condition, from a single participant. Calibration bar = 2 mV, 20 ms. Adapted from Stinear and Byblow (2003a). B. Group mean APB (black bars) and ADM (white bars) MEP amplitudes at rest, and during the 'on' and 'off' phases of imagined and actual thumb abduction. APB MEP amplitude is facilitated relative to rest during the 'on' phase of imagined thumb abduction, and is greater during the 'on' phase than the 'off' phase of imagined and actual thumb abduction. This temporal modulation is not observed in ADM. * $p < 0.05$. For clarity, the significant facilitation of MEP amplitude during actual thumb abduction in both muscles, relative to rest, is not indicated. Adapted from Stinear and Byblow (2004). C. Group mean intracortical inhibition of APB (black bars) and ADM (white bars) at rest, and during the 'on' and 'off' phases of imagined thumb abduction. Note that 100% indicates complete MEP inhibition. Intracortical inhibition is significantly less during the 'on' phase than the 'off' phase of imagined thumb abduction, for APB only. * $p < 0.05$. Adapted from Stinear and Byblow (2004). D. Group mean APB (black bars) and ADM (white bars) MEP amplitudes while at rest and listening to the metronome, and during the 'on' and 'off' phases of visual motor imagery (VMI) and kinaesthetic motor imagery (KMI) of thumb abduction. APB MEP amplitude is significantly facilitated during the 'on' phase of KMI, relative to the 'off' phase, while there is no modulation of ADM MEP amplitude. ** $p < 0.001$. Adapted from Stinear et al. (2006a).

also produced by the other three fingers. This is termed 'enslaving', and reflects neural, muscular, and biomechanical coupling between the digits (Slobounov *et al.* 2002; Zatsiorsky *et al.* 2000). When participants imagine flexing their index finger, the TMS-evoked flexion force is greater than when participants are at rest. Furthermore, small increases in TMS-evoked flexion force are also observed in the other digits (Li *et al.* 2004). This indicates that the neural component of enslaving is present during motor imagery. Similarly, the force produced by the index finger is slightly lower when all of the fingers are flexed together than when this digit is flexed on its own. This force decrement is also observed in the TMS-evoked twitch force during imagined flexion of all the fingers, compared to imagined flexion of the index finger alone (Li *et al.* 2004). These studies demonstrate that the neural mechanisms underlying the grading, enslaving, and decrement of force production during single- and multi-digit actions are operational during imagined movement.

Temporal specificity

High temporal resolution is a major strength of TMS. It allows for the time course of changes in corticospinal excitability during motor imagery to be measured within the range of tens of milliseconds, a distinct advantage over fMRI, for example, which offers much lower temporal resolution. Early studies of imagined simple, repetitive finger flexion, or opposition of the thumb and index finger, produced mixed results. Some found significant facilitation of MEPs in the muscles of interest (Stephan and Frackowiak 1996), while others did not (Abbruzzese *et al.* 1996). As these studies did not attempt to deliver the magnetic stimuli at any particular point in the imagined movement cycle, it is likely that only some stimuli were delivered during the imagined activation of the muscles of interest. This could explain the differences in their results.

Subsequent studies asked participants to imagine moving in time with an auditory stimulus, so that TMS could be delivered at particular times within the imagined movement cycle. One of the first of these studies was conducted by Fadiga *et al.* (1999), who asked participants to imagine flexing and extending their elbow in time with a frequency modulated sound. Magnetic stimuli were delivered randomly, between 100 and 300 ms after the onset of each phase of the sound. MEPs recorded from the muscle of interest (biceps brachii, BB) were significantly facilitated during imagined elbow flexion, but not during extension (Fadiga *et al.* 1999). In a second experiment, MEPs recorded from the muscle of interest (opponens pollicis, OP) were significantly facilitated during imagined hand closing, but not during hand opening. These findings demonstrate temporal modulation of corticospinal excitability during motor imagery.

Further studies have delivered more precisely timed stimuli during imagined movement, by first determining the timing of muscle activity during actual performance of a phasic movement paced with an auditory metronome. During imagined performance of the same paced movement, stimuli can then be delivered at specific times relative to the auditory metronome (rather than randomly within a range of times), which correspond to periods of muscle activity or quiescence during actual performance. This approach has been used to show that corticospinal excitability is modulated in a temporally and muscle-specific way. Reciprocal MEP facilitation in wrist flexor and extensor muscles was demonstrated over the course of phasic imagined wrist flexion and extension (Hashimoto and Rothwell 1999; Levin *et al.* 2004). Similarly, Stinear and Byblow (2003a) instructed participants to imagine repeatedly abducting their thumb in time with a 1 Hz auditory metronome. Magnetic stimuli were delivered during the 'on' phase of imagined APB activation (100 ms prior to the metronome beat, when APB is active during actual task performance). In separate trials, stimuli were delivered during the 'off' phase of imagined activation

(250 ms after the metronome beat, when APB is quiescent during actual task performance). APB MEPs were facilitated only during the 'on' phase, while ADM MEPs were unaffected (Stinear and Byblow 2003a, Figure 4.1A, B). These studies show that the facilitation of corticospinal excitability by motor imagery is muscle-specific, and time-locked to the imagined muscle activity. This strongly suggests that the effects of motor imagery on corticospinal excitability are not due to general cognitive arousal. Rather, it supports the idea that the corticospinal system is a common neural substrate for both actual and imagined movements.

Hemispheric specificity

Corticospinal excitability is typically facilitated in the hemisphere contralateral to the imagined limb movement, and there is some evidence of a handedness asymmetry in this facilitation. In right-handed people, MEPs are facilitated to a greater extent in right-hand muscles during their imagined contraction, than they are in left-hand muscles during their imagined contraction (Yahagi and Kasai 1998, 1999; Marconi *et al.* 2007). This hemispheric asymmetry is not observed in left-handed people, possibly due to a smaller degree of functional asymmetry in this group (Yahagi and Kasai 1999).

There is also some evidence that corticospinal excitability is facilitated in the left M1 during motor imagery of right- and left-hand movements. Fadiga *et al.* (1999) found that MEPs recorded from the right OP were facilitated during imagined closing of either hand, and suppressed during imagined opening of either hand. In contrast, MEPs recorded from the left OP were facilitated during imagined closing of the left hand only, and suppressed during imagined opening of the left hand only. The authors interpreted this as evidence of left-hemisphere dominance for motor imagery, in right-handed people (Fadiga *et al.* 1999). This hypothesis gained further support from Liang *et al.* (2008), who also found that imagined left-index finger abduction facilitated MEPs recorded from the right FDI.

Other studies have produced mixed results. Facchini *et al.* (2002) found that corticospinal excitability in either hemisphere was only facilitated by imagined activation of the contralateral hand, and not the ipsilateral hand. Similarly, it has been shown that right APB MEPs are facilitated relative to baseline during imagined abduction of the right thumb, or both thumbs together, but not during imagined abduction of the left thumb alone (Stinear *et al.* 2006b). These studies seem to contradict the observations of Fadiga *et al.* (1999) and Liang *et al.* (2008). However, in the study by Stinear *et al.* (2006b) imagined thumb abduction was paced with a 1 Hz auditory metronome, to explore temporal modulation. Right APB MEPs were significantly larger during the 'on' phase than the 'off' phase of imagined abduction of the right, left, or both thumbs. This temporal modulation of left-corticospinal excitability, during imagined phasic movement of either hand, supports left-hemisphere dominance for motor imagery (Stinear *et al.* 2006b). This study also found no facilitation or temporal modulation of MEPs recorded from the left APB, during imagery of the left, right, or both hands. This was confirmed with a subsequent study of older adults, again showing that motor imagery of left, right, and bimanual movements facilitated, and temporally modulated, corticospinal excitability in the left hemisphere, but not the right hemisphere (Stinear *et al.* 2007).

Differences in the imagined forcefulness of movement, and the timing of stimuli relative to the time-course of imagined movement, may have contributed to the differences in these studies' results. Overall, it appears that corticospinal excitability is facilitated by motor imagery to a greater extent in the left M1 than the right M1. Furthermore, left M1 corticospinal excitability is facilitated, and temporally modulated, during imagined movement of either hand. These findings suggest that the left hemisphere is dominant for both imagined and actual motor activities in right-handed people. The evidence for facilitation and temporal modulation of right M1 corticospinal excitability during imagined left-hand movement is less clear, and requires further investigation.

Explicit motor imagery strategies

Mentally rehearsing a given movement involves imagining the sensory consequences of performing that movement. Imagery can be focused on simulating the somatosensory consequences of the imagined movement, such as proprioception, cutaneous sensation, muscle tension, and stretch. This is termed 'kinaesthetic motor imagery'. Imagery can also be focused on simulating the sight of one's own limbs performing the movement, and this is termed 'visual motor imagery'. While many studies do not report whether participants were specifically instructed to use one strategy or another, some have explicitly instructed participants to imagine the feeling of the movement, rather than seeing themselves moving (Filippi *et al.* 2001; Marconi *et al.* 2007; Stinear *et al.* 2006b, 2007).

Two studies have directly compared the effects of kinaesthetic and visual imagery strategies on corticospinal facilitation. Fourkas *et al.* (2006b) instructed participants to imagine abducting their thumb at a self-selected pace for 10 seconds, using either a visual or kinaesthetic imagery strategy. MEPs were recorded from APB, in response to stimuli delivered between 3 and 3.5 seconds after the start of each 10-second trial. They found that APB MEPs were facilitated during both visual and kinaesthetic imagery of thumb movement. However, the timing of stimulus delivery relative to imagined task performance was not controlled. This was addressed by Stinear *et al.* (2006a), who instructed participants to use a visual or kinaesthetic strategy to imagine abducting their thumb in time with a 1 Hz auditory metronome. TMS was used to evoke MEPs in the APB muscle, during the 'on' and 'off' phases of imagined APB activity, as previously described. MEPs were also recorded at these times relative to the metronome beats while participants remained at rest, or imagined a static visual scene, as control conditions. APB MEPs were facilitated only during the 'on' phase of the imagined movement, and only when participants were using a kinaesthetic imagery strategy. MEPs were not facilitated, or temporally modulated, while imagining thumb movement with a visual imagery strategy, or under either control condition. These results suggest that kinaesthetic motor imagery more strongly facilitates corticospinal facilitation than visual motor imagery (Stinear *et al.* 2006a, Figure 4.1D). This is likely related to the internal generation of somatosensory afferent input that acts on M1 during kinaesthetic motor imagery (Naito *et al.* 2002). Similarly, fMRI has been used to show that cortical activity in sensorimotor areas is greater during kinaesthetic than visual motor imagery, and closely corresponds to the pattern of activity produced by motor execution (Guillot *et al.* 2008). There is also some evidence that chronic deafferentation precludes the use of a kinaesthetic imagery strategy and its facilitation of corticospinal excitability, presumably because the somatosensory consequences of movement can no longer be internally generated (Mercier *et al.* 2008). Together, these studies suggest that kinaesthetic motor imagery engages the sensorimotor network and facilitates corticospinal excitability, to a greater extent than visual motor imagery.

The distinction between visual and kinaesthetic strategies is closely related to the distinction between first- and third-person perspectives during motor imagery. A first-person perspective involves imagining movement from within one's body, and can include both visual and kinaesthetic elements. In contrast, a third-person perspective requires a visual strategy, as it involves seeing either oneself or another person moving, from the outside. The relationships between perspective and visual and kinaesthetic strategies require that participants be carefully instructed to ensure that the desired combination is used (Chapter 3).

The effects of perspective during visual imagery have been explored by Fourkas *et al.* (2006a). Participants were instructed to imagine repeatedly abducting/adducting their dominant index finger, from a first-person egocentric perspective. In a third-person imagery condition, they were instructed to imagine seeing the experimenter performing the same movement. MEPs were recorded from the FDI muscle, with stimuli delivered 3–3.5 seconds after the onset of imagery. This imprecise timing of stimuli is a potential limitation, as previously mentioned. MEPs were also recorded while participants imagined their resting hand, and during visual imagery of a ball moving up and down on a computer monitor, as control conditions. Participants were not specifically instructed to focus on kinaesthetic or visual features during imagery, but presumably visual imagery dominated during third-person imagery of the experimenter's hand moving, and under the control conditions. During first-person imagery, two-thirds of participants reported using a purely visual strategy, while the remaining one-third reported using a combination of visual and kinaesthetic strategies (Fourkas *et al.* 2006a). FDI MEPs were facilitated under the third-person imagery condition, but not during first-person imagery, relative to the static imagery control condition. These results suggest that visual imagery facilitates corticospinal excitability when participants imagine seeing someone else moving, but not when they imagine seeing themselves moving. This is consistent with the findings of Stinear *et al.* (2006a), who also found that visual imagery of one's own movements did not facilitate corticospinal excitability.

Together, these studies suggest that imagery of one's own movement, from a first-person perspective, facilitates corticospinal excitability when the focus is on somatosensory, rather than visual, consequences of movement. The facilitation of corticospinal excitability by visual imagery of someone else's movements may occur via a separate mechanism, such as the 'mirror neuron' system. This system facilitates corticospinal excitability during action observation, with muscle and temporal specificity (for review see Fadiga *et al.* 2005). When observing the actions of others, this system is thought to support the understanding of action goals, the prediction of movement consequences, and the imitation of others (Rizzolatti and Craighero 2004). Some authors have shown comparable facilitation of corticospinal excitability during observation and explicit motor imagery of the same movement (Clark *et al.* 2004; Leonard and Tremblay 2007; Marconi *et al.* 2007). As the 'mirror neuron' system is activated by the sight of another person's actions, it is probably distinct from the mechanism that facilitates corticospinal excitability during explicit kinaesthetic motor imagery of one's own movements.

Other forms of cognitive activity

An important question addressed by some studies is whether corticospinal excitability facilitation is specific to motor imagery, or can also be produced by other forms of cognitive activity. Mental arithmetic and visual imagery of an expanding and shrinking rectangle have been shown to produce no significant facilitation of corticospinal excitability (Abbruzzese *et al.* 1996; Rossi *et al.* 1998; Fadiga *et al.* 1999; Marconi *et al.* 2007). In contrast, a more demanding mental arithmetic task has been shown to facilitate corticospinal excitability, but to a lesser extent than that produced by motor imagery (Rossini *et al.* 1999). A later study showed that, in some participants, mentally counting backwards facilitated corticospinal excitability to a similar extent as motor imagery (Clark *et al.* 2004). This suggests that cognitive activity can influence corticospinal excitability. However, the studies described in the previous section have demonstrated that the effects of explicit motor imagery on corticospinal excitability are temporally modulated and muscle-specific, which argues against a general arousal mechanism.

Summary

Corticospinal excitability is facilitated during explicit motor imagery in a way that parallels the facilitation observed during actual performance: specific to the muscles involved in task performance; graded according to their contribution to the movement; and occurring with a similar time course. Temporal specificity highlights the need for precise timing of stimuli relative to the imagined movement, in order to obtain accurate measures of imagery's effects on the corticospinal system. Furthermore, the left hemisphere appears to play a dominant role in motor imagery, in right-handed people. Together, these observations strongly suggest that the neural mechanisms that modulate corticospinal excitability during voluntary movement are also operational during explicit motor imagery. The specificity of motor imagery's effects on the corticospinal system argues against their attribution to general cognitive factors such as arousal or attention. Finally, kinaesthetic strategies seem to more effectively facilitate corticospinal excitability than visual strategies, at least when explicitly imagining one's own movement. This is an important consideration for future studies, particularly those exploring potential therapeutic applications of motor imagery, and highlights the need to provide participants with specific instructions.

Site of facilitation

The studies described above have shown that MEP amplitude is specifically facilitated by explicit motor imagery, and this is likely due to the modulation of inputs to M1. However, MEP amplitude reflects the excitability of motor neurons at both the cortical and spinal levels, making it difficult to precisely determine the site of facilitation during imagery. This has been specifically addressed by a number of authors, who have assessed intracortical function within M1 and the excitability of the alpha motor neuron pool, during motor imagery.

Intracortical mechanisms

TMS allows the excitability of intracortical neuronal populations within M1 to be measured. These intracortical populations exert both facilitatory and inhibitory effects on the corticospinal system. The MEP elicited by TMS is a compound potential, produced by waves of descending volleys in the corticomotor pathway. At lower stimulus intensities, these waves are mainly produced by trans-synaptic activation of pyramidal neurons, and are called 'indirect' or I-waves. Three or four I-waves are usually produced by TMS, and their latencies and amplitudes can be recorded from epidural cervical spine electrodes (Di Lazzaro et al. 1998). Early I-waves are preferentially evoked when the TMS coil is oriented to produce current flow in an antero-medial direction in the underlying cortex. Later I-waves are preferentially evoked by current flow in a postero-lateral direction (Sakai et al. 1997). Takahashi et al. (2004) used these coil orientations to determine the effects of motor imagery on early and late I-waves. They found that motor imagery of index finger abduction facilitated MEPs composed of later I-waves, to a greater extent than MEPs composed of early I-waves. This differential effect confirms that the facilitation of MEP amplitude by motor imagery is at least partly due to cortical mechanisms, operating within M1.

The facilitation of later I-waves by motor imagery may be due to increased excitation and/or decreased inhibition by intracortical interneurons, and this can be tested with paired-pulse TMS. Briefly, a weak conditioning stimulus is delivered to M1, followed by a test stimulus. The conditioning stimulus activates low-threshold intracortical interneurons, which alter the excitability of corticospinal neurons, making them more or less responsive to the subsequent test stimulus (Kujirai et al. 1993; Chen et al. 1998). When short interstimulus intervals are used (1–5 ms), the MEP produced by the test stimulus has smaller amplitude. This is probably due to the activation of $GABA_A$-ergic inhibitory interneurons (Ziemann et al. 1996; Ilic et al. 2002). When longer interstimulus intervals are used (10–15 ms), a larger amplitude MEP is produced, probably due to the activation of glutamatergic excitatory interneurons (Liepert *et al.* 1997; Ziemann *et al.* 1998). Intracortical inhibitory interneurons are thought to preferentially act on later I-waves (Di Lazzaro *et al.* 1998), which are more sensitive to motor imagery (Takahashi *et al.* 2004). Paired-pulse TMS can therefore provide a more detailed understanding of how motor imagery influences these distinct neuronal populations.

Early studies of intracortical inhibition and facilitation during imagery produced mixed results. Ridding and Rothwell (1999) found that motor imagery of a weak isometric pinch grip had no effect on the intracortical inhibition or facilitation of MEPs recorded from FDI. In contrast, intracortical inhibition was found to be reduced in OP during imagined sequential finger opposition (Abbruzzese *et al.* 1999), and in flexor digitorum superficialis (FDS) during imagined finger flexion (Patuzzo *et al.* 2003), with no detectable effects on intracortical facilitation. All of these studies observed that motor imagery facilitated the MEPs produced by single-pulse TMS, as expected. However, none delivered the magnetic stimuli at specific times during the imagined movements, or recorded MEPs from any other muscles. Therefore, the temporal and muscle specificity of motor imagery's effects on intracortical inhibition were not evaluated.

These issues were addressed in a study by Stinear and Byblow (2004), who asked participants to imagine abducting their thumb in time with a 1 Hz auditory metronome, as described above. MEPs were recorded from APB and ADM, during the 'on' and 'off' phases of actual and imagined task performance. They found that MEPs were facilitated during the 'on' phase of imagined phasic thumb abduction in APB, confirming the temporal and muscle specificity observed in a previous study (Stinear and Byblow 2003a). They also found that the intracortical inhibition acting on APB was lower during the 'on' phase than the 'off' phase of imagined thumb abduction, and this modulation was not observed for ADM (Figure 4.1C). This indicates that the intracortical inhibition acting on corticospinal neurons is downregulated during imagined task performance, in a muscle- and temporally-specific way. This reflects the modulation of intracortical inhibition during physical performance of this type of task (Stinear and Byblow 2003b). In a second experiment, participants imagined small amplitude, low-force index finger flexion, using the same experimental protocol. MEPs were weakly and non-specifically facilitated in both FDI and ADM, during both the 'on' and 'off' phases of imagined movement, and there were no significant effects on intracortical inhibition (Stinear and Byblow 2004). It seems that corticospinal excitability and intracortical inhibition are less clearly modulated by motor imagery of small amplitude, low-force movements. This may explain why Ridding and Rothwell (1999) were unable to detect any change in intracortical inhibition during imagery of a weak isometric pinch grip.

There is also some evidence that the imagined performance of a simple reaction time task increases corticospinal excitability and reduces intracortical inhibition, with the same time-course as that observed during physical performance of this task (Kumru *et al.* 2008). However, the muscle specificity of this effect has not been explored. Furthermore, this study, and that by Patuzzo *et al.* (2003), did not adjust the test stimulus intensity so that non-conditioned MEPs were of similar amplitudes during imagery and baseline conditions. This is important, because the degree of inhibition produced by the conditioning stimulus can vary as a function of the MEP amplitude produced by the test stimulus (Roshan *et al.* 2003). As MEP amplitude is facilitated by motor imagery, the effectiveness of the conditioning stimulus may be reduced under this condition (Kujirai *et al.* 1993). Therefore, matching MEP amplitudes is an important technical consideration, made by the other studies described here (Abbruzzese *et al.* 1999; Ridding and Rothwell 1999; Stinear and Byblow 2004).

These studies indicate that intracortical inhibition is downregulated during motor imagery, and this is a likely mechanism for the observed facilitation of corticospinal excitability. This confirms that changes in MEP amplitude during motor imagery are at least partly due to intracortical mechanisms, within M1. A number of studies have also investigated the effects of motor imagery on spinal motor neuron excitability, and these are reviewed below.

Spinal mechanisms

It is possible that the MEPs elicited by TMS are facilitated during motor imagery due to increases in alpha motor neuron excitability, rather than, or in addition to, increases in corticospinal neuron excitability. Many studies have therefore explored the effects of imagery on the H-reflex or F-wave, which provide measures of alpha motor neuron excitability. As for MEP recordings during motor imagery, background muscle activity must be eliminated as even very low levels of activity can facilitate spinal excitability (Gandevia *et al.* 1997).

The H-reflex is evoked by transcutaneous electrical stimulation of a mixed peripheral nerve. At lower intensities, stimulation preferentially activates Ia afferent fibres that make monosynaptic connections with the alpha motor neuron pool, evoking an H-reflex that can be recorded with EMG (Capaday 1997). Higher stimulus intensities activate alpha motor neuron axons and motor units, recorded in the EMG as the M-wave. Most studies have found no effect of motor imagery on H-reflex amplitude recorded from upper limb muscles (Abbruzzese *et al.* 1996; Stephan and Frackowiak 1996; Yahagi *et al.* 1996; Kasai *et al.* 1997; Hashimoto and Rothwell 1999; Patuzzo *et al.* 2003). However, H-reflex amplitude is influenced by descending excitatory inputs to the alpha motor neuron pool, and by descending pre-synaptic inhibition of Ia afferent input. Changes in H-reflex amplitude cannot be attributed to one source of input or the other, and their effects may even 'cancel out', leaving the amplitude unchanged. More recently Cowley *et al.* (2008) observed soleus muscle H-reflex facilitation during imagined plantarflexion in just under half of their participants. In these participants, imagined plantarflexion was also associated with wrist flexor H-reflex facilitation (Cowley *et al.* 2008). This indicates that the increase in spinal excitability was not specific to the muscle or limb. Instead, it may reflect the functional coupling between ankle- and wrist-movement representations at the level of the cortex (Baldissera *et al.* 2002; Borroni *et al.* 2004; Byblow *et al.* 2007).

F-waves provide an alternative method for measuring the excitability of the alpha motor neuron pool. Here, transcutaneous electrical stimulation of a peripheral nerve activates motor neuron axons, propagating action potentials in the orthodromic direction to the muscle, where an M-wave can be measured. At high stimulus intensities, which produce a maximal M-wave, action potentials also propagate antidromically to the spinal cord and can depolarize the alpha motor neuron axon hillock, causing a second orthodromic action potential. This is detected as an F-wave, after the M-wave. F-waves are only elicited from a small proportion of the alpha motor neuron pool, and their latency, amplitude, and chronodispersion provide useful clinical information (Panayiotopoulos and Chroni 1996). F-waves' advantage in the study of motor imagery is that they are not affected by pre-synaptic inhibition of Ia afferent input. F-wave parameters, such as amplitude and persistence, are therefore thought to reflect the excitability of the alpha motor neuron pool. Most studies have found no differences between F-waves elicited at rest and during motor imagery (Facchini *et al.* 2002; Patuzzo *et al.* 2003; Stinear and Byblow 2003a; Stinear *et al.* 2006a, b), though see also Liang *et al.* (2008). Rossini *et al.* (1999) found that motor imagery may facilitate F-wave amplitude, with some muscle specificity, but that both motor imagery and mental arithmetic increase F-wave persistence, suggesting a general effect of cognitive activity. These studies recorded only 10–30 F-waves under each experimental condition; and while this may be adequate for determining F-wave latency (Nobrega *et al.* 2004), it may be insufficient for detecting changes in amplitude.

On balance, there is currently no strong evidence for modulation of spinal excitability that could account for the observed muscle- and temporally-specific modulation of MEPs during motor imagery. Further investigation is required, recording a larger number of F-waves in response to stimuli that are precisely timed with respect to imagined task performance.

Summary

Overall, these studies indicate that the facilitation of MEPs by motor imagery is mainly due to increased corticospinal excitability, rather than increased excitability at the spinal level. The increase in corticospinal excitability is at least partly due to reduced intracortical inhibition, and this reduction is muscle- and temporally-specific, as for actual movement. While the effects of motor imagery on spinal excitability remain unclear, the source of any modulation at this level is most likely cortical.

Inhibition of motor output during motor imagery

Given that imagined and actual movement have similar effects on corticospinal and intracortical excitability, one may wonder whether there are specific mechanisms preventing the execution of imagined movement. Is there an active inhibitory process, which takes place in parallel with motor imagery, in order to prevent execution? Or do imagined and executed movements lie on a continuum, with the facilitation of corticospinal excitability by motor imagery remaining sub-threshold for execution?

Participants in the studies described here were trained to perform motor imagery while keeping the target muscles completely relaxed. Other studies have shown that MEPs are suppressed in muscles that are being volitionally relaxed (Stinear and Byblow 2003b; Begum *et al.* 2005), and that increased GABA$_A$-ergic intracortical inhibition is at least partly responsible (Liepert *et al.* 1998; Stinear and Byblow 2003b; Buccolieri *et al.* 2004). This suggests that participants may be engaged in two processes during motor imagery experiments: imagined performance of a particular movement and volitional relaxation of the target muscles. This volitional relaxation may recruit inhibition within M1, lowering corticospinal excitability during motor imagery so that it remains subthreshold for execution. However, there is little support for this hypothesis in the literature to date. A general inhibitory mechanism might be expected to suppress MEP amplitudes recorded from muscles not engaged by the imagined task, but this has not been reported. Instead, MEPs recorded from control muscles remain at resting levels (e.g. Rossini *et al.* 1999; Stinear and Byblow 2003a; Stinear *et al.* 2006a, Figure 4.1B, D). Similarly, when motor imagery is paced with an auditory metronome, MEPs recorded from the target muscle during the 'off' phase of the imagery task have the same or slightly higher amplitude as those recorded at rest, showing no sign of active inhibition (Stinear and Byblow 2003a, 2004; Stinear *et al.* 2006a, Figure 4.1B). Furthermore, intracortical inhibition within M1 is reduced during motor imagery, making this an unlikely mechanism for the prevention of execution (Abbruzzese *et al.* 1999; Patuzzo *et al.* 2003; Stinear and Byblow 2004, Figure 4.1C).

One study reported a decrease in MEP and F-wave amplitude after volitional relaxation of APB for 3 hours, which was not observed if participants imagined abducting their thumb once per second for the same period of time (Taniguchi *et al.* 2008). This may suggest that the effects of volitional relaxation and motor imagery on spinal excitability effectively cancel each other out. However, this study did not include control conditions, where participants simply rested or engaged in another cognitive activity for 3 hours, and the muscle specificity of these effects was not explored. Furthermore, recordings were made before and after motor imagery, and therefore provide no information about the mechanisms preventing motor output during motor imagery.

Therefore, while motor imagery facilitates corticospinal excitability with muscle- and temporal-specificity, there is currently no clear evidence that this occurs against a background of volitional inhibition of corticospinal excitability.

A number of studies have shown that motor imagery facilitates corticospinal excitability to a lesser extent than execution of the same movement (Rossini *et al.* 1999; Stinear and Byblow 2003a, 2004; Clark *et al.* 2004; Leonard and Tremblay 2007; Kumru *et al.* 2008, Figure 4.1A, B). This suggests that imagery and execution are on a continuum, with imagined movements inadvertently generating muscle activity when the facilitation of corticospinal excitability crosses a threshold for activating the alpha motor neuron pool. The weight of evidence currently favours this explanation, rather than an active inhibitory process, for the lack of corticomotor output during motor imagery. However, there are a range of other possibilities that have not yet been investigated. For example, corticomotor output could be actively inhibited at the spinal level by descending input from non-M1 sources, such as premotor cortex and the brainstem. This could counteract any descending corticospinal excitation arising from motor imagery, maintaining the excitability of the alpha motor neuron pool at resting levels during motor imagery. Further investigation is required to determine whether motor output is prevented during motor imagery by the facilitation of inhibitory pathways in parallel with the corticospinal pathway.

Conclusion

There is a reasonably sound body of evidence in support of subthreshold modulation of corticospinal excitability during motor imagery. This modulation is muscle specific, producing graded facilitation of muscle representations according to their contribution to the movement being imagined, with the same time-course as actual performance. The facilitation of corticospinal excitability during motor imagery is associated with specific reductions in intracortical inhibition. The sources of input to M1 producing this modulation likely include fronto-parietal network activity, and possibly the cerebellum and basal ganglia. The roles of these structures in motor imagery are reviewed in Chapter 3.

The effects of motor imagery on the corticospinal system appear to be most potent during explicit kinaesthetic imagery of one's own movements. Explicit motor imagery and actual performance of a given task engage primary motor cortex in a similar way, and may lie on a continuum of corticospinal activation. However, the possibility that motor output is actively inhibited by alternative descending pathways requires further investigation.

References

Abbruzzese, G., Assini, A., Buccolieri, A., Marchese, R., and Trompetto, C. (1999). Changes of intracortical inhibition during motor imagery in human subjects. *Neuroscience Letters, 263*, 113–6.

Abbruzzese, G., Trompetto, C., and Schieppati, M. (1996). The excitability of the human motor cortex increases during execution and mental imagination of sequential but not repetitive finger movements. *Experimental Brain Research, 111*, 465–72.

Baldissera, F., Borroni, P., Cavallari, P., and Cerri, G. (2002). Excitability changes in human corticospinal projections to forearm muscles during voluntary movement of ipsilateral foot. *Journal of Physiology, 539*, 903–11.

Begum, T., Mima, T., Oga, T. *et al.* (2005). Cortical mechanisms of unilateral voluntary motor inhibition in humans. *Neuroscience Research, 53*, 428–35.

Borroni, P., Cerri, G., and Baldissera, F. (2004). Excitability changes in resting forearm muscles during voluntary foot movements depend on hand position: a neural substrate for hand-foot isodirectional coupling. *Brain Research, 1022*, 117–25.

Buccolieri, A., Abbruzzese, G., and Rothwell, J.C. (2004). Relaxation from a voluntary contraction is preceded by increased excitability of motor cortical inhibitory circuits. *Journal of Physiology*, **558**, 685–95.

Byblow, W.D., Coxon, J.P., Stinear, C.M. *et al.* (2007). Functional connectivity between secondary and primary motor areas underlying hand-foot coordination. *Journal of Neurophysiology*, **98**, 414–22.

Capaday, C. (1997). Neurophysiological methods for studies of the motor system in freely moving human subjects. *Journal of Neuroscience Methods*, **74**, 201–18.

Chen, R., Tam, A., Bütefisch, C. *et al.* (1998). Intracortical inhibition and facilitation in different representations of the human motor cortex. *Journal of Neurophysiology*, **80**, 2870–81.

Clark, S., Tremblay, F., and Ste-Marie, D. (2004). Differential modulation of corticospinal excitability during observation, mental imagery and imitation of hand actions. *Neuropsychologia*, **42**, 105–12.

Cowley, P.M., Clark, B.C., and Ploutz-Snyder, L.L. (2008). Kinesthetic motor imagery and spinal excitability: the effect of contraction intensity and spatial localization. *Clinical Neurophysiology*, **119**, 1849–56.

Day, B.J., Dressler, D., Maertens De Noordhout, A. *et al.* (1989). Electric and magnetic stimulation of human motor cortex: surface EMG and single motor unit responses. *Journal of Physiology*, **412**, 449–73.

Di Lazzaro, V., Restuccia, D., Oliviero, A. *et al.* (1998). Magnetic transcranial stimulation at intensities below active motor threshold activates intracortical inhibitory circuits. *Experimental Brain Research*, **119**, 265–8.

Facchini, S., Muellbacher, W., Battaglia, F., Boroojerdi, B., and Hallett, M. (2002). Focal enhancement of motor cortex excitability during motor imagery: a transcranial magnetic stimulation study. *Acta Neurologica Scandinavica*, **105**, 146–51.

Fadiga, L., Buccino, G., Craighero, L., Fogassi, L., Gallese, V., and Pavesi, G. (1999). Corticospinal excitability is specifically modulated by motor imagery: a magnetic stimulation study. *Neuropsychologia*, **37**, 147–58.

Fadiga, L., Craighero, L., and Olivier, E. (2005). Human motor cortex excitability during the perception of others' action. *Current Opinion in Neurobiology*, **15**, 1–6.

Filippi, M.M., Oliveri, M., Pasqualetti, P. *et al.* (2001) Effects of motor imagery on motor cortical output topography in Parkinson's disease. *Neurology*, **57**, 55–61.

Fourkas, A.D., Avenanti, A., Urgesi, C., and Aglioti, S.M. (2006a). Corticospinal facilitation during first and third person imagery. *Experimental Brain Research*, **168**, 143–51.

Fourkas, A.D., Ionta, S., and Aglioti, S.M. (2006b). Influence of imagined posture and imagery modality on corticospinal excitability. *Behavioural Brain Research*, **168**, 190–6.

Gandevia, S.C., Wilson, L.R., Inglis, J.T., and Burke, D. (1997). Mental rehearsal of motor tasks recruits alpha-motoneurones but fails to recruit human fusimotor neurones selectively. *Journal of Physiology*, **505**, 259–66.

Guillot, A., Collet, C., Nguyen, V.A., Malouin, F., Richards, C., and Doyon, J. (2008). Brain activity during visual versus kinesthetic imagery: an fMRI study. *Human Brain Mapping*, DOI: 10.1002/hbm.20658.

Hashimoto, R. and Rothwell, J.C. (1999). Dynamic changes in corticospinal excitability during motor imagery. *Experimental Brain Research*, **125**, 75–81.

Ilic, T.V., Meintzschel, F., Cleff, U., Ruge, D., Kessler, K.R., and Ziemann, U. (2002). Short-interval paired-pulse inhibition and facilitation of human motor cortex: the dimension of stimulus intensity. *Journal of Physiology*, **545**, 153–67.

Kasai, T., Kawai, S., Kawanishi, M., and Yahagi, S. (1997). Evidence for facilitation of motor evoked potentials (MEPs) induced by motor imagery. *Brain Research*, **744**, 147–50.

Kujirai, T., Caramia, M.D., Rothwell, J.C. *et al.* (1993). Corticocortical inhibition in human motor cortex. *Journal of Physiology*, **471**, 501–19.

Kumru, H., Soto, O., Casanova, J., and Valls-Sole, J. (2008). Motor cortex excitability changes during imagery of simple reaction time. *Experimental Brain Research*, **189**, 373–8.

Leonard, G., and Tremblay, F. (2007). Corticomotor facilitation associated with observation, imagery and imitation of hand actions: a comparative study in young and old adults. *Experimental Brain Research*, **177**, 167–75.

Levin, O., Steyvers, M., Wenderoth, N., Li, Y., and Swinnen, S.P. (2004). Dynamical changes in corticospinal excitability during imagery of unimanual and bimanual wrist movements in humans: a transcranial magnetic stimulation study. *Neuroscience Letters, 359*, 185–9.

Li, S., Latash, M.L., and Zatsiorsky, V.M. (2004). Effects of motor imagery on finger force responses to transcranial magnetic stimulation. *Brain Research. Cognitive Brain Research, 20*, 273–80.

Liang, N., Murakami, T., Funase, K., Narita, T., and Kasai, T. (2008). Further evidence for excitability changes in human primary motor cortex during ipsilateral voluntary contractions. *Neuroscience Letters, 433*, 135–40.

Liang, N., Ni, Z., Takahashi, M. *et al.* (2007). Effects of motor imagery are dependent on motor strategies. *Neuroreport, 18*, 1241–5.

Liepert, J., Classen, J., Cohen, L.G., and Hallett, M. (1998). Task-dependent changes of intracortical inhibition. *Experimental Brain Research, 118*, 421–6.

Liepert, J., Schwenkreis, P., Tegenthoff, M., and Malin, J.P. (1997). The glutamate antagonist riluzole suppresses intracortical facilitation. *Journal of Neural Transmission, 104*, 1207–14.

Marconi, B., Pecchioli, C., Koch, G., and Caltagirone, C. (2007). Functional overlap between hand and forearm motor cortical representations during motor cognitive tasks. *Clinical Neurophysiology, 118*, 1767–75.

Mercier, C., Aballea, A., Vargas, C.D., Paillard, J., and Sirigu, A. (2008). Vision without proprioception modulates cortico-spinal excitability during hand motor imagery. *Cerebral Cortex, 18*, 272–7.

Naito, E., Kochiyama, T., Kitada, R. *et al.* (2002). Internally simulated movement sensations during motor imagery activate cortical motor areas and the cerebellum. *The Journal of Neuroscience, 22*, 3683–91.

Nobrega, J.A., Pinheiro, D.S., Manzano, G.M., and Kimura, J. (2004). Various aspects of F-wave values in a healthy population. *Clinical Neurophysiology, 115*, 2336–42.

Panayiotopoulos, C.P., and Chroni, E. (1996). F-waves in clinical neurophysiology: a review, methodological issues and overall value in peripheral neuropathies. *Electroencephalography and Clinical Neurophysiology, 101*, 365–74.

Patuzzo, S., Fiaschi, A., and Manganotti, P. (2003). Modulation of motor cortex excitability in the left hemisphere during action observation: a single- and paired-pulse transcranial magnetic stimulation study of self- and non-self-action observation. *Neuropsychologia, 41*, 1272–8.

Pelgrims, B., Andres, M., and Olivier, E. (2005). Motor imagery while judging object-hand interactions. *Neuroreport, 16*, 1193–6.

Quartarone, A., Bagnato, S., Rizzo, V. *et al.* (2005). Corticospinal excitability during motor imagery of a simple tonic finger movement in patients with writer's cramp. *Movement Disorders, 20*, 1488–95.

Ridding, M.C. and Rothwell, J.C. (1999). Afferent input and cortical organisation: a study with magnetic stimulation. *Experimental Brain Research, 126*, 536–44.

Rizzolatti, G., and Craighero, L. (2004). The mirror-neuron system. *Annual Review of Neuroscience, 27*, 169–92.

Roshan, L., Paradiso, G.O., and Chen, R. (2003). Two phases of short-interval intracortical inhibition. *Experimental Brain Research, 151*, 330–7.

Rossi, S., Pasqualetti, P., Tecchio, F., Pauri, F., and Rossini, P.M. (1998). Corticospinal excitability modulation during mental simulation of wrist movements in human subjects. *Neuroscience Letters, 243*, 147–51.

Rossini, P.M., Rossi, S., Pasqualetti, P., and Tecchio, F. (1999). Corticospinal excitability modulation to hand muscles during movement imagery. *Cerebral Cortex, 9*, 161–7.

Rothwell, J.C. (1991). Physiological studies of electric and magnetic stimulation on the human brain. *Electroencephalography and Clinical Neurophysiology, 43*, 268–78.

Sakai, K., Ugawa, Y., Terao, Y., Hanajima, R., Furubayashi, T., and Kanazawa, I. (1997). Preferential activation of different I waves by transcranial magnetic stimulation with a figure-of-eight-shaped coil. *Experimental Brain Research, 113*, 24–32.

Slobounov, S., Johnston, J., Chiang, H., and Ray, W. (2002). The role of sub-maximal force production in the enslaving phenomenon. *Brain Research,* **954,** 212–9.

Stephan, K.M., and Frackowiak, R.S. (1996). Motor imagery-anatomical representation and electrophysiological characteristics. *Neurochemical Research,* **21,** 1105–16.

Stinear, C.M. and Byblow, W.D. (2003a). Motor imagery of phasic thumb abduction temporally and spatially modulates corticospinal excitability. *Clinical Neurophysiology,* **114,** 909–14.

Stinear, C.M., and Byblow, W.D. (2003b). Role of intracortical inhibition in selective hand muscle activation. *Journal of Neurophysiology,* **89,** 2014–20.

Stinear, C.M., and Byblow, W.D. (2004). Modulation of corticospinal excitability and intracortical inhibition during motor imagery is task-dependent. *Experimental Brain Research,* **157,** 351–8.

Stinear, C.M., Byblow, W.D., Steyvers, M., Levin, O., and Swinnen, S.P. (2006a). Kinesthetic, but not visual, motor imagery modulates corticomotor excitability. *Experimental Brain Research,* **168,** 157–64.

Stinear, C.M., Fleming, M.K., and Byblow, W.D. (2006b). Lateralization of unimanual and bimanual motor imagery. *Brain Research,* **1095,** 139–47.

Stinear, C.M., Fleming, M.K., Barber, P.A., and Byblow, W.D. (2007). Lateralization of motor imagery following stroke. *Clinical Neurophysiology,* **118,** 1794–801.

Takahashi, M., Sugawara, K., Hayashi, S., and Kasai, T. (2004). Excitability changes in human hand motor area dependent on afferent inputs induced by different motor tasks. *Experimental Brain Research,* **158,** 527–32.

Taniguchi, S., Kimura, J., Yamada, T. *et al.* (2008). Effect of motion imagery to counter rest-induced suppression of F-wave as a measure of anterior horn cell excitability. *Clinical Neurophysiology,* **119,** 1346–52.

Tremblay, F., Tremblay, L.E., and Colcer, D.E. (2001). Modulation of corticospinal excitability during imagined knee movements. *Journal of Rehabilitation Medicine,* **33,** 230–4.

Yahagi, S., and Kasai, T. (1998). Facilitation of motor evoked potentials (MEPs) in first dorsal interosseous (FDI) muscle is dependent on different motor images. *Electroencephalography and Clinical Neurophysiology,* **109,** 409–17.

Yahagi, S., and Kasai, T. (1999). Motor evoked potentials induced by motor imagery reveal a functional asymmetry of cortical motor control in left- and right-handed human subjects. *Neuroscience Letters,* **276,** 185–8.

Yahagi, S., Shimura, K. and Kasai, T. (1996). An increase in cortical excitability with no change in spinal excitability during motor imagery. *Perceptual and Motor Skills,* **83,** 288–90.

Zatsiorsky, V.M., Zong-Ming, L., and Latash, M.L. (2000). Enslaving effects in multi-finger force production. *Experimental Brain Research,* **131,** 187–95.

Ziemann, U., Chen, R., Cohen, L.G., and Hallett, M. (1998). Dextromethorphan decreases the excitability of the human motor cortex. *Neurology,* **51,** 1320–4.

Ziemann, U., Lonnecker, S., Steinhoff, B.J., and Paulus, W. (1996). Effects of antiepileptic drugs on motor cortex excitability in humans: a transcranial magnetic stimulation study. *Annals of Neurology,* **40,** 367–78.

Section 2

Neurophysiological correlates of motor imagery

Chapter 5

Electroencephalographic characteristics during motor imagery

Christa Neuper and Gert Pfurtscheller

Introduction

There is a long history of research on neural correlates of mental imagery using the scalp-recorded electroencephalogram (EEG) as a dependent measure. Early research in this area has been directed, for example, at determining whether the occipital alpha rhythm would be specifically attenuated during the generation of visual imagery (Short 1953; Mundy-Castle 1957), or whether the central mu rhythm would be blocked with mere thinking of performing a movement (Klass and Bickford 1957; Chatrian *et al.* 1959; Gastaut *et al.* 1965). Over the last decades, evidence has accumulated that self-generated imagery in different modalities results in activity patterns at corresponding primary sensory or motor regions. Davidson and Schwartz (1977) compared the occipital and sensorimotor EEG activities in the alpha band during self-generated visual versus kinaesthetic imagery, and reported that visual imagery elicited greater relative occipital activation than kinaesthetic imagery. In later studies, a suppression of the posterior alpha band activity during visual imagery has been confirmed in EEG (Marks and Isaaks 1995) and in magnetoencephalography (MEG) as well (Salenius *et al.* 1995).

Analogously, early clinical studies have shown that motor imagery (MI) can activate the corresponding primary sensorimotor areas. Gastaut *et al.* (1965), for example, observed a blocking of the mu rhythm when subjects with limb amputation mobilized the phantom limb mentally. Later on, studies in able-bodied subjects found a similar cortical activity close to the sensorimotor hand area during execution and imagination of hand movement with DC potential measurements (Beisteiner *et al.* 1995) and based on dipole source analysis of electric and magnetic fields (Lang *et al.* 1996). Using a dense array of closely spaced EEG electrodes, Pfurtscheller and Neuper (1997) substantiated that oscillations, generated in or close to primary sensorimotor areas, can be affected by mental activity. When an individual imagines performing a right- or left-hand movement, for example, a similar locally restricted desynchronization (ERD) over the contralateral hand area can be observed, as is typically found during planning or preparation of a real movement. Such a pattern of sensorimotor EEG activity related to MI can also be found in patients with impaired motor function (Neuper and Pfurtscheller 1999; Neuper *et al.* 2006). To date, a number of more recent electrophysiological studies support motor cortex participation in MI (e.g., EEG: McFarland *et al.* 2000; Caldara *et al.* 2004; Neuper *et al.* 2005; Pfurtscheller *et al.* 2005; Carrillo-de-la-Pena *et al.* 2006; MEG: Mellinger *et al.* 2007).

Also, over the last decade, reports based on functional magnetic resonance imaging (fMRI) demonstrated that primary motor and premotor areas are involved not only in the execution of limb movement but also in imagination thereof (Porro *et al.* 1996; Lotze *et al.* 1999; deCharms *et al.* 2004; Dechent *et al.* 2004; see also Chapter 3). It is difficult, however, to determine the dynamic aspect of movement-related activity of these areas based on such imaging techniques that rely on physiological phenomena, which lack the necessary fast time response. In contrast, electrophysiological methods, such as scalp-recorded EEG and MEG or intracranial electrical recordings, offer this possibility, though at the cost of reduced spatial resolution. These methods directly detect neuronal activity on a milliseconds scale by measuring electric potential or magnetic field distributions resulting from postsynaptic potentials.

Cortical activity associated with actual and also mental motor preparation and execution can be detected at the scalp surface in two different ways. One way is simply averaging EEG/MEG activity to reveal movement-related potentials (MRPs) – or the corresponding MEG fields – occurring before, during, and after execution (cf. Kornhuber and Deecke 1965; Cui *et al.* 1999) or mental simulation (Cunnington *et al.* 1997; Caldara *et al.* 2004) of a motor act. The other way is to quantify event-related changes in specific frequency bands. Event-related desynchronization (ERD) defines an amplitude (power) decrease of a rhythmic component, whereas event-related synchronization (ERS) characterizes an amplitude (power) increase (Pfurtscheller and Lopes da Silva 1999). These responses are classically processed by way of band-pass filtering, squaring amplitude values, and averaging over trials. The absolute band power is converted into relative power changes with respect to a reference time interval and ERD/ERS is typically expressed as a percentage value (for more details of ERD/ERS quantification, see Graimann and Pfurtscheller 2006).

MRPs represent the responses of cortical neurons due to changes in the afferent activity. ERD/ERS patterns, in contrast, are mainly due to feedback loops of the complex neural networks in the brain. More specifically, they reflect changes in the activity of local interactions between main neurons and interneurons that control the frequency components of the ongoing EEG. For example, it is known from electrophysiological investigations and computational models (Suffczynski *et al.* 1999) that EEG activities in the alpha frequency band can be generated by two interacting populations, such as the thalamocortical relay and reticular nucleus neurons, that form a feedback loop (for more details on the neurophysiological mechanisms underlying the ERD and ERS phenomena, see Lopes da Silva 2006).

Movement-related potentials

MRPs can be utilized to track the time course of the functional processes involved in real and imagined movements. MRPs associated with voluntary movement, typically show a slowly increasing negative potential, beginning between one and two seconds prior to movement. This negative potential most likely reflects motor preparatory processes. Such pre-movement potentials, the so-called 'Bereitschaftspotential' or readiness potential (RP; Kornhuber and Deecke 1965), preceding self-paced movements, and the contingent negative variation (CNV; Walter *et al.* 1964), preceding externally cued movements, belong to the family of slow cortical potentials. These are slow shifts of the EEG originating in the upper layers of the cortex. Negative slow cortical potentials reflect a long-lasting depolarization of the dendritic network and, in general, indicate a preparatory state of the underlying cortical circuits. Note that in areas where the convexity of the cortex results in an inversion of the cortical dipole directions, such as in the interhemispheric sulcus, inversion of the polarity of slow cortical potentials may be found. This is the case, for example, when studying hand versus foot area activation (e.g., Böcker *et al.* 1994).

Two major components can be distinguished in MRPs preceding voluntary movement (Cunnington *et al.* 1996). The early component consists of a slowly increasing negative potential, showing a bilateral and relatively widespread distribution across the scalp with an amplitude maximum over the vertex (position Cz). This early-stage pre-movement potential is probably caused by activity in several areas, including primary motor regions, but the anterior portion of the supplementary motor area (SMA), known as the pre-SMA, is suggested to be the major source of this component (Cunnington *et al.* 2005). The early pre-movement activity is considered to reflect activity associated with processes of movement preparation. The late component, consisting of a more rapidly increasing negative potential, begins within 500 ms prior to movement. This late component is thought to reflect activity associated with movement execution, arising predominantly from the primary motor cortex, since its localization appears to follow the somatotopic organization of the sensorimotor strip, varying from lateral sources for finger to medial sources for foot movement (Boschert *et al.* 1983).

Cunnington *et al.* (1996) studied MRPs associated with the preparation of an actual versus imagined, externally paced, motor sequence. Interestingly, the early component of the MRPs associated with imagined movements was found not to differ in amplitude, onset time, or topography compared with real movements. This finding has led to the suggestion that imagery and execution involve similar processes of preparing and encoding actions prior to initiation, most likely controlled by the SMA. The peak amplitude of the late potential, however, was higher during preparation of an actual motor response than in the preparation for motor imagination. More recently, Caldara *et al.* (2004), evaluated separately the preparation and the execution periods of overt and covert movements. The paradigm included randomly mixed actual and imagined trials of an externally paced sequence of finger key presses. By using high-resolution EEG recordings and source localization methods, the authors showed that the difference between actual and mental motor acts takes place at the late stages of the preparation period and mainly consists of modulations of the activity of primary motor structures.

Studies using event-related and time-resolved fMRI techniques examined the role of the SMA, in particular the pre-SMA, throughout the preparation, readiness, and execution of actual and imagined actions (for a review, see Cunnington *et al.* 2005). These studies provide converging evidence that the pre-SMA plays a common role in encoding or representing actions prior to voluntary movements, during MI, and also during the observation of others' actions. Therefore, the SMA is very likely involved in preparing and encoding actions prior to movement initiation, whether or not these actions are executed.

A recent study applied dynamic causal modelling to determine the connectivity between SMA and primary motor cortex, in fMRI data sets obtained during motor execution (ME) and imagery (Kasess *et al.* 2008). The results suggest that the SMA may actively inhibit activity of the primary motor cortex in order to prevent movement execution during MI. This would provide a possible explanation for the reported reduced activity in primary motor areas during MI as compared to movement execution (Lotze *et al.* 1999). Altogether, these findings underline the importance of a feedback circuit from primary motor cortex to the SMA for the preparation and control of overt and covert actions. A more detailed consideration of the inhibitory mechanisms during MI can be found in Chapter 6, in this book.

Evidence in favour of the activation of the primary motor cortex during MI (according to the so-called 'functional equivalence hypothesis'; Jeannerod 2001) comes from studies analysing the lateralized readiness potential (LRP). The LRP is an index of brain lateralization derived from the readiness potential, and associated with response preparation in choice reaction tasks that require left- and right-hand responses. It is usually computed by subtracting event-related potential (ERP) activity at C3 minus C4 for the right responses, and C4 minus C3 for the left responses, respectively (Coles 1989). In this way, non-motor contribution is removed from this index of lateralized activity. The origin of the LRP in the primary motor cortex has been supported by dipole estimation (Leuthold and Jentzsch 2002) and MEG measurements (Praamstra *et al.* 1999). Studies with simple simulated and executed movement tasks have shown that the mental rehearsal of a movement elicited such a lateralized activity at central scalp sites (Galdo-Alvarez and

Carrillo-de-la-Pena 2004; Carrillo-de-la-Pena *et al.* 2008). Interestingly, an inversion of LRP for foot responses was observed at both times – when the movements were performed or just imagined (Carrillo-de-la-Pena *et al.* 2006). These results provide convincing evidence that MI can give rise to the generation of a LRP, indicating activation of primary motor structures during MI.

ERD/ERS patterns

It is well-established that preparation, execution, and also imagination of movement produce a circumscribed desynchronization (ERD) localized over sensorimotor areas, with maxima in the alpha band (mu rhythm, ~10 Hz) and beta band (~20 Hz) (Jasper and Penfield 1949; Chatrian *et al.* 1959; Pfurtscheller and Neuper 1997). The mu ERD is most prominent over the contralateral Rolandic region during motor preparation and extends bilaterally symmetrical with movement initiation. ERD during hand MI is very similar to the pre-movement ERD, i.e., it is locally restricted to the contralateral sensorimotor areas (Neuper and Pfurtscheller 1999). Since ERD of alpha band and beta frequency components can be viewed as an electrophysiological correlate of an activated cortical network, prepared to process information with an increased excitability of cortical neurons (Lopes da Silva and Pfurtscheller 1999), the pre-movement ERD and the ERD during MI may reflect a similar type of readiness or presetting of neural networks in sensorimotor areas (Neuper and Pfurtscheller 2001a). This means that according to the time course and spatial pattern of ERD/ERS, MI can be compared to motor preparation rather than ME.

It is important to note that mu desynchronization is not a unitary phenomenon. If different frequency bands within the range of the extended alpha band are analysed, two distinct patterns of desynchronization can be observed (Pfurtscheller *et al.* 2000a). Lower mu desynchronization (in the range of about 8–10 Hz) is obtained during almost any type of motor task. It is topographically widespread over the entire sensorimotor cortex and probably reflects general motor preparation and attentional processes. Upper mu desynchronization (in the range of about 10–12 Hz), in contrast, is topographically restricted and typically reflects the somatotopic representation of the different body parts in the sensorimotor strip, with the foot/leg area located close to the midline, the more lateral hand/arm motor area, and the face area located laterally on the convex side of the cerebral hemisphere (motor homunculus). The lower mu frequency component often displays a similar ERD with hand and foot movement, while the higher components show a different pattern with an ERD during hand movement and an ERS with foot movement. This type of reactivity of different mu components, suggesting a functional dissociation between upper and lower mu components, was found for movement execution and imagery as well (Neuper and Pfurtscheller 2001a).

Localized desynchronization of the mu rhythms in a motor task may be accompanied by an increase of synchronization (ERS) in the 10-Hz band over areas not engaged in the task (Pfurtscheller and Neuper 1994; Pfurtscheller *et al.* 1996a; Neuper and Pfurtscheller 2001a). Pfurtscheller *et al.* (2006) studied several MI tasks, such as cue-based left hand, right hand, foot, or tongue MI using a dense array of EEG recordings over sensorimotor and adjacent regions. Basically, hand MI activates neural networks in the cortical hand representation area, which is manifested in the hand area mu ERD. Such a mu ERD was found in all able-bodied subjects with a clear contralateral dominance. The midcentral ERD, in the case of foot MI, was weak and not found in every subject. The reason for this may be that the foot representation area is located within the mesial wall. It is very interesting, however, that foot as well as tongue MI enhanced the hand area mu rhythm. In addition, tongue MI induced mu oscillations in or close to the foot representation area.

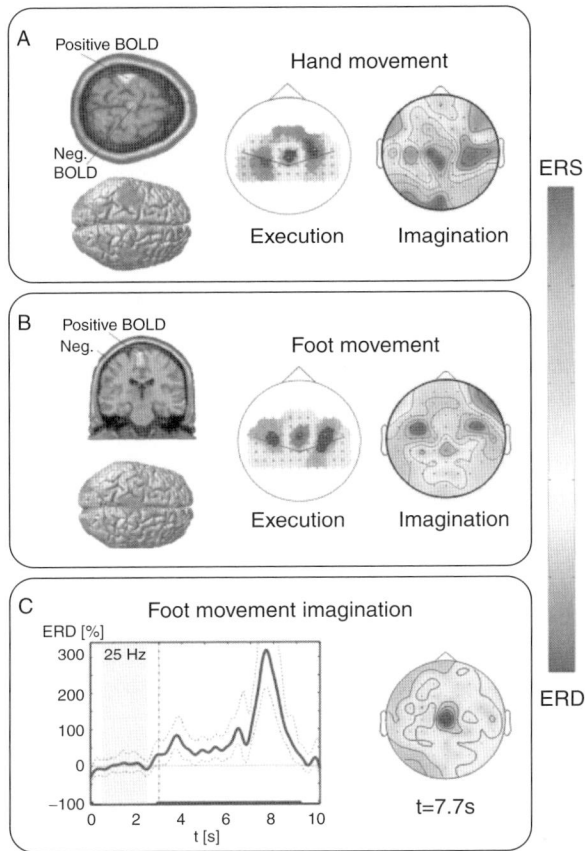

Fig. 5.1 Examples of activation patterns obtained with functional magnetic resonance imaging (fMRI) and EEG (ERD/ERS) during execution and imagination of hand (A) and foot movements (B). Note the correspondence between the focus of the positive BOLD signal and ERD, and between the negative BOLD signal and ERS, respectively. C: Topoplot and time course of the beta rebound in the foot motor imagery task for a representative subject (illustrating a group effect). The dominant frequency of the beta rebound (25 Hz) and the latency of its maximum (7.7 s) are indicated. The subject started imagery at second 3 and stopped it at second 7. See colour plate section.

Examples demonstrating a hand area ERD and foot area ERS during hand movement/imagery and hand area ERS and foot area ERD during foot movement/imagery, respectively, can be seen in Figure 5.1A, B.

Because the mu rhythm typically occurs in the absence of processing sensory information or motor output, it was conceived to reflect a cortical 'idling' or 'nil-work' state (Mulholland 1995). Therefore, it has been hypothesized that the 10-Hz ERS is produced by deactivated cortical areas and may represent idling or inhibitory cortical activity (Pfurtscheller *et al.* 1996a). More recently, it has been shown that mu ERS likely reflects more than an idling state (for a review, see Pineda 2005). Exemplarily, an alpha (i.e., upper mu) power increase has been found to be related to context-dependent inhibition of extended sensorimotor networks (Hummel *et al.* 2002).

To describe the observation that ERD and ERS occur at the same moment in time in different scalp locations, the term 'focal ERD/surround ERS' was introduced by Lopes da Silva and colleagues (Suffczynski *et al.* 1999; Lopes da Silva 2006). The focal mu desynchronization in the upper alpha frequency band may reflect a mechanism responsible for selective attention focused to a motor subsystem. This effect may be accentuated by top-down control inhibiting activation in other cortical areas, not directly involved in the specific motor task. In this process, the interplay between thalamo-cortical modules and the inhibitory reticular thalamic nucleus neurons may play an important role (Lopes da Silva 1991, 2006). Thus, the antagonistic activation pattern can be interpreted to reflect a kind of lateral inhibitory processing in thalamo-cortical circuits, due to focused attention during preparation of an actual or mental motor act (Neuper and Pfurtscheller, 2001a).

Further support for the phenomenon of 'focal ERD/surround ERS' comes from regional blood flow (rCBF) and fMRI studies. A decrease of cerebral blood flow was reported in the somatosensory cortical representation area of one body part, whenever attention was directed to a distant body part (Drevets *et al.* 1995). A similar decrease of the BOLD signal (negative BOLD) was observed in the hand motor area, when the subject imagined or executed toe movements (Ehrsson *et al.* 2003). In this case attention was withdrawn from the hand and directed to the foot zones, resulting in a positive BOLD response in the foot representation area. This antagonistic behaviour in hemodynamic (fMRI) and bioelectrical (EEG) responses during hand and foot movement is visualized in Figure 5.1A, B. It has to be noted, that for the fMRI a task-related paradigm (covert movements over 2 seconds) and for the EEG measurements an event-related paradigm (overt or covert movements in intervals of approximately 10 seconds) was used.

Alternatively, the antagonistic pattern of hand and foot MI may be understood in context of the complex interlimb coordination. The existence of an inhibitory relationship between the foot and hand motor cortex has been suggested, for example, based on cortical mapping using focal transcranial magnetic stimulation (TMS; Baldissera *et al.* 2002). In this regard, Marconi *et al.* (2007) recently reported that imagined ankle movements markedly reduced excitability in the hand cortical representation. This inhibitory effect, observed in healthy subjects, was not present in individuals after amputation of a lower limb. The coordination of upper and lower limb movements cannot be accounted for by direct connections between the hand and foot cortical representations in primary motor areas (Huntley and Jones 1991), but rather by a distributed cortico-cortical network that includes also the premotor and supplementary motor areas (Debaerea *et al.* 2001).

Beta rebound

Since the pioneering work of Jasper and Penfield (1949) it is well known that motor areas typically generate oscillations with components around 20 Hz, which are blocked before the initiation of voluntary movements. This blocking is restricted to the cortical area representing the corresponding part of the limb, as supported in electrocorticographic (ECoG; Arroyo, *et al.* 1993; Crone *et al.* 1998) and neuromagnetic (MEG) measurements (Salmelin and Hari 1994; Salmelin *et al.* 1995). More specifically, the sources of the beta components are mostly centred in the anterior bank of the central sulcus, whereas the mu rhythm (10 Hz) generators are concentrated near the post-central gyrus (Salmelin and Hari 1994). Part of these beta oscillations are blocked or desynchronized not only during planning and execution, but also during imagination of a motor action (Pfurtscheller and Neuper 1997).

After the motor act, the beta band activity recovers very fast (within one second) and short-lasting beta bursts appear over those areas that had displayed ERD earlier (Pfurtscheller *et al.* 1996b). Such localized beta oscillations, described as 'beta rebound', can also be observed following somatosensory stimulation (Salmelin and Hari 1994; Salenius *et al.* 1997; Neuper and Pfurtscheller 2001b). Interestingly, the beta rebound induced by median nerve stimulation can be suppressed by various tasks involving motor cortex activation, including also mental MI (Salenius *et al.* 1997; Schnitzler *et al.* 1997; Neuper *et al.* 2001b). This interference supports the idea that MI utilizes the same cortical networks in primary motor areas, which are responsible for the generation of the beta oscillations (Schnitzler *et al.* 1997). There is general agreement that the beta rebound reflects a short-lasting state of deactivation or even active inhibition of motor cortex networks (Salmelin *et al.* 1995; Pfurtscheller *et al.* 1996b). Further support for this assumption is provided by studies, which show that the excitability level of motor cortex neurons is significantly reduced after finger movement (Chen *et al.* 1998) and median nerve stimulation (Chen *et al.* 1999), particularly during the time interval in which the beta rebound takes place.

Recently, Pfurtscheller *et al.* (2005) reported a distinct spatial distribution of beta ERS after different types of MI (i.e., imagination of right/left hand, both feet, and tongue movement). A particularly pronounced beta rebound was found after foot MI with a clear maximum over the vertex (electrode position Cz). An example of a topographic map with the corresponding ERD/ERS time course in the selected beta frequency band for the foot imagery task is displayed in Figure 5.1C. Of special interest is that this study, though involving only mental imagery tasks, confirms previous findings of a larger beta rebound induced by voluntary movement/stimulation of the foot rather than the hand (Neuper and Pfurtscheller 2001b).

A possible explanation would be that the SMA contributes to the production of the midcentral beta ERS. Because of the proximity between the foot motor area and the SMA (Tanji 1996), oscillatory activity generated in these areas can probably not be differentiated from scalp EEG recordings (Ikeda *et al.* 1992). It may be speculated that the termination of motor cortex activity (i.e., 'resetting'), independent of whether it follows the actual execution or just imagination of a movement, may involve at least two networks – one in the primary motor area and another one in the SMA. Evidence for a beta rebound generated in the SMA during a motor act comes from ECoG recordings in epileptic patients (Ohara *et al.* 2000). In the case of a hand movement, networks in both areas are able to generate beta oscillations, showing slightly different frequencies (Pfurtscheller *et al.* 2000b; Neuper and Pfurtscheller 2001b). Execution or imagination of both feet movement may involve both the SMA and the two cortical foot representation areas. Taking into account the close proximity of these cortical areas, associated with the fact that the response of the corresponding networks in both areas may be synchronized, it is likely that a large-amplitude beta rebound occurs after foot movement imagery. Summarizing, the midcentrally located beta rebound may be interpreted as an electrophysiological correlate of a simultaneous 'resetting' of overlapping neural networks in the foot representation areas and the SMA.

As noted earlier, studies analysing MRPs typically support an important contribution from the SMA to this potential. Both executed as well as imagined movements have been shown to be associated with SMA activation (Jankelowitz and Colebatch 2002). A recent study focused on the engagement of the primary motor area during overt execution and imagery of hand versus foot movements (Carrillo-de-la Pena *et al.* 2006). LRPs were obtained during both, while subjects physically executed or mentally simulated the motor task. As expected by the somatotopic organization of the primary motor cortex, the LRP was the opposite polarity when foot, rather than hand, movements were prepared. This may be explained by the location of the hand area in the crown and foot area in the medial wall of the motor cortex. Interestingly, the inversion of polarity was also found for the imagery task. Since it is well documented that the LRP is generated in the primary motor brain region, the reported finding strongly supports the involvement of primary motor structures.

Visual-motor versus kinaesthetic imagery

There are at least two different strategies that people may use when they are asked to imagine a motor act (Annett 1995; Milton *et al.* 2008). They may, for example, either imagine a self-performed action with 'interior view' or, alternatively, imagine seeing themselves or another person performing actions by producing a 'mental video'. The first type of imagery, also called internal imagery, is supposed to involve kinaesthetic feelings of the movement. The second type of imagery produces a visual representation of the moving limb, either from the first-person view or from a third-person perspective. The latter is also referred to as external imagery. In the absence of explicit instructions, the preferred mode of mental imagery in adult subjects is visual rather than kinaesthetic (Hall and Martin 1997; Gregg *et al.* 2007).

Brain-imaging methods have shown that visual-motor and kinaesthetic imagery activate overlapping as well as distinct cortical regions (Solodkin *et al.* 2004; Guillot *et al.* 2009). Therefore, it is of interest whether the different ways how subjects perform MI are associated with dissimilar electrophysiological activation patterns (i.e., in terms of time, frequency, and spatial domains). A recent study, using a within-subject design, compared the EEG patterns associated with either kinaesthetic or visual-MI (Neuper *et al.* 2005). To create kinaesthetic motor imagery (MIK), participants were instructed to imagine the experience of clenching softly a ball with their right hand. Visual-motor imagery (MIV) was induced by instructing the subjects to visualize grasping movements of a right hand from a third-person perspective. In order to facilitate the respective imagination task, it was preceded by a corresponding 'real' task, i.e., ME or visual observation (OOM) of physical hand movements.

The goal of that study was to identify relevant features of the ongoing multi-channel EEG (i.e., electrode locations and reactive frequency components) that represent the specific mental processes. To this end, a neural network classifier, the distinction sensitive learning vector quantization (DSLVQ) algorithm (Pregenzer and Pfurtscheller 1999), which is an extended version of Kohonen's learning vector quantization algorithm (LVQ), was applied. This method, which is well established in the brain–computer interface field, uses a weighted distance function and adjusts the influence of different input features through supervised learning. This procedure was performed for each subject to distinguish dynamic episodes of specific processing (ME, visual motor/kinaesthetic imagery, observation of movement) from hardly defined EEG patterns during resting periods.

The results reveal the highest classification accuracies (i.e., detection rates), in average close to 80 %, for the real conditions (i.e., ME and OOM), both at the corresponding representation areas. Albeit the great variability between participants during the imagery tasks, the classification accuracies obtained for the MIK (66 %) were in average better than the results of the MIV (56 %). For the recognition of both, the execution (ME) and the MIK of right-hand movement, electrodes close to position C3 provided the best input features (Figure 5.2). Whereas the focus of activity during OOM was found close to parieto-occipital cortical areas, MIV did not reveal a clear spatial pattern and could not be successfully detected in single trial EEG classification.

These data confirm previous studies that MI, specifically when creating kinaesthetic feelings, can be used to 'produce' movement-specific and locally restricted patterns of the oscillatory brain activity. This has important implications for the operation of brain–computer interface (BCI) devices and for the use of MI in neurorehabilitation (for a review, see Pfurtscheller and Neuper 2001; Pfurtscheller *et al.* 2008; see also Chapter 14 in this book). It can be expected that specific instructions on how to imagine actions may contribute to enhance activation in primary sensori-motor cortical areas and, therewith, to improve BCI control. The potential that subjects may be

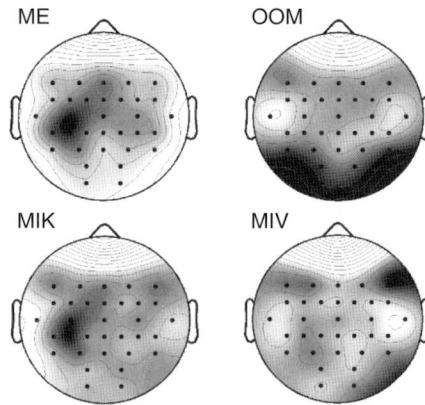

Fig. 5.2 Topographical map of grand average classification accuracies (N=14) plotted at the corresponding electrode positions (linear interpolation), separately for the four experimental conditions (ME, OOM, MIK, MIV). Black areas indicate the most relevant electrode positions for the recognition of the respective task. Scaling was adjusted to minimum and maximum values obtained for each condition (ME (min/max %): 53/76; OOM (min/max %): 56/77; MIK (min/max %): 51/64; MIV (min/max %):51/61). Modified from Neuper *et al.* (2005).

able to learn to increase motor cortex activation during 'feedback-regulated' imagined movements has been demonstrated in previous studies using online EEG classification (see e.g., Neuper *et al.* 1999) as well as real-time fMRI (deCharms *et al.* 2004).

Stroke patients

The finding that the imagination of body limb movements can activate primary motor areas opens promising perspectives on the restoration of movement (and acquisition of motor skills) through mental rehearsal for patients with motor dysfunctions. For example, the use of MI is currently considered as one therapeutic approach to recover motor impairment (hemiparesis) after stroke (Stevens and Stoykov 2003; Sharma *et al.* 2006). The advantage of this method is that any patient can independently, whether residual muscle activity is available or not, undergo training. The only requirement is voluntary mental activity. One drawback, however, is the missing of proper screening and monitoring tools, which allow for an objective quantification of the therapy-based improvement (Sharma *et al.* 2006).

Movement-related ERD/ERS has been studied in a variety of neurological disorders affecting the sensorimotor system such as Parkinson's disease, multiple sclerosis, and stroke. In these disorders, the extent of abnormality in the pattern of ERD/ERS turned out to be related to the severity of the underlying pathology (for a review, see Leocani and Comi 2006). Already Pfurtscheller *et al.* (1981) provided evidence that sensorimotor EEG activity of stroke patients is correlated to the execution of hand movements. More recently, movement-related reactivity of mu and beta rhythms has been investigated in subacute (Platz *et al.* 2000) and chronic stages after ischemic stroke (Gerloff *et al.* 2006). Certain features of mu and beta ERD found in the mentioned studies, such as earlier appearance and increased expression over the ipsilateral sensorimotor or frontal regions, may be interpreted in terms of compensation to motor impairment, or as the result of a lack of cortical inhibition upon areas which should not be actively involved in the task (cf. Leocani and Comi 2006).

As the imagery-related changes in sensorimotor brain oscillations can be easily recorded from scalp electrodes placed over central head regions, they provide the possibility to quantify and monitor MI-related brain activity in stroke patients. A recent study examined EEG recordings of hemiparetic stroke patients during left- and right-hand MI in order to determine whether time-frequency maps of ERD/ERS and single-trial classification (by means of the DSLVQ method) are suited to keep record of the changing brain activity after stroke (Scherer *et al.* 2007). Seven right-handed patients with right-sided (cortical and/or subcortical) ischemic brain lesion participated in this preliminary study. All participants suffered from hemiparesis of the left-upper extremity after their first-time stroke, which had occurred between 2 and 36 months prior to the study. A cue-based experimental paradigm was used to collect EEG recordings of left- and right-hand ME and MI. Considering the severity of the hemiparesis, subjects were asked to compress a soft rubber ball for approximately 2 seconds during ME, and to imagine performing the same motor task without any movement attempt during MI.

Figure 5.3 shows the grand-average time-frequency ERD/S maps and a summary of the single trial classification results, separately for the left-hand (affected side) and right-hand (unaffected side) motor tasks. We used single trial DSLVQ classification to determine the most sensitive frequency components apt to discriminate between a resting state and the execution or the imagination of hand movements. Relevant ERD patterns were found over the left (undamaged) hemisphere and the midline central area. The right (damaged) hemisphere did not show significant changes related to the experimental task. Although imagery and execution differed slightly with respect to the frequency bands involved, most significant changes were found in the frequency components 8–12 Hz and 14–22 Hz, respectively.

The DSLVQ classification results confirm that it is possible to detect imagined movements of the intact as well as affected hand from single trial EEG with relatively high accuracy. The average classification performance (determined at the best classification time point) was between 74 and 79 % for the different conditions. The DSLVQ feature relevance values show clear reactivity in the mu and beta band at the undamaged hemisphere (electrode position C3). But, due to the lesion, it was not possible to classify the oscillatory brain activity of the damaged side (electrode position C4). A comparison of the identified frequency components associated with the right (intact)-hand tasks with data from healthy subjects (cf. Neuper *et al.* 2005) reveals quite similar activity in the mu and beta range for both groups. The reduced imagery-related activity of the affected side can be traced back to a reduced baseline spectral density and is in accordance with previous studies that showed a reduced movement-related alpha and beta ERD over the damaged hemisphere (Platz *et al.* 2000).

Of interest is that ME and MI of the affected (left) hand induced very similar patterns in the ipsilateral undamaged hemisphere as obtained with right-hand MI. To some extent, also the midline central area shows frequency specific activation. These results are in line with neuroimaging studies that revealed activation of homologous areas in the unaffected hemisphere during movement of the affected hand (Feydy *et al.* 2002).

Gerloff *et al.* (2006) studied ERD of mu and beta rhythms to finger extension movements in right-handed patients in the chronic stages after a left-capsular infarct. Compared with normal subjects, patients had a higher beta ERD (16–20 Hz) over the right-central region, both preceding and during movement execution. Increased activation of the right-frontal region, as indicated by beta ERD, was also found with positron emission tomography (PET) in the same subjects. Moreover, the patients showed increased coherence, an indicator of functional cortico-cortical connections, between the right-frontal and the midline-frontal region. Altogether, these findings suggest increased effort requiring additional recruitment of ipsilateral sensorimotor and premotor areas and increased cross-talk with midline frontal regions involved in motor control

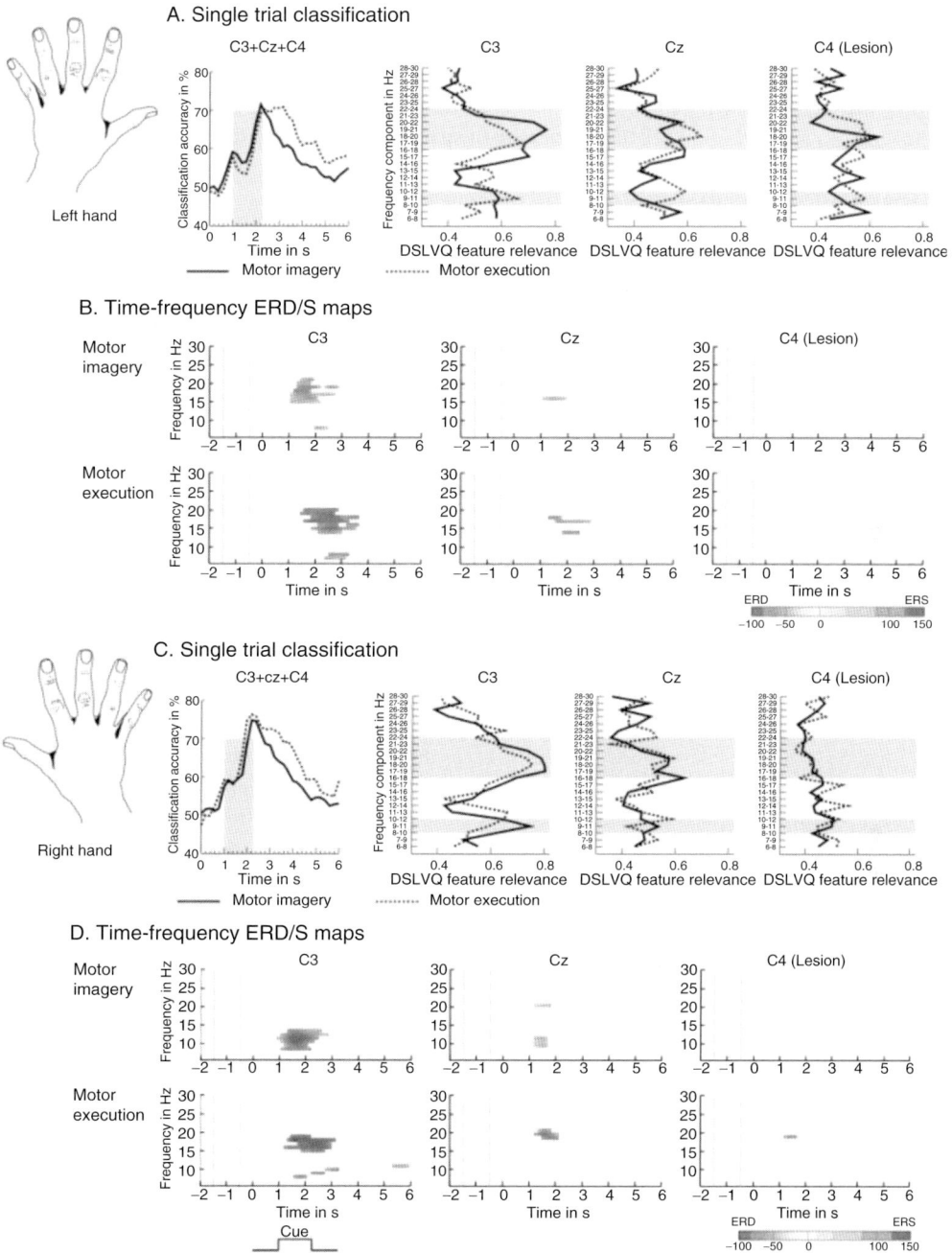

Fig. 5.3 Results of single trial classification, depicted in the form of time curves of DSLVQ classification accuracies for the combination of channels C3, Cz, and C4 and diagrams representing the corresponding feature relevance values of overlapping frequency bands for the 3 channels, separately for left-hand (A) and right-hand (C) motor tasks. Grand-average time-frequency ERD/S maps (confidence level α=0.05) for electrode locations C3 (undamaged), Cz and C4 (damaged hemisphere) are shown for left (affected)-hand (B) and right (unaffected)-hand motor imagery and execution (D). Modified from Scherer et al. (2007). See colour plate section.

(Gerloff *et al.* 2006). However, an important point to consider is that the side of stroke may play a role for the activation of neural circuits in primary motor areas by MI. The cognitive mechanisms underlying MI appear to be more strongly affected in patients with right-hemisphere rather than left-hemisphere stroke (Stinear *et al.* 2007). This effect may be related to the right-hemisphere's specialization for the processing of spatial cues, the latter being closely involved in the representation of movement.

The reported findings suggest that ERD/ERS analyses, in particular methods of single-trial classification, are useful tools to monitor MI-related brain activity in stroke patients and, therewith, contribute to quantify the effectiveness of MI as a rehabilitation method after stroke. Using a BCI system, it is even possible to provide immediate feedback for the patient. Mentally induced increase (ERS) and/or decrease (ERD) of sensorimotor rhythms may be reinforced, for example, when the appropriate EEG changes are used as a trigger to induce assisted movements, for example, performed with the help of an orthotic hand attached to the patient's own (Birbaumer *et al.* 2006). Another possibility would be providing feedback by presenting a virtual body part whose movement is controlled by the output signal of the BCI (Pfurtscheller and Neuper 2006). In the latter case, the act of observing the hand movement itself may lead to an activation of the sensorimotor brain activity (Pineda 2005; Neuper *et al.* 2009).

Summary and concluding remarks

Based on the concept of functional equivalence of actual and mental motor acts, mental imagery of motor behaviour plays an important role in motor skill learning and in recovery of motor abilities after neurological damage. Brain imaging methods like fMRI have made it possible to identify the brain regions that are activated during MI, and there is now compelling evidence that MI involves to a large extent the same cortical areas that are activated during actual motor preparation and execution. The main advantage of fMRI is its ability to identify the involved brain structures with high spatial resolution. But the poor temporal resolution of the hemodynamic response makes it difficult to address questions concerning the functional organization of the involved regions of cortical activation.

Electrophysiological techniques such as EEG and MEG provide direct measures of the neuronal activity with high temporal resolution. Therefore, these methods can be used to study the dynamic aspect of movement-related activity of the involved areas. By measuring movement-related potentials and event-related changes of brain oscillations in different frequency bands, it is possible to study the time course of short-lasting changes of neuronal activity in distinct time windows before, during, and after an executed or imagined motor action. The studies reviewed in the previous sections consistently corroborate a functional equivalence between movement preparation/execution and kinaesthetic MI, and support the role of a feedback circuit from primary motor cortex to the SMA for the preparation and control of overt and covert actions. Taken together, these studies also provide converging evidence of modern brain imaging methods like fMRI and classical EEG techniques. For example, the preparation of actual or imagined motor actions is associated with increased neural activation within the SMA, as indexed by negative potential shifts and increased hemodynamic responses. Another example is the antagonistic behaviour in hemodynamic (fMRI) and bioelectric (EEG) responses during imagery of voluntary movements of different body parts, showing specific activation increase (indexed by ERD and positive BOLD responses) in somatotopically organized sections of the primary motor cortex, and a decrease of activation (10 Hz-ERS, negative BOLD) in 'unattended' motor areas. There is no doubt that conventional EEG recordings have too poor spatial resolution to provide detailed data on the anatomical structure of the neural networks mediating the imagery experience. Therefore, the use of multimodal techniques (e.g., combining fMRI and EEG) appears particularly promising to study the neuronal processes involved in mental MI.

The main advantages of EEG recordings are related to its high temporal resolution and the specific information reflected in the time course of EEG data. Recent studies have demonstrated that imagery-related brain activity can be detected in real-time from the ongoing EEG. Imagery of distinct limb movements (e.g., right hand vs. left hand; hand vs. foot movement) has been shown to represent an efficient mental strategy to operate an external device, such as a spelling system or a neuroprosthesis, based on brain signals (Neuper *et al.* 2006; Pfurtscheller *et al.* 2008; see also Chapter14 in this book). Moreover, the mentioned findings have important implications for the use of mental rehearsal of movements in neurorehabilitation after stroke. Newly developed protocols based on mentally rehearsing movements and EEG neurofeedback represent a promising approach to assessing the motor system because they can activate and 'reinforce' sensorimotor networks that the lesions affected.

Acknowledgements

A part of the studies reviewed here was supported by the 'Steiermärkische Landesregierung', Project NeuroCenter Styria (GZ: A3-16 B 74-05/1), Graz, Austria.

References

Annett, J. (1995). Motor imagery: perception or action? *Neuropsychologia, 33*, 1395–1417.

Arroyo, S., Lesser, R.P., Gordon, B., Uematsu, S., Jackson, D., and Webber, R. (1993). Functional significance of the mu rhythm of human cortex: an electrophysiological study with subdural electrodes. *Electroencephalography and Clininical Neurophysiology, 87*, 76–87.

Baldissera, F., Borroni, P., Cavallari, P., and Cerri, G. (2002). Excitability changes in human corticospinal projections to forearm muscles during voluntary movement of ipsilateral foot. *Journal of Physiology, 539*, 903–11.

Beisteiner, R., Höllinger, P., Lindinger, G., Lang, W., and Berthoz, A. (1995). Mental representations of movements. Brain potentials associated with imagination of hand movements. *Electroencephalography and Clinical Neurophysiology, 96*, 183–93.

Birbaumer, N., Weber, C., Neuper, C., Buch, E., Haapen, K. and Cohen, L. (2006). Physiological regulation of thinking: brain-computer interface (BCI) research. *Progress in Brain Research, 159*, 369–91.

Böcker, K.B.E., Brunia, C.H.M., and Cluitmans, P.J.M. (1994). A spatio-temporal dipole model of the readiness potential in humans. II. Foot movement. *Electroencephalography and Clinical Neurophysiology, 91*, 286–94.

Boschert, J., Hink, R.F., and Deecke, L. (1983). Finger movement versus toe movement-related potentials: further evidence for supplementary motor area (SMA) participation prior to voluntary action. *Experimental Brain Research, 52*, 73–80.

Caldara, R., Deiber, M.P., Andrey, C., Michel, C.M., Thut, G., and Hauert, C.A. (2004). Actual and mental motor preparation and execution: a spatiotemporal ERP study. *Experimental Brain Research, 159*, 389–99.

Carrillo-de-la-Peña, M.T., Galdo-Álvarez, S., and Lastra- Barreira, C. (2008). Equivalent is not equal: Primary motor cortex (MI) activation during motor imagery and execution of sequential movements. *Brain Research, 1226*, 134–43.

Carrillo-de-la-Pena, M.T., Lastra-Barreira, C., and Galdo-Alvarez, S. (2006). Limb (hand vs. foot) and response conflict have similar effects on event-related potentials (ERPs) recorded during motor imagery and overt execution. *European Journal of Neuroscience, 24*, 635–43.

Chatrian, G.E., Petersen, M.C., and Lazarte, J.A. (1959). The blocking of the Rolandic wicket rhythm and some central changes related to movement. *Electroencephalography and Clinical Neurophysiology, 11*, 497–510.

Chen, R., Corwell, B., and Hallett, M. (1999). Modulation of motor cortex excitability by median nerve and digit stimulation. *Experimental Brain Research*, **129**, 77–86.

Chen, R., Yaseen, Z., Cohen, L.G., and Hallett, M. (1998). Time course of corticospinal excitability in reaction time and self-paced movements. *Annals of Neurology*, **44**, 317–25.

Coles, M.G.H. (1989). Modern mind-brain reading: psychophysiology, physiology and cognition. *Psychophysiology*, **26**, 251–69.

Crone, N.E., Miglioretti, D.L., Gordon, B., Sieracki, J.M., Wilson, M.T., and Uematsu, S. (1998). Functional mapping of human sensorimotor cortex with electrocorticographic spectral analysis I: alpha and beta event-related desynchronization. *Brain*, **121**, 2271–99.

Cui, R.Q., Huter, D., Lang, W., and Deecke L. (1999). Neuroimage of voluntary movement: topography of the Bereitschaftspotential, a 64-Channel DC current source density study. *NeuroImage*, **9**, 124–34

Cunnington, R., Iansek, R., Bradshaw, J.L., and Phillips, J.G. (1996). Movement-related potentials associated with movement preparation and motor imagery. *Experimental Brain Research*, **111**, 429–36.

Cunnington, R., Iansek, R., Johnson K.A., and Bradshaw, J.L. (1997). Movement-related potentials in Parkinson's disease. Motor imagery and movement preparation. *Brain*, **120(8)**, 1339–53.

Cunnington, R., Windischberger, C., and Moser, E. (2005). Premovement activity of the pre-supplementary motor area and the readiness for action: studies of time-resolved event-related functional MRI. *Human Movement Science*, **24**, 644–56.

Davidson, R.J. and Schwartz, G.E. (1977). Brain mechanisms subserving self-generated imagery: electrophysiological specificity and patterning. *Psychophysiology*, **14**, 598–602.

Debaerea, F., Swinnena, S.P., Béatseb, E., Sunaertb, S., Van Heckeb, P., and Duysensc, J. (2001). Brain areas involved in interlimb coordination: a distributed network. *NeuroImage*, **14**, 947–58.

deCharms, C., Christoff, K., Glover, G.H., Pauly, J.M., Whitfield, S., and Gabrieli, J.D. (2004). Learned regulation of spatially localized brain activation using real-time fMRI. *NeuroImage*, **21**, 436–43.

Dechent, P., Merboldt, K.D., and Frahm, J. (2004). Is the human primary motor cortex involved in motor imagery? *Cognitive Brain Research*, **19**, 138–144.

Drevets, W., Burton, H., Videen, T., Snyder, A., Simpson, J.J., and Raichle, M. (1995). Blood flow changes in human somatosensory cortex during anticipated stimulation. *Nature*, **373(6511)**, 198–9.

Ehrsson, H.H., Geyer, S., and Naito, E. (2003). Imagery of voluntary movement of fingers, toes, and tongue activates corresponding body-part-specific motor representations. *Journal of Neurophysiology*, **90**, 3304–16.

Feydy, A., Carlier, R., Roby-Brami, A., *et al.* (2002). Longitudinal study of motor recovery after stroke: recruitment and focusing of brain activation. *Stroke*, **33**,1610–7.

Galdo-Álvarez, S., and Carrillo-de-la-Peña, M.T. (2004). ERP evidence of MI activation without motor response execution. *Neuroreport*, **15**, 2067–70.

Gastaut, H., Naquet, R., and Gastaut, Y. (1965). A study of the mu rhythm in subjects lacking one or more limbs. *Electroencephalography and Clinical Neurophysiology*, **18**, 720–21.

Gerloff, C., Bushara, K., Sailer, A., *et al.* (2006). Multimodal imaging of brain reorganization in motor areas of the contralesional hemisphere of well recovered patients after capsular stroke. *Brain*, **129**, 791–808.

Graimann, B. and Pfurtscheller, G. (2006). Quantification and visualization of event-related changes in oscillatory brain activity in the time-frequency domain. *Progress in Brain Research*, **159**, 79–97.

Gregg, M., Hall, C., and Butler, A. (2007). The MIQ-RS: a suitable option for examining movement imagery ability. *Evidence-Based Complementary and Alternative Medicine,* Available at: http://ecam. oxfordjournals.org/cgi/content/full/nem170v1.

Guillot A., Collet C., Nguyen V.A., Malouin F., Richards C., and Doyon J. (2009). Brain activity during visual versus kinaesthetic imagery: an fMRI study. *Human Brain Mapping*, **30**, 2157–72.

Hall, C.R. and Martin, K.A. (1997). Measuring movement imagery abilities: a revision of the movement imagery questionnaire. *Journal of Mental Imagery*, **21**, 143–54.

Hummel, F., Andres, F., Altenmuller, E., Dichgans J., and Gerloff, C. (2002). Inhibitory control of acquired motor programmes in the human brain. *Brain*, **125**, 404–20.

Huntley, G.W. and Jones, E.G. (1991). Relationship of intrinsic connections to forelimb movement representations in monkey motor cortex: a correlative anatomic and physiological study. *Journal of Neurophysiology*, **66**, 390–413.

Ikeda A., Lüders, H.O., Burgess, R.C., and Shibasaki, H. (1992). Movement-related potentials recorded from supplementary motor area and primary motor area. *Brain,* **115**, 1017–43.

Jankelowitz, S.K. and Colebatch, J.G. (2002). Movement-related potentials associated with self-paced, cued and imagined arm movements. *Experimental Brain Research*, **147**, 98–107.

Jasper, H.H. and Penfield, W. (1949). Electrocorticograms in man: effect of the voluntary movement upon the electrical activity of the precentral gyrus. *European Archives of Psychiatry and Clinical Neurosciences*, **183**, 163–74.

Jeannerod, M. (2001). Neural simulation of action: a unifying mechanism for motor cognition. *NeuroImage*, **14**, 103–9.

Kasess, C.H., Windischberger, C., Cunnington, R., Lanzenberger, R., Pezawas, L., and Moser, E. (2008). The suppressive influence of SMA on M1 in motor imagery revealed by fMRI and dynamic causal modeling. *NeuroImage*, **40**, 828–37.

Klass, S.G. and Bickford, R.G. (1957). Observations on the Rolandic Arceau rhythm. *Electroencephalography and Clinical Neurophysiology*, **9**, 570.

Kornhuber, H.H. and Deecke, L. (1965). Hirnpotentialaenderungen bei Willkuerbewegungen und passiven Bewegungen des Menschen: Bereitschafts-potential und reafferente Potentiale. *Pfluegers Archives*, **284**, 1–17.

Lang, W., Cheyne, D., Hollinger, P., Gerschlager, W., and Lindinger G. (1996). Electric and magnetic fields of the brain accompanying internal simulation of movement. *Cognitive Brain Research,* **3**, 125–9.

Leocani, L. and Comi, G. (2006). Movement-related event-related desynchronization in neuropsychiatric disorders. *Progress in Brain Research*, **159**, 351–66.

Leuthold, H. and Jentzsch, I. (2002). Distinguishing neural sources of movement preparation and execution: an electrophysiological analysis. *Biological Psychology* **60**, 173–98.

Lopes da Silva, F.H. (1991). Neural mechanisms underlying brain waves: from neural membranes to networks. *Electroencephalography and Clinical Neurophysiology*, **79**, 81–93.

Lopes da Silva, F.H. (2006). Event-related neural activities: what about phase? *Progress in Brain Research*, **159**, 3–17.

Lopes da Silva, F.H. and Pfurtscheller, G. (1999). Basic concepts on EEG synchronization and desynchronization, in G. Pfurtscheller and F.H. Lopes da Silva (ed.), *Event-Related Desynchronization*. Handbook of Electroencephalography and Clinical Neurophysiology. Revised Series, Vol.6, pp. 3–11. Amsterdam: Elsevier.

Lotze, M., Montoya, P., Erb, M., *et al.* (1999). Activation of cortical and cerebellar motor areas during executed and imagined hand movements: an fMRI study. *Journal of Cognitive Neuroscience,* **11**, 491–501.

Marconi, B., Koch, G., Pecchioli, C., Cavallari, P., and Caltagirone, C. (2007). Breakdown of inhibitory effects induced by foot motor imagery on hand motor area in lower-limb amputees. *Clinical Neurophysiology*, **118**(11), 2468–78.

Marks, D.F. and Isaaks, A.R. (1995). Topographic distribution of EEG activity accompanying visual and motor imagery in vivid and non-vivid imagers. *British Journal of Psychology*, **86**, 271–82.

McFarland, D.J., Miner, L.A., Vaughan, T.M., and Wolpaw, J.R. (2000). Mu and beta rhythm topographies during motor imagery and actual movements. *Brain Topography*, **12**, 177–86.

Mellinger, J., Schalk, G., Braun, C., *et al.* (2007). An MEG-based brain–computer interface (BCI). *NeuroImage*, **36**, 581–93.

Milton, J., Small, S.L., and Solodkin, A. (2008). Imaging motor imagery: methodological issues related to expertise. *Methods*, **45**, 336–41.

Mulholland, T. (1995). Human EEG, behavioral stillness and biofeedback. *International. Journal of Psychophysiology*, **19**, 263–79.

Mundy-Castle, A.C. (1957). The electroencephalogram and mental activity. *Electroencephalography and Clinical Neurophysiology*, **9**, 643–55.

Neuper, C., Mueller-Putz, G.R., Scherer, R., and Pfurtscheller, G. (2006). Motor imagery and EEG-based control of spelling devices and neuroprostheses. *Progress in Brain Research*, **159**, 393–409.

Neuper, C. and Pfurtscheller, G. (1999) Motor imagery and ERD, in G. Pfurtscheller and F.H. Lopes da Silva (ed.), *Event-Related Desynchronization*. Handbook of Electroencephalography and Clinical Neurophysiology. Revised Edition Vol. 6. pp. 303–25. Amsterdam: Elsevier.

Neuper, C. and Pfurtscheller, G. (2001a). Event-related dynamics of cortical rhythms: frequency-specific features and functional correlates. *International Journal of Psychophysiology*, **43**, 41–58.

Neuper, C. and Pfurtscheller, G. (2001b). Evidence for distinct beta resonance frequencies in human EEG related to specific sensorimotor cortical areas. *Clinical Neurophysiology*, **112**, 2084–97.

Neuper, C., Scherer, R., Reiner, M., and Pfurtscheller, G. (2005). Imagery of motor actions: differential effects of kinaesthetic and visual-motor mode of imagery in single-trial EEG. *Cognitive Brain Research*, **25**, 668–77.

Neuper, C., Scherer, R., Wriessnegger, S., and Pfurtscheller, G. (2009). Motor imagery and action observation: modulation of sensorimotor brain rhythms during mental control of a brain-computer interface. *Clinical Neurophysiology*, **120**, 239–47.

Neuper, C., Schlögl, A., and Pfurtscheller, G. (1999). Enhancement of left-right sensorimotor EEG differences during feedback-regulated motor imagery. *Journal of Clinical Neurophysiology*, **16**, 373–82.

Ohara, S., Ikeda, A., Kunieda, T., *et al.* (2000). Movement-related change of electrocorticographic activity in human supplementary motor area proper. *Brain*, **123**, 1203–15.

Pfurtscheller, G., Brunner, C., Schlögl, A., and Lopes da Silva, F.H. (2006). Mu rhythm (de)synchronization and EEG single-trial classification of different motor imagery tasks. *NeuroImage*, **31**,153–9.

Pfurtscheller, G. and Lopes da Silva, F.H. (1999). Event-related EEG/MEG synchronization and desynchronization: basic principles. *Clinical Neurophysiology*, **110**, 1842–57.

Pfurtscheller, G., Müller-Putz, G., Scherer, R., and Neuper, C. (2008). Rehabilitation with brain-computer interface systems. *IEEE Computer Science*, **41**, 58–65.

Pfurtscheller, G. and Neuper, C. (1994). Event-related synchronization of mu rhythm in the EEG over the cortical hand area in man. *Neuroscience Letters*, **174**, 93–6.

Pfurtscheller, G. and Neuper, C. (1997). Motor imagery activates primary sensorimotor area in humans. *Neuroscience Letters*, **239**, 65–8.

Pfurtscheller, G. and Neuper, C. (2001). Motor imagery and direct brain-computer communication, *Proceedings IEEE (Special Issue); Neural Engineering: Merging Engineering & Neuroscience*, **89**, 1123–34.

Pfurtscheller, G. and Neuper, C. (2006). Future prospects of ERD/ERS in the context of brain–computer interface (BCI) developments. *Progress in Brain Research*, **159**, 433–7.

Pfurtscheller, G., Neuper, C., and Krausz, G. (2000a). Functional dissociation of lower and upper frequency mu rhythms in relation to voluntary limb movement. *Clinical Neurophysiology*, **111**, 1873–9.

Pfurtscheller, G., Neuper, C., Pichler-Zalaudek, K., Edlinger, G., and Lopes da Silva, F.H. (2000b). Do brain oscillations of different frequencies indicate interaction between cortical areas in humans? *Neuroscience Letters*, **286**, 66–8.

Pfurtscheller, G., Neuper, C., Brunner, C., and Lopes da Silva, F.H. (2005). Beta rebound after different types of motor imagery in man. *Neuroscience Letters*, **378**, 156–9.

Pfurtscheller, G., Sager, W., and Wege, W. (1981). Correlations between CT scan and sensorimotor EEG rhythms in patients with cerebrovascular disorders. *Electroencephalography and Clinical Neurophysiology*, **52**, 473–85.

Pfurtscheller, G., Stancák, A., and Neuper, C. (1996a). Event-related synchronization (ERS) in the alpha band – an electrophysiological correlate of cortical idling: a review. *International Journal of Psychophysiology*, **24**, 39–46.

Pfurtscheller, G., Stancák, A., and Neuper, C. (1996b). Post-movement beta synchronization. A correlate of an idling motor area? *Electroencephalography and Clinical Neurophysioloy*, **98**, 281–93.

Pineda, J.A. (2005). The functional significance of mu rhythms: translating 'seeing' and 'hearing' into 'doing'. *Brain Research,* **50**, 57–68.

Platz, T., Kim, I.H., Pintschovius, H., *et al.* (2000). Multimodal EEG analysis in man suggests impairment-specific changes in movement-related electric brain activity after stroke. *Brain*, **123**, 2475–90.

Porro, C.A., Francescato, M.P., Cettolo, V., *et al.* (1996). Primary motor and sensory cortex activation during motor performance and motor imagery: a functional magnetic resonance imaging study. *Journal of Neuroscience,* **16**, 7688–98.

Praamstra, P., Schmitz, F., Freund, H.J., Schnitzler, A. (1999). Magneto-encephalographic correlates of the lateralized readiness potential. *Cognitive Brain Research,* **8**, 77–85.

Pregenzer, M. and Pfurtscheller, G. (1999). Frequency component selection for an EEG-based brain to computer interface. *IEEE Transactions on Rehabilitation Engineering*, **7**, 413–9.

Salenius, S., Kajola, M., Thompson, W.L., Kosslyn, S., and Hari, R. (1995). Reactivity of magnetic parieto-occipital alpha rhythm during visual imagery. *Electroencephalography and Clinical Neurophysiology*, **95**, 453–62.

Salenius, S., Schnitzler, A., Salmelin, R., Jousmäki, V., and Hari, R. (1997). Modulation of human cortical Rolandic rhythms during natural sensorimotor tasks. *NeuroImage*, **5**, 221–8.

Salmelin, R., Hämäläinen, M., Kajola, M., Hari, R. (1995). Functional segregation of movement related rhythmic activity in the human brain. *NeuroImage*, **2**, 237–43.

Salmelin, R. and Hari, R. (1994). Characterization of spontaneous MEG rhythms in healthy adults. *Electroencephalography and Clinical Neurophysiology*, **91**, 237–48.

Scherer, R., Mohapp, A., Grieshofer, P., Pfurtscheller, G., and Neuper, C. (2007). Sensorimotor EEG patterns during motor imagery in hemiparetic stroke patients. *International Journal of Bioelectromagnetism*, **9**, 155–62.

Schnitzler, A., Salenius, S., Salmelin, R., Jousmäki, V., and Hari, R. (1997). Involvement of primary motor cortex in motor imagery: a neuromagnetic study. *NeuroImage*, **6**, 201–8.

Sharma, N., Pomeroy, V.M., and Baron, J.C. (2006). Motor imagery: a backdoor to the motor system after stroke? *Stroke*, **37**, 1941–52.

Short, P.L. (1953). The objective study of mental imagery. *British Journal of Psychology*, **44**, 38–51.

Solodkin, A., Hlustik, P., Chen, E.E. and Small, S.L. (2004). Fine modulation in network activation during motor execution and motor imagery. *Cerebral Cortex,* **14**, 1246–55.

Stevens, J.A. and Stoykov, M.E. (2003). Using motor imagery in the rehabilitation of hemiparesis. *Archives in Physical Medicine and Rehabilitation,* **84**, 1090–2.

Stinear, C., Fleming, M., Barber, P., and Byblow, W. (2007). Lateralization of motor imagery following stroke. *Clinical Neurophysiology*, **118**, 1794–1801.

Suffczynski, P., Pjin, J., Pfurtscheller, G., and Lopes da Silva, F. (1999). Event-related dynamics of alpha band rhythms: a neuronal network model of focal ERD/surround ERS, in G. Pfurtscheller and F. Lopes da Silva (ed.), *Event-Related Desynchronization*. Handbook of Electroencephalography and Clinical Neurophysiology, Vol. 6, pp.67–85. Amsterdam: Elsevier.

Tanji, J. (1996). New concepts of the supplementary motor area. *Current Opinion in Neurobiology*, **6**, 782–7.

Walter, W.G., Cooper, R., Aldridge, V.J., McCallum, W.C., and Winter, A.L. (1964). Contingent negative variation: an electric sign of sensorimotor association and expectancy in the human brain. *Nature*, **203**, 380–4.

Chapter 6

Electromyographic activity during motor imagery

Aymeric Guillot, Florent Lebon, and Christian Collet

Introduction

In this section, we concentrate on understanding the peripheral muscular activity which may occur during the mental representation of an action. A great amount of experimental data has already been focused on the physiological mechanisms involved during motor imagery (MI), and most especially on how the descending motor commands are inhibited. Two major hypotheses have been favoured to explain the inconsistent results regarding the activation or absence of activation of muscle activity, hence considering MI either as an isolated rehearsal in the central nervous system or as a mental process engaging both alpha skeletomotor and gamma fusimotor motoneurones (Gandevia 1999). Among the theories that have been proposed to explain the MI-related effects in enhancing motor performance, the psychoneuromuscular theory (Carpenter 1894), earlier, postulated that mental rehearsal may produce electrical impulses in the target nerves and muscles, MI being thus a mirror image of the actual activity. Jacobson (1931, 1932) provided the first scientific evidence of this idea by reporting that MI of bending the arm produced small contraction within the flexor arm muscles. According to this theory, such physiological responses are thought to generate slight neuromuscular feedback, strong enough to improve subsequent motor performance through priming of the motor pathways. There is yet ongoing discussion in the chapter, however, regarding whether muscle activation during MI is currently associated with improved motor performance. Especially, the inflow processing theory argued that such muscular activity may be sufficient to provide effective proprioceptive feedback to the central nervous system. Conversely, the outflow processing theory may consider this residual muscular activity as a consequence of imagery mainly, rather than pure imagery benefits (Lutz 2003). A great number of experiences reporting autonomic responses during imagined performance (for review, Guillot and Collet 2005; see also Chapter 7, in this book) provided further evidence that changes occur at the level of the central nervous system, and thus MI effects do not result from peripheral feedback only. Altogether, the hypothesis stating that covert muscle activation may substantially contribute to motor performance enhancement should not be completely eliminated. Hence, the aim of this chapter was to review the main studies supporting these two hypotheses, and thus to gain more insight into the electromyographic (EMG) activity recorded during MI.

Absence of EMG activity during MI

Muscular quiescence has been observed in many MI studies involving different arm and foot motor sequences. While demonstrating the effectiveness of MI in the enhancement of muscle strength, Yue and Cole (1992) as well as Ranganathan et al. (2004) did not find any muscle activity in the trained digit abductor and elbow flexor. Similar results were also reported in leg muscles by Decety *et al.* (1993), in a study using nuclear magnetic resonance spectroscopy. Other researches further failed to find any muscular activity during imagined palmar flexion and wrist dorsiflexion (Naito *et al.* 2002), flexor digitorum superficialis muscles (Lotze *et al.* 1999), forearm flexion (Yahagi *et al.* 1996), elbow flexor muscles (Herbert *et al.* 1998), arm movements (Gentili *et al.* 2006; Lim *et al.* 2006; Personnier *et al.* 2007), volleyball and squat performance (Shick 1970; Mulder *et al.* 2005), and abduction of the big toe (Mulder *et al.* 2004).

Interestingly, and especially in neuroimaging studies, some investigators recorded EMG activity before the participants engaged in MI practice. The goal of such separate EMG studies was to ensure that the participants were able to perform the MI task without actually moving before scanning sessions (Michelon *et al.* 2006), while EMG data may also be provided during scanning sessions *per se*. For example, Lotze *et al.* (2003) and Kleber *et al.* (2007) did observe an absence of EMG activity in finger extensors during MI in amateur and professional violinists, as well as in muscles involved in imagined singing. In such cases, EMG recordings served as demonstrating that variations of cerebral blood flow were related to mental work and not to movements that could have accompanied MI. Similarly, no increase of EMG activity was recorded during imagination of a simple or complex finger flexion/extension task (Gerardin *et al.* 2000), nor during mental simulation of foot movements (Lafleur *et al.* 2002; Jackson *et al.* 2003). Here again, such findings may attest that brain activations recorded during MI cannot be attributed to actual micro-movements. Finally, some experiments also looked for muscular quiescence as a precondition to engagement in MI practice (Hanakawa *et al.* 2003, 2008; Zijdewind *et al.* 2003).

At first glance, the findings of the studies mentioned above may rule out the neuromuscular or afference-based peripheral explanation as no proprioceptive feedback was available during the imagery experience. Caution should be exercised with the interpretation of the data, however, as a wide range of experimental studies provided evidence of a subliminal muscular activity during imagined performance.

EMG activity during MI

As suggested by Washburn (1916), earlier, and further substantiated by several authors (Jacobson 1931, 1932; Shaw 1938; McGuigan 1978; Epstein 1980; Wehner *et al.* 1984), an activity of the same muscles has been observed during both MI and overt movement execution. As evidence, the magnitude of the activation was reduced by comparison to that observed during actual execution. Especially, Suinn (1980) showed that downhill skiers triggered the same muscles that those activated during the different portions of the course. Similar observations were reported in different types of motor skills including swimming, rowing, waterski and basketball (Bird, 1984), squeezing a rubber ball (Livesay and Samaras 1998), as well as during karate and juggling performance (Harris and Robertson 1986; Jowdy and Harris 1990). Bonnet *et al.* (1997) further showed that EMG activity may be modulated by the lateralization and the intensity of the simulated foot pressure, albeit the magnitude of the signal was 20 times less than during actual contraction. Using microneurographic recordings in six spindle afferents innervating extensor muscles in the forearm and tibialis anterior, Gandevia *et al.* (1997) demonstrated that not only MI did activate the alpha motoneurones, but that the skeletomotor discharge was also accompanied by recruitment of spindle afferents if the covert contraction was sufficiently strong. The cortical regions mediating MI should thus be capable of recruiting spinal motoneurones within the spinal cord during the mental rehearsal of an overt action. This latter finding is in agreement with the controversial assumption that imagined movements produce qualitatively similar, but quantitatively lesser, drive to muscles than the actual execution; thus resulting in sensory feedback that may also, in return, contribute to the activation of motor areas.

Interestingly, the content of mental representation has also been found to correlate with the magnitude and the location of EMG patterns. Especially, and even though inconsistent results were first reported by Vigus and Williams (1985), MI in a first-person perspective resulted in greater EMG activity than MI in a third-person perspective (Hale 1982; Harris and Robinson 1986). Similarly, increased EMG activity was observed when the participants included assertions to behaviour, such as somatomotor and visceral responses in their MI content, as compared to imagery primarily including information about the stimulus context, i.e., the content of the scenario (Bakker et al. 1996; Boschker 2001; Lutz and Lindner 2001). Boschker (2001) confirmed that muscular activity was greater in the active than in the passive arm, and that imagining lifting a heavy dumbbell resulted in increased EMG magnitude than MI of a lighter object. These results were corroborated by the findings of Slade et al. (2002). Overall, these findings indicate a significant increase in EMG activity when MI was performed in a first-person perspective. They also suggest that the physiological responses reflect the spatial differentiation and the quantitative characteristics of the image. More recently, Guillot et al. (2007) have reported a pattern of EMG activity during MI in all agonist, synergist, and antagonist muscles involved in the movement, as a function of both the weight to be lifted and the muscle contraction type. Especially, they found that the subliminal muscular responses during MI of concentric, isometric, and eccentric contractions overall mirrored the configuration of the EMG activity recorded during actual practice. By providing evidence of a modulation of the EMG power spectrum frequency during different types of imagined muscle contractions, Lebon et al. (2008) further supported the hypothesis of a specific motor programme performed as a function of muscle contraction type during MI. To date, however, the pattern of muscular activation has not been found to match the triphasic sequence generated during actual motor performance, hence challenging the inflow processing explanation (Murphy et al. 2008). With regards the functional equivalence between MI and motor performance (Holmes and Collins 2001; Guillot and Collet 2008), imagery benefits may thus be explained with reference to the central representational theory (Mulder et al. 2004; Murphy et al. 2008).

Finally, some authors postulated that the intensity of EMG activity recorded during MI may be related to the individual ability to form an accurate mental representation of the motor skill. Hecker and Kazcor (1988), Boschker (2001), as well as Mulder et al. (2005) failed to confirm such hypothesis, however, as no relationship between muscular activity and imagery ability, as evaluated through psychological tests and MI questionnaires, was observed. Similarly, results by Dickstein et al. (2005) undermined such relationship, and Guillot et al. (2007) did not provide evidence that the participants producing more specific patterns of EMG activity were better imagers than those who produced lower EMG responses. By contrast, Lutz (2003) found positive correlations between EMG activity and imagery vividness as measured by psychological tests and subjective self-estimation of MI quality. These latter results were however quite equivocal as only four out of nine correlations were either marginally or statistically significant in their first experiment, while no relationship was found in their second study. Hence, future experimental research is necessary to re-examine in greater details whether the correlation between MI accuracy and peripheral muscular activity, whenever observed, may be considered effective and reliable.

What explanation for such inconsistencies?

As mentioned in the earlier paragraphs, the wealth of literature has provided several inconsistent results regarding the concomitant EMG activity in the muscles participating in the movement during MI. Recent data by Li et al. (2004) and Dickstein et al. (2005) are in agreement with such observation. First, by investigating the effects of MI on spinal segmental excitability,

Li *et al.* (2004) observed finger flexors EMG and torque reflex responses in only four out of nine participants. Second, Dickstein *et al.* (2005) reported that EMG was sometimes, but not always, recorded in both healthy individuals and post-stroke hemiparetic patients. They did not find any systematic discernable EMG activity in the monitored muscles. Many confounding factors may be considered to explain such variability in experimental findings. These range from methodological issues and experimental conditions to data reliability and interpretation.

First, there is strong evidence that the results may be impacted by differences in experimental designs as well as in methodological issues (for reviews, see Türker 1993; Kleissen *et al.* 1998). While useful recordings may be obtained through surface EMG electrodes if appropriate precautions are taken, intramuscular electrodes should be preferred, especially when the activity is recorded in small peripheral or deep muscles. With the exception of the study by Gandevia *et al.* (1997), however, the MI-related experiments, dealing with this research area, have been performed using surface electrodes recordings. Accordingly, many authors argued that as during motor preparation (Mellah *et al.* 1990), preparatory fibres could primarily be involved during MI too; and that the activity of deep and tonic fibres may not be systematically observed with usual surface EMG recordings (Jeannerod, 1994, 2006; Jeannerod and Frak 1999). The slow metabolic rate of these fibres may also explain why nuclear magnetic resonance techniques failed to detect any overt muscular changes during imagined performance. In addition, the EMG signal during mental practice through surface electrodes may have been affected by specific methodological parameters, for example, electrode geometry, distance between active fibres and electrodes, or even location of the muscle; hence supporting, at least partially, possible inconsistencies among the different studies. Discrepancies may also result from the reliability of the EMG measures in the context of different studies investigating similar recording sites, which is highly dependent upon electrode surface location. Accordingly, the surface EMG signal displayed some variability, even though it is difficult to conclude the lack of consistency due to metrologic problems (Clark *et al.* 2007). As a matter of fact, the reproducibility and reliability of recordings have been shown in a wide range of experiments, but the lack of precision in the description of some experimental designs may not be sufficient to ensure the validity of the interpreted data.

Differences related to mental representation content and MI instructions given by the experimenters may also contribute to understand why EMG activity was not systematically reported. Especially, we previously gathered data regarding the impact of using the first- versus third-person imagery perspective on subliminal muscular responses. We further underlined the difference within the use of MI scripts including the description of the context as compared to the somatomotor responses accompanying mental rehearsal (see Ranganathan *et al.* 2002). Finally, we highlighted the effect of the muscular contraction type and the intensity of the mental effort. In each case, EMG responses, whenever observed, were found specific to the mental representation content. These data may suggest that using different types of MI or differentiating the content of the mental images may result either in a task-dependent EMG response pattern, or, conversely, in muscular quiescence. Such confounding factors should thus be taken into consideration before interpreting the muscle activation or absence of activation during MI, and further need to be controlled in future experimental designs.

Excitability of spinal reflex pathways

In view of the results, described above, changes in excitability of the motor pathways during MI should also be expected, thus providing further information on the involved mechanisms underlying the mental representation of overt movements. First, many experiments were designed to investigate the monosynaptic reflex responses (H- and T-reflex amplitudes) following direct nerve stimulation or tendinous stretch during MI. Bonnet *et al.* (1997) showed that imagined foot pressure resulted in an increase of both spinal reflex excitability, which was only slightly weaker than the reflex facilitation elicited by the physical execution of the same movement. They also found that T-reflexes were much more facilitated than H-reflexes and that response amplitude were also dependent upon the side and force of the imagined movement. As the T-reflex is triggered by a tendon tap (to elicit neuromuscular spindles stretch and response), it supports the assumption of a selective increase in the excitability of gamma motoneurons and spindle activation during MI. Gandevia *et al.* (1997) and Gandevia (1999) also provided evidence that the H-reflex increased independently of altered skeletomotor activity during MI, hence suggesting that mental rehearsal may activate descending inputs to spinal reflex circuits. In addition, Hale *et al.* (2003) argued that the H-reflex may be modulated by MI practice rather than by the intensity of the mental effort. Such results are equivocal, however, as Oishi *et al.* (1994) and Oishi and Maeshima (2004) reported a depression in H-reflex amplitude during MI of speed skating in elite athletes, such decrease being interpreted as resulting from descending neural mechanisms which may reduce motor neuron excitability. Further, Kaneko *et al.* (2003) also found that the H-reflex response did not differ between rest and MI conditions in both healthy individuals and orthopaedic patients with splints. Second, the excitability of the corticospinal pathways may also be tested by using transcranial magnetic stimulation (see Chapter 4 in this book), hence leading to the measurement of the motor evoked potentials in the muscles involved in the actual or imagined movement (Pascual-Leone *et al.* 1995; Abbruzzese *et al.* 1999). A wide range of experimental studies did consistently support the assumption that MI may increase corticospinal activity (e.g., Rossini *et al.* 1999; Stinear and Byblow 2003; Clark *et al.* 2004; Li *et al.* 2004). Accordingly, Hashimoto and Rothwell (1999) showed that evoked responses were larger in the flexor muscles during imagined wrist flexion, while the opposite was true for the extensor muscles. Furthermore, MI was found to increase the corticospinal activity during mental rehearsal, by influencing specifically the muscles directly responsible for the execution (Fadiga *et al.* 1999). Stinear *et al.* (2006) also demonstrated that only kinaesthetic imagery did produce muscle-specific and temporally modulated facilitation of the corticospinal pathway, while visual imagery did not have similar effect. In contrast, Fourkas *et al.* (2006) recently reported that kinaesthetic imagery did not lead to higher facilitation than visual imagery, albeit excitability was found to fluctuate with hand posture congruency, especially during kinaesthetic imagery (the imagery task was performed in two conditions in which the imagined and the actual hand could be either congruent or incongruent, and a lack of excitability was recorded during incongruent kinaesthetic imagery). The discrepancy between these two studies may be explained by differences in the experimental design, especially by the stimulus intensity over the primary motor cortex. Also, the nature of the MI instructions may have contributed to differentiating the findings of the two studies. In the study by Fourkas *et al.* (2006), the visual imagery instructions were more specifically designed to achieve visual imagery in a first-person perspective, i.e., using an egocentric reference frame. By contrast, Stinear *et al.* (2006) requested the participants to 'imagine seeing their thumb moving in time with the metronome', so that the third-person imagery perspective was not completely excluded. Such difference would suggest that performing first- versus third-person visual imagery perspectives may result in different modulation of the corticospinal excitability, although this still remains a hypothesis awaiting further experimental investigation. Also, while Mercier *et al.* (2008) suggested that vision without proprioception modulates corticospinal excitability during MI, Fourkas *et al.* (2008) later reported that muscles may show increased task-dependent corticospinal facilitation associated with individual level of physical expertise. Finally, Sohn *et al.* (2003) demonstrated that MI of suppressing movement (also called negative imagery) resulted in altered corticospinal excitability using transcranial magnetic stimulation.

The hypothesis of motor inhibition

MI has consistently been defined as the mental rehearsal of a motor act without any overt movement. This means that the neural commands for muscular contractions are blocked at some level of the motor system by active inhibitory mechanisms. Jeannerod (1994) early postulated that incomplete inhibition of the motor command would provide a valid explanation to account for these muscular discharges. Interestingly, and consistent with this assumption, Schwoebel et al. (2002) showed that a brain-damaged patient failed to inhibit the motor consequences of MI, and thus fully 'executed the imagined action', hence highlighting uninhibited movements during mental rehearsal. The neural generators of inhibitory signals, however, have not yet been clearly identified in the MI literature (Michelon et al. 2006). Two main hypotheses were offered to explain such processes. First, the inhibitory mechanisms have been thought to be effective before the information elaborated within the associate cortices is sent to the primary motor cortex. Especially, and as reviewed by Jeannerod (2006), this inhibition may have originated from the prefrontal cortical areas, in line with the implication of these regions in behavioural inhibition (Garavan et al. 1999; Watanabe et al. 2002). By investigating the impairment of the inhibitory function of the prefrontal cortex, the studies by Marshall et al. (1997) and Brass et al. (2001) support this assumption. Such hypothesis would not be compatible, however, with the activation of the primary motor cortex per se during MI (see Chapter 3 in this book). The activation of the prefrontal cortex during mental rehearsal may thus be linked to the selection of the appropriate representation, rather than to some inhibitory processes (Shallice 1988). Especially, if the inferior frontal cortex may participate in suppressing the motor executive mechanisms during MI, other factors might also be involved (Deiber et al. 1998). Furthermore, the comparison of brain activation during MI in healthy individuals and in patients with spinal cord injury did not confirm the role of the inferior frontal cortex in the volitional movement suppression (Alkadhi et al. 2005). At the cortical level, some other data in damaged patients suggested that the disruption of a fronto-parietal articulation due to bilateral parietal damage may also account for the failure of action inhibition (Schwoebel et al. 2002), hence confirming the critical role that the parietal cortex may play in the generation of the mental representation. Also, recent experimental studies have highlighted the potential implication of the ventromedial prefrontal and superior temporal cortices (de Lange et al. 2007), as well as the supplementary motor area (Kasess et al. 2008). A second potential explanation is proposed by Bonnet et al. (1997) and Jeannerod (2006) who state that the inhibitory mechanisms are localized downstream of the motor cortex, possibly at the spinal cord or brainstem level. Accordingly, Lotze et al. (1999) postulated that the posterior cerebellum might play a crucial role in the inhibition of the motor command (see also Lotze and Halsband 2006). Inhibitory processes at the intraspinal level have also been proposed (Prut and Fetz 1999; Jeannerod 2006; McMillan et al. 2006). Indeed, a superimposed global inhibition is thought to be propagated from the premotor cortex to the spinal cord, inhibitory delay patterns suppressing the tendency to initiate movement.

An alternative explanation was offered by Burle et al. (2002) who interpreted the subthreshold EMG activity as partial errors that are detected and aborted by the central nervous system before the overt response threshold is reached. Even though their experimental work did not focus on imagery per se, such interpretation might be well suited for MI in which execution is aborted and the idea of action is not readily transformed into action (Dickstein et al. 2005). Even though there is strong evidence that MI and motor preparation do not differ substantially and may even be closely related, Michelon et al. (2006) underlined that MI does not necessarily need to perform a motor simulation, i.e., include the mapping of the effector-specific commands required to achieve the movement. Bonnet et al. (1997) also argued that it would be more appropriate to compare MI and action, rather than motor preparation, hence considering MI as the intention to stop movement execution. This assumption is undermined by other researchers, who rather suggest that MI is more closely related to pre-executive processes of a movement than its actual execution (e.g. Hanakawa *et al.* 2008). Altogether, motor inhibition is thought to be clearly different in the two cases, as motor preparation is specifically characterized by inhibitory mechanisms acting at the spinal level well before the time to act, especially in order to protect motoneurons against a premature action triggering (see also Duclos *et al.* 2008). As recently suggested by Hanakawa *et al.* (2008), the issue of MI versus motor inhibition will thus require further clarification.

Conclusive contribution of EMG data to the understanding of MI

This chapter aimed to focus on the muscular activity accompanying the mental representation of an overt movement. Results were found inconsistent and thus prevent to draw a definitive conclusion regarding this issue. When observed, the modification of EMG pattern seems more than an epiphenomenon, even though it remains difficult to interpret. Jeannerod (1995) early proposed that studies investigating MI in deafferented patients may be of particular interest, especially by ruling out the role of spindle afferents, even if EMG discharges were recorded. By investigating MI of hand movement in a deafferented patient holding the dominant hand in a compatible or incompatible posture while imagining the movement, Mercier *et al.* (2008) recently demonstrated, however, that afferent feedback may play a crucial role in modulating MI processes. In addition, research has not yet concluded that the increase in muscular activity fully contributes to performance enhancement. Moreover, reports of increased EMG activity during MI have usually failed to demonstrate a simultaneous physical performance improvement, and low correlation was observed between increased muscular activity and level of expertise, either for physical or imagined performance. As suggested by Guillot and Collet (2005), and on the basis of the discrepancies reviewed in this section, we may conclude that EMG recordings should not be considered a strong reliable indicator of MI vividness and accuracy, and that caution should therefore be exercised before interpretation of any activation or absence of activation of muscle activity during MI. Hence, agreement about the exact mechanisms has still to be reached, in particular, to give a straightforward understanding of the inhibitory processes involved in the suppression of the motor command during MI.

References

Abbruzzese, G., Assini, A., Buccolieri, A., Marchese, R., and Trompetto, C. (1999). Changes of intracortical inhibition during motor imagery in human subjects. *Neuroscience Letters*, **263**, 113–16.

Alkadhi, H., Brugger, P., Boendermarker, S.H. *et al.* (2005). What disconnection tells about motor imagery: evidence from paraplegic patients. *Cerebral Cortex*, **15**, 131–40.

Bakker, F.C., Boschker, M.S., and Chung, T. (1996). Changes in muscular activity while imaging weight-lifting using stimulus or response propositions. *Journal of Sport and Exercise Psychology*, **18**, 313–24.

Bird, E.I. (1984). EMG quantification of mental rehearsal. *Perceptual and Motor Skills*, **59**, 899–906.

Bonnet, M., Decety, J., Jeannerod, M., and Requin, J. (1997). Mental simulation of an action modulates the excitability of spinal reflex pathways in man. *Cognitive Brain Research*, **5**, 221–8.

Boschker, M.S.J. (2001). *Action-Based Imagery: on the Nature of Mentally Imagined Motor Actions.* Amsterdam: Ipskamp Printpartners.

Brass, M., Zysset, S., and von Cramon, Y. (2001). The inhibition of initiative response tendencies. *Neuroimage*, **14**, 1416–23.

Burle B., Possamaï, C.A., Vidal F., Bonnet, M., and Hasbroucq, T. (2002). Executive control on the Simon effect: an electromyographic and distributional analysis. *Psychological Research*, **66**, 324–36.

Carpenter, W.B. (1894). *Principles of Mental Physiology*. Fourth edition. New York: Appleton.

Clark B.C., Cook S.B., and Ploutz-Snyder L.L. (2007). Reliability of techniques to assess human neuromuscular function in vivo. *Journal of Electromyography and Kinesiology*, **17**, 90–101.

Clark S., Tremblay, F., and Ste-Marie, D. (2004). Differential modulation of corticospinal excitability during observation, mental imagery and imitation of hand actions. *Neuropsychologia*, **42**, 993–6.

de Lange, F.P., Roelofs, K., and Toni, I. (2007). Increased self-monitoring during imagined movements in conversion paralysis. *Neuropsychologia*, **45**, 2051–58.

Decety, J., Jeannerod, M., Durozard, D., and Baverel, G. (1993). Central activation of autonomic effectors during mental simulation of motor actions in man. *Journal of Physiology*, **461**, 549–63.

Deiber, M.P., Ibanez, V., Honda, M., Sadato, N., Raman, R., and Hallett, M. (1998). Cerebral processes related to visuomotor imagery and generation of simple finger movements studied with positron emission tomography. *Neuroimage*, **7**, 73–85.

Dickstein, R., Gazit-Grunwald, M., Plax, M., Dunsky, A., and Marcovitz, E. (2005). EMG activity in selected target muscles *during* imagery rising on tiptoes in healthy adults and poststroke hemiparetic patients, *Journal of Motor Behavior*, **37**, 475–83.

Duclos, Y., Schmied, A., Burle, B., Burnet, H., and Rossi-Durand, C. (2008). Anticipatory changes in human motoneuron discharge patterns during motor preparation. *Journal of Physiology*, **586**, 1017–28.

Epstein, M. (1980). The relationship of mental imagery and mental rehearsal to performance of a motor task. *Journal of Sport Psychology*, **2**, 211–20.

Fadiga, L., Buccino, G., Craighero, L., Fogassi L., Gallese, V., and Pavesi, G. (1999). Corticospinal excitability is specifically modulated by motor imagery: a magnetic stimulation study. *Neuropsychologia*, **37**, 147–58.

Fourkas, A.D., Avenanti, A., Urgesi, C., and Aglioti, S.M. (2006). Corticospinal facilitation during first and third person imagery. *Experimental brain Research*, **168**, 143–51.

Fourkas, A.D., Bonavolontà, V., Avenanti, A., and Aglioti, S.M. (2008). Kinaesthetic imagery and tool-specific modulation of corticospinal representations in expert tennis players. *Cerebral Cortex*, **18**, 2382–90.

Gandevia, S.C., Wilson, L.R., Inglis, J.T., and Burke, D. (1997). Mental rehearsal of motor tasks recruits alpha-motoneurones but fails to recruit human fusimotor neurones selectively. *Journal of Neurophysiology*, **505**, 259–66.

Gandevia, S.C. (1999). Mind, muscles and motoneurones. *Journal of Science and Medicine in Sport*, **2**, 167–80.

Garavan, H., Ross, T.J., and Stein, E.A. (1999). Right hemispheric dominance of inhibitory control: an event-related functional MRI study. *Proceedings of the National Academy of Sciences*, **96**, 8301–6.

Gerardin, E., Sirigu, A., Lehericy, S. *et al.* (2000). Partially overlapping neural networks for real and imagined hand movements. *Cerebral Cortex*, **10**, 1093–104.

Guillot, A. and Collet, C. (2005). Contribution from neurophysiological and psychological methods to the study of motor imagery. *Brain Research Reviews*, **50**, 387–97.

Guillot, A., Lebon, F., Rouffet, D., Champely, S., Doyon, J., and Collet, C. (2007). Muscular responses during motor imagery as a function of muscle contraction types. *International Journal of Psychophysiology*, **66**, 18–27.

Guillot, A. and Collet, C. (2008). Construction of the motor imagery integrative model in sport: a review and theoretical investigation of motor imagery use. *International Review of Sport and Exercise Psychology*, **1**, 31–44.

Gentili, R., Papaxanthis, C., and Pozzo, T. (2006). Improvement and generalization of arm motor performance through imagery practice. *Neuroscience*, **137**, 761–72.

Hale, B.D. (1982). The effects of internal and external imagery on muscular and ocular concomitants. *Journal of Sport Psychology*, **4**, 379–87.

Hale, B.S., Raglin, J.S., and Koceja, D.M. (2003). Effect of mental imagery of a motor task on the Hoffmann reflex. *Behavioural Brain Research*, **142**, 81–7.

Hanakawa, T., Immisch, I., Toma, K., Dimyan, A., Van Gelderen, P., and Hallett, M. (2003). Functional properties of brain areas associated with motor execution and imagery. *Journal of Neurophysiology*, **89**, 989–1002.

Hanakawa, T., Dimyan, M.A., and Hallett, M. (2008). Motor planning, imagery, and execution in the distributed motor networks: a time-course study with functional MRI. *Cerebral Cortex*, **41**, 1021–31.

Harris, D.V. and Robinson, W.J. (1986). The effect of skill level on EMG activity during internal and external imagery. *Journal of Sport Psychology*, **8**, 105–11.

Hashimoto, R. and Rothwell, J.C. (1999). Dynamic changes in corticospinal excitability during motor imagery. *Experimental Brain Research*, **125**, 75–81.

Hecker, J.E. and Kazcor, L.M. (1988). Application of imagery theory to sport psychology: some preliminary findings. *Journal of Sport and Exercise Psychology*, **10**, 363–73.

Herbert, R.D., Dean, C., and Gandevia, S.C. (1998). Effects of real and imagined training on voluntary muscle activation during maximal isometric contractions. *Acta Physiologica Scandinavica*, **163**, 361–8.

Holmes, P. and Collins, D.J. (2001). The PETTLEP approach to motor imagery: a functional equivalence model for sport psychologists. *Journal of Applied Sport Psychology*, **13**, 60–83.

Jackson, P.L., Lafleur, M.F., Malouin, F., Richards, C.L., and Doyon, J. (2003). Functional cerebral reorganization following motor sequence learning through mental practice with motor imagery. *Neuroimage*, **20**, 1171–80.

Jacobson, E. (1931). Electrical measurement of neuromuscular states during mental activities. *American Journal of Physiology*, **96**, 115–21.

Jacobson, E. (1932). Electrophysiology of mental activities. *American Journal of Psychology*, **44**, 677–94.

Jeannerod, M. (1994). The representing brain: neural correlates of motor intention and imagery. *Behavioural Brain Sciences*, **17**, 187–245.

Jeannerod, M. (1995). Mental imagery in the motor cortex. *Neuropsychologia*, **33**, 1419–32.

Jeannerod, M. (2006). *Motor Cognition*. New York: Oxford University Press.

Jeannerod, M. and Frak, V. (1999). Mental imaging of motor activity in humans. *Current Opinion in Neurobiology*, **9**, 735–9.

Jowdy, D.P. and Harris, D.V. (1990). Muscular responses during mental imagery as a function of motor skill level. *Journal of Sport and Exercise Psychology*, **12**, 191–201.

Kaneko, F., Murakami, T., Onari, K., Kurumadani, H., and Kawaguchi, K. (2003). Decreased cortical excitability during motor imagery after disuse of an upper limb in humans. *Clinical Neurophysiology*, **114**, 2397–2403.

Kasess, C.H., Windischberger, C., Cunnington, R., Lanzenberger, R., Pezawas, L., and Moser, E. (2008). The suppressive influence of SMA on M1 in motor imagery revealed by fMRI and dynamic causal modeling. *Neuroimage*, **40**, 828–37.

Kleber, B., Birbaumer, N., Veit, R., Trevorrow, T., and Lotze, M. (2007). Overt and imagiend singing of an Italian aria. *Neuroimage*, **36**, 1238–46.

Kleissen, R.F.M., Buurke, J.H., Harlaar, J., and Zivold, G. (1998). Electromyography in the biomechanical analysis of human movement and its clinical application. *Gait and Posture*, **8**, 143–58.

Lafleur, M.F., Jackson, P.L., Malouin, F., Richards, C.L., Evans, A.C., and Doyon, J. (2002). Motor learning produces parallel dynamic functional changes during the execution and imagination of sequential foot movements. *Neuroimage*, **2**, 142–57.

Lebon, F., Rouffet, D., Collet, C., and Guillot, A. (2008). Modulation of EMG power spectrum frequency during motor imagery. *Neuroscience Letters*, **435**, 181–5.

Li, S., Kamper, D.G., Stevens, J.A., and Rymer, W.Z. (2004). The effect of motor imagery on spinal segmental excitability. *Journal of Neuroscience*, **27**, 9674–80.

Lim, V.K., Polych, M.A., Holländer, A., Byblow, W.D., Kirk, I.J., and Hamm, J.P. (2006). Kinaesthetic but not visual imagery assists in normalizing the CNV in Parkinson's disease. *Clinical Neurophysiology*, **117**, 2308–14.

Livesay, J.R. and Samaras, M.R. (1998). Covert neuromuscular activity of the dominant forearm during visualization of a motor task. *Perceptual and Motor Skills*, **86**, 371–4.

Lotze, L., Montoya, P., Erb, M. *et al.* (1999). Activation of cortical and cerebellar motor areas during executed and imagined hand movements: an fMRI study. *Journal of Cognitive Neuroscience*, **11**, 491–501.

Lotze, M., Scheler, G., Tan, H.R.M., Braun, C., and Birbaumer, N. (2003). The musician's brain: functional imaging of amateurs and professionals during performance and imagery. *Neuroimage*, **20**, 1817–29.

Lotze, M. and Halsband, U. (2006). Motor imagery. *Journal of Physiology (Paris)*, **99**, 386–95.

Lutz, R. and Lindner, D.E. (2001). Does electromyographic activity during motor imagery predict performance? A test of bioinformational theory and functional equivalences. *Journal of Sport and Exercise Psychology*, **23**, S63.

Lutz, R.S. (2003). Covert muscle excitation is outflow from the central generation of motor imagery. *Behavioural Brain Research*, **140**, 149–63.

Marshall, J.C., Halligan, P.W., Fink, G.R., Wade, D.T., and Frackowiak, R.S.J. (1997). The functional anatomy of a hysterical paralysis. *Cognition*, **64**, B1–8.

McGuigan, F.J. (1978). *Cognitive Psychophysiology: Principles of Covert Behavior*. Englewood Cliffs, NJ: Prentice-Hall.

McMillan, S., Ivry, R.B., and Byblow, W.D. (2006). Corticomotor excitability during a choice-hand reaction time task. *Experimental brain Research*, **172**, 230–45.

Mellah, S., Rispal-Padel, L., and Rivière, G. (1990). Changes in excitability of motor units during preparation for movement. *Experimental Brain Research*, **82**, 178–86.

Mercier, C., Aballea, A., Vargas, C.D., Paillard, J., and Sirigu, A. (2008). Vision without proprioception modulates cortico-spinal excitability during hand motor imagery. *Cerebral Cortex*, **18**, 272–7.

Michelon, P., Vettel, J.M., and Zacks, J.M. (2006). Lateral somatotopic organization during imagined and prepared movements. *Journal of Neurophysiology*, **95**, 811–22.

Mulder, T., Zijlstra, S., Zijlstra, W., and Hochstenbach, J. (2004). The role of motor imagery in learning a totally novel movement. *Experimental Brain Research*, **154**, 211–7.

Mulder, T., de Vries S., and Zijlstra, S. (2005). Observation, imagination and execution of an effortful movement: more evidence for a central explanation of motor imagery. *Experimental Brain Research*, **163**, 344–51.

Murphy, S., Nordin, S.M., and Cumming, J. (2008). Imagery in sport, exercise and dance, in T. Horn (ed.), *Advances in Sport Psychology*, pp. 306–15. Champagne, IL: Human Kinetics.

Naito, E., Kochiyama, T., Kidata, R. *et al.* (2002). Internally simulated movement sensations during motor imagery activate cortical motor areas and the cerebellum. *Journal of Neurosciences*, **22**, 3683–91.

Oishi, K., Kimura, M., Yasukawa, M., Yoneda, T., and Maeshima, T. (1994). Amplitude reduction of H-reflex during mental movement simulation in elite athletes. *Behavioural Brain Research*, **62**, 55–61.

Oishi, K. and Maeshima, T. (2004). Autonomic nervous system activities during motor imagery in elite athletes. *Journal of Clinical Neurophysiology*, **21**, 170–9.

Pascual-Leone, A., Nguyet, D., Cohen, L.G., brasil-Neto, J.P., Cammarota A., and Hallet, M. (1995). Modulation of muscle responses evoked by transcranial magnetic stimulation during the acquisition of new fine motor skills. *Journal of Neurophysiology*, **74**, 1037–45.

Personnier, P., Paizis, C., Ballay, Y., and Papaxanthis, C. (2007). Mentally represented motor actions in normal aging II. The influence of the gravito-inertial context on the duration of overt and covert arm movements. *Behavioural Brain Research*, **186**, 273–83.

Prut, Y. and Fetz, E.E. (1999). Primate spinal interneurons show premovement instructed delay activity. *Nature*, **401**, 590–4.

Ranganathan, V.K., Kuykendall, T., Siemionow, V., and Yue, G.H. (2002). Level of mental effort determines training-induced strength increases. *Society for Neuroscience Abstracts*, **32**, 768.

Ranganathan, V.K., Siemionow, V., Liu, J.Z., Sahgal, V., and Yue, G.H. (2004). From mental power to muscle power-gaining strength by using the mind. *Neuropsychologia,* **42**, 944–56.

Rossini, P.M., Rossi, S., Pasqualetti, P., and Tecchio, F. (1999). Corticospinal excitability modulation to hand muscles during movement imagery. *Cerebral Cortex*, **9**, 161–7.

Schwoebel, J., Boronat, C.B., and Coslett, H.B. (2002). The man who executed 'imagined' movements: evidence for dissociable components of the body schema. *Brain and Cognition*, **50**, 1–16.

Shallice, T. (1988). *From Neuropsychology to Mental Structure*. Cambridge: Cambridge University Press.

Shaw, W.A. (1938). The distribution of muscular action potentials during imaging. *The Psychological Record*, **2**, 195–216.

Shaw, W.A. (1940). The distribution of muscular action potentials to imagined weight lifting. *Archives of Psychology*, **247**, 1–50.

Shick, J. (1970). Effects of mental practice on selected volleyball skills for college women. *Research Quarterly*, **41**, 88–94.

Slade, J.M., Landers, D.M., and Martin, P.E. (2002). Muscular activity during real and imagined movement: a test of inflow explanations. *Journal of Sport and Exercise Psychology*, **24**, 151–67.

Sohn, Y.H., Dang, N., and Hallett, M. (2003). Suppression of corticospinal excitability during motor negative imagery. *Journal of Neurophysiology*, **90**, 2303–9.

Stinear, C.M. and Byblow, W.D. (2003). Motor imagery of phasic thumb abduction temporally and spatially modulates corticospinal excitability. *Clinical Neurophysiology*, **114**, 909–14.

Stinear, C.M., Byblow, W.D., Steyvers, M., Levin, O., and Swinnen, S.P. (2006). Kinaesthetic, but not visual, motor imagery modulates corticospinal excitability. *Experimental Brain Research*, **168**, 157–64.

Suinn, R.M. (1980). Body thinking: psychology for Olympic champions, in R.M. Suinn (ed.), *Psychology in Sports: Methods and Applications*, pp. 306–315. Mineapolis: Burgess.

Türker, K.S. (1993). Electromyography: some methodological problems and issues. *Physical Therapy*, **73**, 698–710.

Vigus, T.L. and Williams, J.L. (1985). The physiological correlates of internal and external imagery. *Unpublished manuscript.*

Washburn, M.F. (1916). *Movement and Mental Imagery: Outlines of a Motor Theory of the Complex Mental Processes*. Boston: Houghton Mifflin.

Watanabe J., Sugiura M., Sato K. *et al.* (2002). The human prefrontal and parietal association cortices are involved in NO-GO performances: an event-related fMRI study. *Neuroimage*, **17**, 1207–16.

Wehner, T., Vogt, S., and Stadler, M. (1984). Task-specific EMG-characteristics during mental training. *Psychological Research*, **46**, 389–401.

Yahagi, S., Shimura, K., and Kasai, T. (1996). An increase in cortical excitability with no change in spinal excitability during motor imagery. *Perceptual and Motor Skills*, **83**, 288–90.

Yue, G. and Cole, K.J. (1992). Strength increases from the motor program: comparison of training with maximal voluntary and imagined muscle contractions. *Journal of Neurophysiology*, **67**, 114–23.

Zijdewind, J., Toering, S.T., Bessen, B., Van-Der-Laan, O., and Diercks, R.L. (2003). Effects of imagery motor training on torque production of ankle plantar flexor muscles. *Muscle Nerve*, **28**, 168–73.

Chapter 7

Autonomic nervous system activities during imagined movements

Christian Collet and Aymeric Guillot

Introduction

At first glance, there is no clear relationship between the mental activity of representing an action and the functioning of the autonomic nervous system (ANS). The process of representing an action is dependent upon high brain functions involving sensorial-motor coupling, mediated by memory systems. The ANS is the part of the nervous system which controls vital functions. Its overall activity is that of maintaining a state of homeostasis in the organism and of performing the adaptation responses when faced with changes in the external and internal milieus. There is thus a long way before being able to link motor imagery activity and the ANS function.

We will first review the evolution of the conceptions related to ANS functioning as this will probably explain why the activity of this part of the nervous system could first be considered being unrelated to high mental processes. Progressively, however, we will examine how autonomic activity can influence mental functions and, in turn, how motor imagery may elicit physiological responses at the peripheral level of the autonomic effectors. The aim is to draw a step-by-step progression from the understanding of the physiological basis of the ANS to its relationships with high mental processes such as motor imagery. We will then detail how these physiological responses may be analysed to not only provide objective evidence that motor imagery is actually performed, but also to serve as a reliable evaluation of its effectiveness.

The classical view of the autonomic nervous system function

The ANS is composed of visceral afferent pathways, integration centres at the level of the brain stem, the hypothalamus, and cerebral cortices. The physiology of the ANS describes different efferent pathways subdivided into sympathetic, parasympathetic, and enteric branches responsible for regulating organs' functions by nervous signals and by releasing neurotransmitters (McCorry 2007). These efferent pathways innerve internal organs, in particular, the cardiac muscle, the smooth muscle, as well as the exocrine and endocrine glands. An important point which will be further developed is that efferent pathways also innerve the skin, i.e., the organ directly located at the interface between the body and the environment. The ANS is also made of afferent pathways, arranged in two patterns, the oligosynaptic circuits mediating reflex adaptation responses of the visceral systems and more complex circuits, with projections to nuclei in the brain stem and the brain. The information is therefore collected and responses are produced, this latter operation affecting, in turn, the systems mentioned above. Taken as a whole, this basic view leads to a system made of two main subdivisions: the orthosympathetic branch aimed at mobilizing energy to face emergency situations (the catabolic function), and the parasympathetic branch with the opposite function, i.e., restoring and maintaining the resources of the organism at a level compatible with life (the anabolic function). This organization leads, however, to the two following main critical positions.

First, at the anatomical level, and with regard to the first contribution by Bichat (1802), the ANS is often considered as being separated from the somatic nervous system. On the one hand, Bichat pointed out the continuous action of a part of the nervous system (leading to the concept of *organic* life), and the intermittent action of the other part (controlling the *animal* life), on the other. This is still expressed by the explicit terms of 'visceral' and 'somatic', respectively. This also makes the distinction between the vegetative life, independently of the will and the consciousness, and the somatic life, which leads to voluntary actions in relation with the environment. As a matter of fact, many authors further underlined that the two systems work together and proposed different theoretical models taking into account the intensity and the directional aspects of the behaviour (Karli 1977; Näätänen 1973). Using an interesting metaphor, Mogenson (1977) compared the ANS to the butlers' pantry of an old house of the nineteenth century, due to its role in the maintenance of the organism functions. Likewise, he compared the central nervous system to the living room where friends are warmly welcomed. The butler's pantry would therefore be needed to welcome someone in the living room just as the ANS is required to enable the central nervous system performing the behaviour.

Second, at the functional level, the ANS is designed to maintain constant the internal milieu by averaging and opposing reciprocal actions of the sympathetic and the parasympathetic branches (Cannon 1915). As traditionally conceived, the sympathetic system has a chain of interconnected ganglia close to the spinal cord, each specifically connecting pre-ganglionic to post-ganglionic fibre to send information to the target organs. Due to such organization, the information is spread across the ganglia chain, resulting in overall activation of the organism. The sympathetic function has thus been described as serving the mobilization of bodily resources, for example increasing cardiac and respiratory frequencies to facilitate oxygen uptake, routing blood from internal organs to somatic muscles, thus providing supplementary energy to both brain and muscles. Conversely, the parasympathetic branch should act to decrease demands, for example bringing the heart rate back to basal level. Hence, the two branches of the ANS have been described as functionally opposing systems, the action of one branch being reciprocally related to the other. As a consequence, this dated view led to consider the main function of the ANS as controlling and regulating the general activation, i.e. only playing the role of a quantitative system mobilizing energy to serve behavioural output. The emergency function of the ANS was incorporated into the general concept of stress or arousal.

Human mental processes and the autonomic nervous system

During the last twenty years of the twentieth century, two fundamental notions have been more precisely highlighted and discussed independently. The well-accepted notion of sympathetic tone was questioned early on by Wallin (Wallin 1981). In human being, direct recordings of the neural sympathetic activity showed specific responses with little crosstalk between ganglia. This finding was later confirmed by Wallin and Fagius (1986) who found that muscular endings are sensitive to variation in blood pressure while skin endings remain silent. Conversely, the opposite observation was found as the sympathetic endings innervating the skin are very sensitive to mental stress, whereas those innervating muscles are not. This result is in favour of separated subsystems within the sympathetic organisation, made of building blocks controlling specific internal functions. Following the fundamental findings by Wallin and Fagius (1986, 1988), Jänig and his colleagues, McLachlan and Häbler, confirmed these first results in a series of review papers between 1992 and 2003. Though the sympathetic component of the ANS is widely concerned with the body's response to stress, they demonstrated that a range of neuroscientific techniques (including the microneurography technique – for a review, see Vallbo *et al.* 2004) started to reveal the specialized properties of the functional pathways in the sympathetic system at molecular, cellular, and integrative levels (Jänig and McLachlan 1992a,b; Jänig and Habler 2000, 2003). Such a hypothesis was also early shared by Kummer (1992), and more recently by Morrison (2001), who stated that 'the early views of the sympathetic nervous system as a monolithic effector activated globally in situations requiring a rapid and aggressive response to life-threatening danger have been eclipsed by an organizational model featuring an extensive array of functionally specific output channels that can be simultaneously activated or inhibited in combinations that result in the patterns of autonomic activity supporting behaviour'. At the same time, Porges (1995a) drew quite the same conclusion with reference to the parasympathetic branch when the neural activity exerted from the dorsal motor nucleus was differentiated from that originating from the nucleus ambiguous. Interestingly, the first was the part of the vegetative vagal function *per se*, while the second was linked mostly with attention processes and emotional reactivity. There is thus evidence of a clear linkage between mental functions, i.e. emotion and attention, and a part of the ANS (Porges 1995b). Finally, Berntson *et al.* (1991) evidenced that the relationships between sympathetic and parasympathetic activities are more complex than the principle of simple reciprocity, as different types of coupling may be observed, including reciprocal function, but also co-activation or uncoupled mode in which a change in one branch leaves the other unchanged. As later shown by Hugdahl (1996), 'Autonomic activity that accompanies attention, orienting and learning has demonstrated that the autonomic nervous system is not simply a 'non-cognitive' and automatic part of brain function'. This was early hypothesized by studying the well-known orienting response. This is defined as the response of both the somatic and the ANS to specific stimuli. The appropriate sensorial receptors record the specific properties of the stimulus which then result in orienting the subject's body in the direction of the stimulus. This can be seen as the behavioural response. Simultaneously, a sympathetic response is elicited, for example increased heart rate or electrodermal activity, these physiological responses being related to alertness. Both somatic and autonomic activities thus show that the stimulus has been perceived and probably processed. Interestingly, the orienting response was related by Sokolov (1963) to the representations of the world in memory. The stimulus novelty is better aimed at eliciting high autonomic responses simultaneously with different bodily reactions ('flight or fight' responses), and should probably be subjected to habituation (Bradley 2009). Conversely, a well-known stimulus would elicit a weak response with greater probability as it is rapidly identified by the sensorial systems and recognized by the perception function as usual information. With reference to brain memory systems, the next step is to consider that any information could be mentally evoked, i.e. in the absence of any overt stimulus, and that the same autonomic responses might be elicited under such conditions, i.e. as a result of a top-down process. An intermediate phase would further suggest that behavioural and physiological responses could be elicited indirectly when the information is pre-cued, for example following the presentation and the observation of pictures or videos. The evocation of the movement by viewing the motor scene would probably elicit the same mental state, as this is usually obtained when somebody actually performs the action (Bolliet *et al.* 2005a).

Sensory intake versus rejection distinction

While the orienting response makes the subject responding to external stimuli as a function of stimulus significance, a similar process is active when he or she observes a motor action. The process elicited by the external stimulus is related to intake, whereas this originated from motor imagery could be seen as rejection. As far as movement observation is concerned, it can be seen as a mixed process because the observation serves the construction of a mental evocation which, in turn, may elicit the representation of the observed scene. Such representation may involve the observer who imagined him(her)self performing the movement. The observer could also imagine the movement using a third-person perspective, in case of imagining another subject performing the action. Bolliet *et al.* (2005a) did not find any difference between the ANS responses recorded during the actual execution of a movement, the self-video tape observation and the video-taped observation of somebody else performing the same movement. This might suggest that the cognitive processes activated during movement execution were involved to the same extent during movement observation, whatever the experimental condition. Another interesting issue is that the autonomic response was shorter when the movement observed was performed at a low intensity level (e.g., lifting a load of about 50% of own best mark) than at a high intensity (load of 90% of own best mark). These results confirmed previous data by Paccalin and Jeannerod (2000) who found consistent changes during two experiments, i.e., when subjects watched an actor lifting a weight with increasing loads or a walking and running performance on a treadmill moving at increasing speed. Accordingly, changes in respiration rate of the observer were proportional to the effort made by the actor and followed the actor's running speed, especially during accelerated running. The respiration rate also increased linearly with the speed of the treadmill. Taken together, these data suggest that observation share some processes with action execution, on the one hand, and with action representation, on the other. Observation is probably based on a process which connects the observed movement onto an internal model of the movement that could then make the subject simulating that action (Iacoboni *et al.* 1999). In turn, a simulated action can elicit perceptual activity which resembles the activity that would have occurred if the action had actually been performed (Hesslow 2002). According to Nyberg *et al.* (2000), perceptual simulation can be elicited by different perceptual activities, including the observation, due to its ability to emulate mental representation of movement simultaneously with its observation. On the basis of these theoretical and empirical contributions, we may conclude that perception, observation, and mental representation share many common mental processes, mainly based upon sensorial perception and information stored within the memory that would thus elicit the same autonomic responses. Consequently, if information has the potential power to trigger autonomic response, when it is actually perceived, the mental representation of the same information should have the same effect when simply imagined. On the side of motor action, the mental representation of a movement should elicit the same central and autonomic activity as that recorded when the movement is actually performed. Meister *et al.* (2004) vividly showed that actually and mentally playing music on a silent keyboard yielded similar activation of the fronto-parietal network. Conklin *et al.* (2000) showed that the imagery of interrupted smoking was associated with increased heart rate of the smoker (also with increased negative mood due to frustration), whereas the imagery of completed smoking elicited the opposite autonomic response with more positive psychological satisfaction.

The autonomic nervous system: a witness of mental and motor imagery

Motor imagery is usually defined as a dynamic mental state during which the representation of a given motor act is internally rehearsed in working memory without any overt motor output (Decety 1996). More recently, Stevens (2005) defined this construct as 'a class of images of one's own bodily movements which are used to simulate or plan for subsequent action', thus underlining the close relationship between movement imagination and preparation. One may add to this definition that the mental image is self-formed by the subject who does not need any external help to generate the representation of the action (e.g., a kind of pre-cueing which could serve the construction of the mental image). The motor image originates from an internal model of movement, resulting from mental operations of generating sequential actions or recalled from procedural memory in which the action planning is stored. Motor skills require being planned and programmed before being physically executed (Paillard 1982). If this is an obvious function of the central nervous system, motor preparation also involves the ANS for providing energy that makes movement execution possible. The ANS has features that make this system the natural 'first principle' from which initiation of action can arise (Peters 2000). In studying how elite pistol shooters prepare themselves just before shooting, Tremayne and Barry (2001) recorded electrodermal and cardiac activities. Electrodermal activity varied as a function of arousal before the shot, attesting the regulation of energy exertion to the specific task requirements. Another interesting result is that the pre-shot electrodermal levels were lower for the best performances, as compared with the worst shots. These variations in electrodermal activity were paralleled by a pre-shot cardiac deceleration, which was longer and more systematic for best than poor shots. As previously mentioned (Porges 1995a), cardiac deceleration has clearly been linked with attention processes (see also, for review, Jennings and Van der Molen 2005; Bradley 2009). These critical findings underline that reliable information is obtained from the ANS activity, the first being related to variations of arousal, and the second being associated with more qualitative processes such as focusing attention. These two variations are interpreted in terms of two separate, although closely linked, processes – arousal and vigilance (Näätänen 1973). This was well-illustrated by studying the autonomic correlates of motor preparation in elite weightlifters, who clearly subdivided the concentration phase into a period of vigilance, immediately followed by a period of increased arousal (Collet et al. 2006). These two concentration phases resulted in specific variations of cardiac activity, bradycardia being first observed (phasic activity), before the heart rate increased progressively as an index of body resources mobilization (tonic activity). As a matter of fact, behaviour might result from programming motor commands at both the somatic and the autonomic levels of the central nervous system, and is therefore co-programmed, as previously suggested by Mogenson (1977). Consequently, motor imagery can be the first stage of movement as preparing the execution can include mental sequences during which several parts of the movement or even the entire movement is rehearsed. Thus, the action previously imagined has a high probability to make the sympathetic activity increasing. The first effect of motor imagery is to make the ANS mobilizing energy as if the movement would be actually performed. Hence, it becomes quite difficult to distinguish between movement preparation and mental representation of movement. In a study involving elite air rifle shooters, Deschaumes-Molinaro et al. (1992) showed that the concentration phase before shooting elicited autonomic responses very close to those recorded during the forthcoming actual shooting. The almost identical nature of ANS responses during the concentration and the actual shooting periods provided evidence that elite shooters recalled memorized routines of shooting by imagining the forthcoming motor sequences, with the aim to better control the execution stages using motor imagery. Furthermore, it was very interesting to establish that the performance was higher when the autonomic response of the concentration period fitted with that of the execution (Deschaumes-Molinaro et al. 1991). Autonomic activity was recorded from several physiological indices including heart rate and respiratory frequencies, electrodermal activity and skin temperature, and was quantified using classical measurement of response amplitude and duration. Each measurement performed during the concentration period was divided by the corresponding value recorded during actual execution. In other words, and as responses from each phase were closely correlated, the resulting ratio was always around 1. Autonomic responses were then processed in a way that data from each elite shooter resulted in a single autonomic index made of the mean of all ratios. Shooters of the highest level exhibited the ratio closest to 1. In case of poor performance, the ratio was less than 1, suggesting that the average autonomic response was weaker during the concentration period than during the execution. As a consequence, the quality of motor imagery preceding shooting was evaluated as being insufficient to provide efficient behavioural output. Alternatively, autonomic response analysis was considered an important factor of the final motor performance analysis and could be used to control mental rehearsal during training sessions.

By analysing elite shooters' autonomic responses, we already underlined that motor imagery performed during the preparation phase elicited tonic changes attesting to variations in arousal. This was also evidenced in a more simple motor activity like walking. Decety *et al.* (1991) measured cardiac and respiratory activity during actual and mental locomotion as a function of increasing speeds. Wuyam *et al.* (1995) also used locomotion on a treadmill to examine the variation elicited by motor imagery on respiration rate. In both experiments, heart rate and respiratory frequency increased proportionately with the mental effort of the imagery experience. The same autonomic variables served at evaluating the mental effort attached to the motor imagery of swimming over a distance of 100m (Beyer *et al.* 1990). Both variables increased during the motor imagery session as compared to the control condition, i.e. rest. Overall, there are many other experimental results in which motor imagery performance correlated with variations of autonomic indicators. Bolliet *et al.* (2005b) showed high and rapid tonic variations in heart rate in a group of elite weightlifters. The heart rate increased by about a mean of 30% as early as the athletes were called by the referee for lifting. When the weightlifters were requested to imagine the same situation, a similar pattern of physiological variation was observed, although to a lesser extent. Interestingly, changes in heart rate were paralleled by those in skin resistance, which decreased during the same period, and were thus interpreted as an index of increasing arousal. This autonomic response to imagined movement was also found by Wang and Morgan (1992) in the same type of task (imagining lifting dumbbells), albeit with different autonomic indicators – respiration rate and systolic blood pressure showing increased values by comparison to the control condition. Fusi *et al.* (2005) also confirmed that imagined walking led to a significant, albeit small (less than 10%), increase in ventilation and oxygen consumption, and to larger increases (up to 40%) in respiratory rate, which was paralleled by a non-significant trend towards a decline of tidal volume. Based on the results mentioned above, there is now sufficient experimental matter to provide evidence of a close correlation between motor imagery and ANS variations. Two studies by Oishi (Oishi and Maeshima 2004; Oishi *et al.* 2000) drew the same conclusion, with larger changes in heart rate and respiration. Both also provided evidence to the sensitivity of the electrodermal activity, a less-used index from the ANS than those usually recorded, for example from the cardio-respiratory function.

The particular case of electrodermal activity (EDA)

The electrodermal activity (EDA) is one of the oldest physiological indices as it was recorded for the first time at the end of the nineteenth century, and was believed to provide information about mental states (Féré 1888; Tarchanoff 1890). Early called galvanic skin response, the term 'electrodermal' is now preferred for describing the electrical changes of the skin, using skin conductance or skin resistance (one being the reverse of the other) with the international units, Siemens and Ohm, respectively. This physiological variable is of particular interest. On the one hand, variations of EDA result from the activity of the eccrine sweat glands, and, on the other, EDA is under the control of the sympathetic branch only. There is no parasympathetic innervation of sweat glands, certainly because the reverse action of sweating is simply obtained when the command to the sympathetic endings has stopped. As depending upon the sympathetic nervous sub-system, sweat glands activity thus reflects the general arousal and changes in arousal due to emotional-significant stimuli, which could have both internal and external origins. Increase in EDA is represented by increase in skin conductance or decrease in skin resistance, and often parallels cardiovascular arousal (increases in heart rate and blood pressure).

Motor preparation and motor activity are generally accompanied by an increase in EDA (Critchley 2002), as motor imagery is. These motor-related autonomic responses are mediated, in part, by commands from the central nervous system, which make the sympathetic arousal varying according to the information significance. Results by Vissing (1997) confirmed that sympathetic activation of skin is predominantly influenced by central motor commands. Thus, EDA is a sensitive psycho-physiological index of changes in autonomic sympathetic arousal that are integrated with sensory-motor, emotional, and cognitive states. In the studies by Oishi *et al.* (Oishi and Maeshima 2004; Oishi *et al.* 2000), a significant decrease in skin resistance was associated with increased heart rate and respiration rates as early as the motor imagery session started, when compared to the control condition. After acknowledging the close correlation between motor imagery and its peripheral functional substrate, we can also examine the use of the ANS variables in the evaluation of motor learning, particularly when learning procedures include motor imagery. The question of evaluating the individual ability to form accurate mental images of an overt action with the help of autonomic variables will also be asked. Roure *et al.* (1998) integrated motor imagery sessions within learning sequences with the aim to improve a complex motor skill. The authors recorded EDA along the training sessions. The participants were assigned into three groups: the physical training group, the imagery-training group, and the control group. The subjects of the imagery group were asked for additional imagery training. However, the combination of mental and physical work in the motor imagery group was comparable to that of the physical group in order to have equal amount of training and equal time of exposure to the task. The participants of the motor imagery group significantly outperformed those of the physical group during the retention test, while the performance of the control group remained stable.

Using Autonomic Nervous System (ANS) responses to evaluate motor imagery

The role of motor imagery in motor learning was evidenced for a long time (Feltz and Landers 1983), and later confirmed many times (see Lotze and Halsband 2006, for review). However, few studies have been based upon the use of ANS responses to control and evaluate the effectiveness of motor imagery during learning. The study by Papadelis *et al.* (2007) revealed significantly higher performance level of the imagery-training group than the control group, thus supporting the efficiency of motor imagery when integrating into training sessions. Heart rate and respiratory rate significantly increased during imagery sessions as compared to rest. While cardio-respiratory recording was considered a witness of mental rehearsal, however, little was known regarding how these variables evolve along the learning process. Roure *et al.* (1998) were interested in this issue during the learning of a complex motor skill. After a first test devised to determine the basal performance level of each participant, the training period included a series of 15 motor imagery sessions, until the retention test. The authors also recorded several autonomic variables during mental training sessions, and used the EDA to control motor imagery quality and adjust the resulting load each subject could undergo during one session of mental rehearsal (Roure *et al.* 1999). As the autonomic response pattern recorded during motor imagery resembled that observed during actual execution, this was taken as reference for mental rehearsal. Thus, response amplitude and duration recorded during each mental trial should match those of the actual execution: this was taken as criteria for efficient mental work. In case of difference, the subjects were advised to change the focus of attention during motor imagery training and were given recommendations about important cues on which attention should be oriented to improve execution. In addition, response amplitude and duration were also used to adjust the number of successive mental repetitions, i.e., to control the mental load of a training session. Motor imagery requires high mental demand and cannot be continued for too much time. Consequently, as early as response duration and amplitude decreased, in course of time disappearing suddenly, the experimenters considered the mental abilities to be exceeded. Although the subjects were engaged in mental work and told that they tried to imagine the movement, the physiological response analysis attested that the mental work was no more effective during these trials. In other words, autonomic responses were a mean to evaluate the efficiency of mental rehearsal and then to adapt mental training to each subject's ability. After 15 training sessions, the retention test was performed. Interestingly, the authors reported that actual response duration and amplitude decreased simultaneously to the motor skill improvement. This was interpreted as a sign of motor automation, the more automated the skill, the weak the mental load resulting from actual execution. Consequently, as autonomic response that correlates to motor imagery matches that recorded during actual execution, it should also decrease across time as an indicator of movement automation. During the post-test, a significant decrease was observed in autonomic responses as compared to the pre-test. Electrodermal response duration in the group that engaged in motor imagery practice decreased from 12s to 8s, whereas the same response remained stable in the control group, about 10s. As expected, this pattern was associated with better skilled performance on the one hand, and with decrease in the resulting strain due to movement automation, on the other (Roure *et al.* 1999).

More recently, autonomic responses also served to pre-select participants having individual imagery ability ranging from good to excellent. Guillot *et al.* (2008) hypothesized that difference in motor imagery abilities were supported by structural differences in the central nervous system. To test this assumption, they compared the pattern of cerebral activations in 13 skilled and 15 unskilled imagers during both physical execution and motor imagery of a sequence of finger movements. Differences in motor imagery abilities were assessed using a combination of some well-established tools, i.e. motor imagery questionnaire as well as mental chronometry tests (according to the well-known principle of isochrony – for a review, see Guillot and Collet 2005). To have a more objective evaluation of motor imagery abilities, however, they also included measurements of the ANS activity directly associated with mental chronometry sessions. Pooled together, these evaluations can be considered a thorough procedure in selecting the best imagers, and autonomic activity analysis brings additional information to usual tests based on questionnaires mainly.

Another question that has been early addressed to the psycho-physiological ANS responses to imagined exercise is related to the imagery perspectives, i.e. internal imagery versus external (Wand and Morgan 1992). Surprisingly, among the amount of central investigations (using fMRI or other techniques), this concern was belatedly raised in the 2000 (Solodkin *et al.* 2004; Guillot *et al.* 2009; see also Olsson *et al.* 2008). Despite the extensive overlap of neural networks mediating visual and kinaesthetic imagery, Solodkin *et al.* (2004) highlighted the role of the connection of the superior parietal lobule to the supplementary motor area in both types of motor imagery. In the same way, Guillot *et al.* (2009) provided evidence that motor-related regions and the inferior and superior parietal lobules were the common neural substrate of visual and kinaesthetic imagery. However, visual imagery activated predominantly the occipital regions and the superior parietal lobules, whereas kinaesthetic imagery yielded more activity in motor-associated structures and the inferior parietal lobule. The study by Wang and Morgan (1992) provided evidence of autonomic changes during motor imagery that were identical to those observed during actual exercise, as previously mentioned. However, oxygen consumption, respiratory rate, respiratory exchange ratio, heart rate, and diastolic blood pressure were similar during internal and external imagery. Such inconsistencies may come from the different time scales between the central and peripheral changes. Central processes assessed by fMRI are nearly in real-time whereas peripheral responses exhibit temporal inertia due to the transmission of commands to the effectors, and to the physiological change itself at the level of the effectors, for example variation in blood pressure. Few experiences have thus been conducted to address this question and new experimental designs, involving other ANS variables such as electrodermal activity, should probably challenge this interesting issue.

The effects of mental practice on motor performance could be explained by the existence of a top-down mechanism based on the activation of a central representation of movements, since the autonomic activation during motor imagery seems to be centrally controlled (Decety *et al.* 1993; Fusi *et al.* 2005). Far from the dated view related to ANS functioning, peripheral indicators from autonomic effectors provide evidence of a close correlation with cognition. The sympathetic outflow to the heart is modulated by the activity of the anterior cingulate cortex, and the cardiovagal activity is under the control of the ventral medial prefrontal cortex (Wong *et al.* 2007). These two cortical structures are known to control both emotional states and cognition. To the same extent, higher control of EDA is mediated by neural networks involving prefrontal, insular, parietal cortices, and limbic structures including cingulate and medial temporal lobe with the amygdala and the hippocampus (Critchley 2005). The neural substrate for these peripheral autonomic responses is associated with motivational and affective states which, in turn, mediate motor imagery. Taken as a whole, recording EDA, as well as other autonomic variables at the peripheral level, provides an opened window on high brain functions (Collet and Guillot 2009). These indices can obviously contribute to the study of motor imagery among various other neurophysiological and psychological methods (Guillot and Collet 2005).

Although the relationships between motor imagery and the ANS have been established, an important question remains as motor commands to somatic effectors are inhibited during motor imagery, while those targeted autonomic effectors are not. There is thus a potential dissociation of efferences within the process of co-programming that needs to be clarified.

Somatic and autonomic motor commands inhibition during motor imagery

Defining motor imagery as the representation of movement without any overt action supposes that the imager remains motionless. Thus, no physiological activity should be recorded in the muscles involved in the rehearsed action, although this has been widely discussed (see Chapter 6 in this book). To investigate the changes of the motoneuron excitability during mental simulation of a voluntary movement, Oishi and Maeshima (2004) recorded the soleus H-reflex. The amplitude of H-reflex was almost constant before motor imagery initiation but was drastically reduced just after the motor imagery started, and lasted until the end of motor imagery. They concluded that the descending neural mechanisms that reduce motoneuron excitability are activated when full, vivid motor imagery is performed. The neural commands for muscular contractions are probably blocked at some level of the motor system that inhibits motor execution. However, a slight electromyographic (EMG) activity has often been observed during the imagination of movement. Such changes may result from tonic contractions while subjects performed motor imagery, and should thus be considered artefacts. However, Jeannerod (1994) early postulated that incomplete inhibition of the motor command would provide a valid explanation to account for these muscular discharges. Recent data are in favour of this latter hypothesis. When considering the different types of muscular contraction (isometric, concentric, and eccentric), Guillot *et al.* (2007) provided evidence of selective changes in EMG activity. Imagining an eccentric contraction elicited a significant weaker activity than all other conditions. Interestingly, the changes in the EMG pattern mirrored those observed during physical movement, thus supporting the hypothesis of a selective effect of motor imagery at the level of muscular activity, and of an incomplete inhibition of the motor command. Although ANS response amplitude and duration are usually reduced when the movement is mentally performed by comparison to its actual execution, the ANS activity is far to be inhibited (Collet and Guillot 2009). The rationale for the absence of inhibition of autonomic commands is probably related to the anticipated function of the ANS. Autonomic motor programming would anticipate both the need for energetic mobilization required by the planned movement and the amount of activity needed in the motor pathways to perform the movement. The combination of the motor command inhibition with the absence of inhibition of the ANS responses leads to suppose a relative independence of somatic and autonomic commands at the level of the central motor system or, at least, a dissociation of somatic and autonomic co-programming during motor imagery. This assumption is a working hypothesis waiting for further experimental investigation, but there is high probability that autonomic responses accompanying mental representation may serve as reference because they constitute a set of information provided to the sensorial systems as internal feedbacks. Autonomic responses act as somatic markers which give information to the individual and help him (her) in decision making (Damasio 1996). Finally, with reference to early theories related to biofeedback (Schwartz 1976), learning to self-regulate these patterns of autonomic responses may serve subjective experience and enhance the effectiveness of biofeedback procedures by training the individuals to integrate and coordinate specific patterns of cognitive, autonomic, and motor responses.

At the level of chemical modifications, Wuyam *et al.* (1995) also reported a reduction in end-tidal $P_{(CO2)}$. While there is ample evidence that residual micro-contractions may accompany motor imagery, even when the instruction is to remain motionless, recent data do not lead to the conclusion that motor imagery has changed peripheral metabolic parameters. This issue was early addressed by Decety *et al.* (1993), who measured muscle metabolism directly by nuclear magnetic resonance spectroscopy while motor imagery was carried out.

Cardio-respiratory activity was also monitored during both actual and mental leg exercise, and was increased simultaneously with muscle metabolic parameters during actual exercise: drop in phosphocreatine (PCr), increase in inorganic phosphate (Pi) concentrations, and fall in intracellular pH to 6.65. End-tidal $P_{(CO2)}$ was unaltered. Under the motor imagery condition, cardio-respiratory activity was comparable to that elicited during actual exercise. Conversely, the metabolic parameters remained unchanged. The end-tidal $P_{(CO2)}$ decreased progressively to about 18% of the resting value during mental simulation due to greater elimination of CO_2 during hyperventilation without increase in CO_2 production. This result was later confirmed by Fusi *et al.* (2005). Monitoring of autonomic changes thus demonstrated that the cardio-respiratory activation during motor imagery was greater than that required by the increase in metabolic demands. These results are also in favour of dissociation between somatic and autonomic commands. Research should now progress in the direction of a better understanding of the processes of motor commands inhibition in association with ANS commands. Whereas a large amount of research focused on demonstrating the close correlation between actual and imagined execution, research should now be perhaps reoriented to provide insight to the structural and functional neural substrate differentiating motor representation of movement from its actual execution, just before the motor commands are sent within the motor pathways.

Conclusion

Motor imagery is one of the more sophisticated mental operations making the subjects engage in predictive activities, drawing plans, and anticipating the possible consequences of being actualized. To react appropriately in social relationships, we also have a tendency to simulate how others think of us through mental imagery. These brain operations are accompanied by a set of physiological modifications which may be recorded at the level of peripheral effectors. These may be used by researchers to evaluate such mental states indirectly, thus constructing an inferential model of brain functioning. Among them, variables from the ANS have a good reliability because they correlate mental functioning in a specific way. Until the two past decades, the ANS was rather considered to control general physiological changes related to variations in arousal. If this basic function still remains to serve behaviours related to survival, the modern view of its anatomical organization has enlarged its function to a more complex social regulation: 'The evolution of the autonomic nervous system provides an organizing principle to interpret the adaptive significance of mammalian affective processes including courting, sexual arousal, and the establishment of enduring social bonds' (Porges 1998). Each mental operation, including motor imagery, is thus reflected within a part of our nervous system which is inaccessible to our will and consciousness, but reveals a part in the form of specific and structured physiological variations.

References

Berntson, G.G., Cacioppo, J.T., and Quigley, K.S. (1991). Autonomic determinism: the modes of autonomic control, the doctrine of autonomic space and the laws of autonomic constraint. *Psychological Review*, **98**, 459–87.

Beyer, L., Weiss, T., Hansen, E., Wolf, A., and Seidel, A. (1990). Dynamics of central nervous activation during motor imagination. *International Journal of Psychophysiology*, **9**, 75–80.

Bichat, M.F.X. (1802). *General Anatomy Applied to Physiology and Medicine*. Paris: Brosson, Gabon and Cie.

Bolliet, O., Collet, C., and Dittmar, A. (2005a). Observation of action and autonomic nervous system responses. *Perceptual and Motor Skills*, **101**, 195–202.

Bolliet, O., Collet, C., and Dittmar, A. (2005b). Actual versus simulated preparation in weightlifting: a neurovegetative study. *Applied Psychophysiology and Biofeedback*, **30**, 11–20.

Bradley, M.M. (2009). Natural selective attention: orienting and emotion. *Psychophysiology*, **46**, 1–11.

Cannon, W.B. (1915). *Bodily Changes in Pain, Hunger, Fear and Rage*. New York: Appleton.

Collet, C., Guillot, A., Bolliet, O., and Dittmar, A. (2006). Neurovegetative correlates of preparation in weightlifting. *International Journal of Sports Physiology and Performance*, **1**, 373–85.

Collet, C. and Guillot, A. (2009). Peripheral responses elicited by motor imagery: a window on central and peripheral nervous system relationships related to motor inhibition, in S.P. Weingarten and H.O. Penat (eds), *Cognitive Psychology Research Developments*, 245–59.

Conklin, C.A., Tiffany, S.T., and Vrana, S.R. (2000). The impact of imagining completed versus interrupted smoking on cigarette craving. *Experimental and Clinical Psychopharmacology*, **8**, 68–74.

Critchley, H.D. (2002). Electrodermal responses: what happens in the brain? *Neuroscientist*, **8**, 132–42.

Damasio, A.R. (1996). The somatic marker hypothesis and the possible functions of the prefrontal cortex. *Philosophical Transactions of the Royal Society B: Biological Sciences*, **351**, 1413–20.

Decety, J., Jeannerod, M., Germain, M., and Pastène, J. (1991). Vegetative response during imagined movement in proportional to mental effort. *Behavioural Brain Research*, **42**, 1–5.

Decety, J., Jeannerod, M., Durozard, D., and Baverel, G. (1993). Central activation of autonomic effectors during mental simulation of motor actions in man. *Journal of Physiology (London)*, **461**, 549–63.

Decety, J. (1996). The neurophysiological basis of motor imagery. *Behavioural Brain Research*, **77**, 45–52.

Deschaumes-Molinaro, C., Dittmar, A., and Vernet-Maury E. (1991). Relationship between mental imagery and sporting performance. *Behavioural Brain Research*, **45**, 29–36.

Deschaumes-Molinaro, C., Dittmar, A., and Vernet-Maury, E. (1992). Autonomic nervous system response patterns correlate with mental imagery. *Physiology and Behaviour*, **51**, 1021–7.

Feltz, D.L., and Landers, D.M. (1983). The effects of mental practice on motor skill learning and performance: a meta-analysis. *Journal of Psychology*, **5**, 25–57.

Féré, C. (1888). Note about the modifications of electrical tension in the human body. *Comptes rendus de la Société de Biologie*, **5**, 217–19.

Fusi, S., Cutuli, D., Valente, M.R., Bergonzi, P., Porro, C.A., and Di Prampero, P.E. (2005). Cardioventilatory responses during real or imagined walking at low speed. *Archives Italiennes de Biologie*, **143**, 223–8.

Guillot, A. and Collet, C. (2005). Contribution from neurophysiological and psychological methods to the study of motor imagery. *Brain Research Review*, **50**, 387–97.

Guillot, A., Collet, C., Nguyen, V.A., Malouin, F., Richards, C., and Doyon, J. (2008). Functional neuroanatomical networks associated with expertise in motor imagery. *NeuroImage*, **41**, 1471–83.

Guillot, A., Lebon, F., Rouffet, D., Champely, S., Doyon, J., and Collet C. (2007). Muscular responses during motor imagery as a function of muscle contraction types. *International Journal of Psychophysiology*, **66**, 18–27.

Guillot, A., Collet, C., Nguyen, V.A., Malouin, F., Richards, C., and Doyon, J. (2009). Brain activity during visual versus kinaesthetic imagery: an fMRI study. *Human Brain Mapping*, **30**, 2157–72.

Hesslow, G. (2002). Conscious thought as simulation of behaviour and perception. *Trends in Cognitive Science*, **6**, 242–7.

Hugdahl, K. (1996). Cognitive influences on human autonomic nervous system function. *Current Opinion in Neurobiology*, **6**, 252–8.

Iacoboni, M., Woods, R.P., Brass, M., Bekkering, H., Mazziotta, J.C., and Rizzolatti, G. (1999). Cortical mechanisms of human imitation. *Science*, **286**, 2526–8.

Jänig, W. and McLachlan E.M. (1992a). Characteristics of function-specific pathways in the sympathetic nervous system. *Trends in Neuroscience*, **15**, 475–81.

Jänig, W. and McLachlan E.M. (1992b). Specialized functional pathways are the building blocks of the autonomic nervous system. *Journal of the Autonomic Nervous System*, **41**, 3–13.

Jänig, W. and Häbler, H.J. (2000). Specificity in the organization of the autonomic nervous system: a basis for precise neural regulation of homeostatic and protective body functions. *Progress in Brain Research*, **122**, 351–67.

Jänig, W. and Häbler, H.J. (2003). Neurophysiological analysis of target-related sympathetic pathways – from animal to human: similarities and differences. *Acta Physiologica Scandinavica*, **177**, 255–74.

Jeannerod, M. (1994). The representing brain: neural correlates of motor intention and imagery. *Behavioural Brain Sciences*, **17**, 187–245.

Jennings, J.R. and van der Molen, M.W. (2005). Preparation for speeded action as a psychophysiological concept. *Psychological Bulletin*, **131**, 434–59.

Karli, P. (1977). Aggressive behaviour, in M. Blanc (ed.), Neurobiology Research. pp. 231–55. Paris: Seuil, Points Science.

Lotze, M. and Halsband, U. (2006). Motor imagery. *Journal of Physiology (Paris)*, **99**, 386–95.

Kummer, W. (1992). Neuronal specificity and plasticity in the autonomic nervous system. *Anatomischer Anzeiger (Annals of anatomy)*, **174**, 409–17.

McCorry, L.K. (2007). Physiology of the autonomic nervous system. *American Journal of Pharmaceutical Education*, **71**, article 78, 1–11.

Meister, I.G., Krings, T., Foltys, H., Müller, M., Töpper, R., and Thron, A. (2004). Playing piano in the mind – an fMRI study on music imagery and performance in pianists. *Cognitive Brain Research*, **19**, 219–28.

Mogenson, G.J. (1977). The Neurobiology of Behaviour: An Introduction. Hillsdale: Lawrence Erlbaum Associates.

Morrison, S.F. (2001). Differential control of sympathetic outflow. *American Journal of Physiology: Regulatory, Integrative and Comparative Physiology*, **281**, R683–98.

Näätänen, R. (1973). The inverted-U relationship between activation and performance: a critical review, in S. Kornblum (ed.), *Attention and Performance IV*. pp. 155–74. New York: Academic Press.

Nyberg, L., Habib, R., McIntosh, A.R., and Tulving, E. (2000). Reactivation of encoding-related brain activity during memory retrieval. *Proceedings of the National Academies of Science USA*. **97**, 11120–4.

Olsson, C.J., Jonsson, B., Larsson, A., and Nyberg, L. (2008). Motor representations and practice affect brain systems underlying imagery: an FMRI study of internal imagery in novices and active high jumpers. *The Open Neuroimaging Journal*, **2**, 5–13.

Oishi, K. and Maeshima, T. (2004). Autonomic nervous system activities during motor imagery in elite athletes. *Journal of Clinical Neurophysiology*, **21**, 170–9.

Oishi, K., Kasai, T., and Maeshima, T. (2000). Autonomic response specificity during motor imagery. *Journal of Physiological Anthropology and Applied Human Science*, **19**, 255–61.

Paccalin, C. and Jeannerod, M. (2000). Changes in breathing during observation of effortful actions. *Brain Research*, **862**, 194–200.

Paillard, J. (1982). Apraxia and the neuro-physiology of motor control. *Philosophical Transactions of the Royal Society of London, (biology)*, **B298**, 111–34.

Papadelis, C., Kourtidou-Papadeli, C., Bamidis, P., and Albani, M. (2007). Effects of imagery training on cognitive performance and use of physiological measures as an assessment tool of mental effort. *Brain and Cognition*, **64**, 74–85.

Peters, M. (2000). The importance of autonomic nervous system function for theories of cognitive brain function. *Brain and Cognition,* **42,** 93–4.

Porges, S.W. (1995a). Orienting in a defensive world: mammalian modifications of our evolutionary heritage. A Polyvagal Theory. *Psychophysiology*, **32**, 301–18.

Porges, S.W. (1995b). Cardiac vagal tone: a physiological index of stress. *Neuroscience and Biobehavioral Reviews*, **19**, 225–33.

Porges, S.W. (1998). Love: an emergent property of the mammalian autonomic nervous system. *Psychoneuroendocrinology*, **23**, 837–61.

Roure R., Collet C., Deschaumes-Molinaro C., *et al*. (1998). Autonomic nervous system responses correlate with mental rehearsal in volleyball training. *European Journal of Applied Physiology and Occupational Physiology*, **78**, 99–108.

Roure, R., Collet, C., Deschaumes-Molinaro, C., Delhomme, G., Dittmar, A., and Vernet-Maury, E. (1999). Imagery quality estimated by autonomic response is correlated to sporting performance enhancement. *Physiology and Behavior*, **66**, 63–72.

Schwartz, G.E. (1976). Self-regulation of response patterning: implications for psychophysiological research and therapy. *Biofeedback and Self Regulation*, **1**, 7–30.

Sokolov, E.N. (1963). *Perception and the conditioned reflex*. London: Pergamon Press.

Solodkin, A., Hlustik, P., Chen, E.E., and Small, S.L. (2004). Fine modulation in network activation during motor execution and motor imagery. *Cerebral Cortex*, **14**, 1246–55.

Stevens, J.A. (2005). Interference effects demonstrate distinct roles for visual and motor imagery during the mental representation of human action. *Cognition*, **95**, 329–50.

Tarchanoff, G. (1890). About galvanic skin response from the excitation of sensorial organs and different psychic activities. *Pflügers Archives*, **46**, 46–55.

Tremayne, P. and Barry, R.J. (2001). Elite pistol shooters: physiological patterning of best vs. worst shots. *International Journal of Psychophysiology*, **41**, 19–29.

Vallbo, A.B., Hagbarth, K.E., and Wallin, B.G. (2004). Microneurography: how the technique developed and its role in the investigation of the sympathetic nervous system. *Journal of Applied Physiology*, **96**, 1262–9.

Vissing, S.F. (1997). Differential activation of sympathetic discharge to skin and skeletal muscle in humans. *Acta Physiologica Scandinavica (Suppl.)*, **639**, 1–32.

Wallin, B.G. (1981). Sympathetic nerve activity underlying electrodermal and cardiovascular reactions in man. *Psychophysiology*, **18**, 470–6.

Wallin, B.G. and Fagius, J. (1986). The sympathetic nervous system in man: aspects derived from microelectrodes recordings. *Trends in Neurosciences*, **2**, 63–7.

Wallin, B.G. and Fagius, J. (1988). Peripheral sympathetic neural activity in conscious humans. *Annual Review of Physiology*, **50**, 565–76.

Wang, Y. and Morgan, W.P. (1992). The effect of imagery perspectives on the psychophysiological responses to imagined exercise. *Behavioural Brain Research*, **52**, 167–74.

Wuyam, B., Moosavi, S.H., Decety, J., Adams, L., Lansing, R.W., and Guz, A. (1995). Imagination of dynamic exercise produced ventilatory responses which were more apparent in competitive sportsmen. *Journal of Physiology (London)*, **482**, 713–24.

Wong, S.W., Massé, N., Kimmerly, D.S., Menon, R.S., and Shoemaker, J.K. (2007). Ventral medial prefrontal cortex and cardiovagal control in conscious humans. *NeuroImage*, **35**, 698–708.

Chapter 8

Neurophysiological substrates of motor imagery ability

Aymeric Guillot, Magali Louis, and Christian Collet

Introduction

The previous chapters were designed to provide insight into the nature and the origin of motor imagery. This chapter will be based on such approaches, but will primarily focus on the use of physiological recordings that correlate with imagery accuracy and ability. Even though motor imagery might improve the performance and learning of a variety of motor tasks (for reviews, see Feltz and Landers 1983; Guillot and Collet 2008), the power of imagination is roughly dependent on the individual capacity to elicit efficient mental images. However, the ability to effectively produce accurate mental images is not universal and is subjected to wide individual differences (Isaac and Marks 1994). In other words, all individuals have the capacity to form mental images, but not to the same degree (Hall *et al.* 1998). While some subjects have trouble in forming the mental image of a movement, others might generate a very accurate mental representation of the same action. As suggested by Murphy *et al.* (2008), 'one's ability to imagine is probably the most well-acknowledged individual difference variable in imagery studies, as compared either to age, gender, level of participation or years of experience'. Accordingly, there is now ample evidence that the imagery-related benefits are dependent upon the individual imagery abilities. For example, we and other researchers have demonstrated that individuals encountered greater difficulty in using kinaesthetic imagery than visual imagery during the early learning stage of a new motor skill, but with practice they became more efficient at performing imagery in both modalities (Hardy and Callow 1999; Guillot *et al.* 2004). This section is thus specifically designed to summarize literature providing an objective assessment of motor imagery. As reported in a review by Guillot and Collet (2005b), a wide range of techniques can be used to measure individual imagery ability. Each of them will be taken into account in the present chapter. Even though there are few neuroimaging data, we will first focus on the pattern of brain activations in participants with good and poor motor imagery abilities. Then, we will consider the large amount of experimental data in which both behavioural and peripheral physiological recordings were monitored.

The concept of motor imagery ability

What is motor imagery ability and how can we measure it? At first glance, this is a fairly basic but important question. The apparent answer is that people are able to form vivid mental representation of a movement, and can describe the characteristics of this motor act, by providing, for example, the key-components of the mental image they are attempting to form. The correct answer, however, is not quite that simple, and research findings illustrate a more complex picture. Moreover, forming vivid and accurate mental representations remains a systematic problem that must be resolved by the experimenter. First, in the last decade, a very important number of data have been designed to show whether both motor learning and neurorehabilitation may benefit from motor imagery practice. A large amount of these experimental studies, however, did not give satisfactory information with regards to the procedure of imagery use. Furthermore, these studies did not indicate whether motor imagery was controlled, and whether the compliance of the participants with imagery instructions was well understood. Such methodological issues are sufficient to hinder the conclusions that one can reach. A valid and thorough testing procedure thus appears imperative to guarantee the individual imagery ability of the participants. Second, the concept of motor imagery ability and quality (or accuracy) refers to the content of the image. Hence, vividness and controllability are the two dimensions most often discussed (Murphy and Jowdy 1992; Moran 1993; Richardson 1994; Morris *et al.* 2005; Vealey and Greenleaf 1998). Vividness defines the intrinsic characteristics of the image, i.e. its clarity and richness, while controllability describes the ability to manipulate and transform the mental image, as well as its maintenance over time (Denis *et al.* 1985; Moran 1993). Also, the accuracy illustrates how imagery reflects the reality of the mental content. Finally, it is now well-established that the ease or difficulty that individuals encounter in preserving the temporal characteristics of the motor performance must be considered (for reviews, see Guillot and Collet 2005a; Malouin *et al.* 2008), as it may have considerable impact on subsequent motor performance duration (Louis *et al.* 2008). Before considering the neurophysiological substrates of motor imagery accuracy, we would like to review the four components of imagery quality mentioned above. One should also keep in mind that research illustrated the importance of teaching the correct technique to participants to improve the quality of their imagery experience (Murphy *et al.* 2008). Furthermore, it has been suggested that a reciprocal relationship may exist between imagery use and ability (Vadocz *et al.* 1997), i.e. participants with high imagery abilities are more likely to use motor imagery, while performing imagery subsequently bolsters imagery ability.

Vividness, controllability, and exactness

Vividness is probably the imagery ability dimension which has been the most extensively examined by researchers. Imagery is often defined as perceiving, but in the absence of the immediate appropriate sensory stimulation (Kosslyn *et al.* 2001). Accordingly, the imagery experience consists on forming the mental image of an earlier perceptual event (although it is possible to anticipate an event and to imagine something that has not been actually perceived). Vivid motor imagery will thus characterize a mental representation using detailed sensory cues, for example coloured and dynamic images of the movement, significant feeling and sensations of muscle contractions, accurate movement-related auditory information, or defined tactile sensations. Ideally, such mental simulation is very close to the actual experience of the movement itself, hence simultaneously increasing the exactness of motor imagery. The dimensions of imagery ability were well-described by Morris *et al.* (2005), and further assess the reality of the imagery experience as they depict the perceptual stimulation (for the structural and functional similarities between imagery and perception, see also Chapters 1 and 2 in this book). The controllability refers to the manipulation and the transformation of the image content. Such dimension is particularly important during mental rotation, as the participants have to mentally rotate a perceptual stimulus. As mental rotation is an incremental process, this might suggest that participants transform objects in their mind similarly as during actual practice (Wraga *et al.* 2003). One should keep in mind that mental images can 'easily' be transformed inadequately, and may thus alter the exactness of the imagery experience. In a well-known review of literature, Thompson and Kosslyn (2000) described the four operations of the nervous system that occur during imagery: generation, inspection, maintenance, and transformation of the image. In fact, imagery often consists of proposing images from stored information. Then, one must identify the shapes and spatial relations of these images. Finally, images should be maintained and even transformed, while passing through multiple positions. Whereas the vividness and the exactness of the imagery experience might predominantly refer to the generation and inspection of the image, controllability would be primarily linked to the maintenance and transformation of the perceptual image.

Temporal aspects of motor imagery

While the interest of researchers on motor imagery speed manipulation has been a recent development, a handful of experimental studies have now examined the similarities and differences between motor imagery duration and the time needed to physically execute the same action. In a well-known study using image-scanning paradigm, Kosslyn *et al.* (1978) provided evidence that more time was required to mentally scan longer distances. Similar chronometric patterns were also reported when mental scanning of representations was extracted from verbal descriptions (Denis *et al.* 1995). Interestingly, Cocude *et al.* (1999) demonstrated that participants with high visuospatial abilities were more efficient than those with poor ones. Regarding motor imagery *per se*, a similar temporal equivalence has been established through a large variety of motor tasks (e.g., Decety *et al.* 1989; Maruff and Velakoulis 2000), albeit not being systematic and still dependent on many external influencing factors (for review, see Guillot and Collet 2005a). On the basis of these findings, investigators have concluded that motor imagery is a valuable technique in improving motor performance, but only when motor imagery reflects every aspect (including speed) of the actual movement (Guillot and Collet 2005a; Calmels *et al.* 2006). More importantly, Louis *et al.* (2008) demonstrated that changing motor imagery speed (voluntarily or not) was sufficient to elicit changes in the timing of actual movements. Their results also indicated a similar outcome for highly automated motor tasks, such as in sport skills for which action timing has already been fixed and controlled for years, hence highlighting the importance of controlling motor imagery speed. The authors further pointed that caution should be exercised before generalizing the necessity to imagine in real-time, as there are some instances where slow or fast imagery could also be beneficial. Altogether, both years of experience and motor imagery skill are thought to influence the individual's ability to reach and increase the temporal equivalence between actual and imagined durations (e.g., Reed 2002).

Measurement of motor imagery ability and accuracy

Self-report questionnaires and psychological evaluations

A substantial paper by Hall *et al.* (1985) reviewed the first experimental data dealing with the question of imagery ability measurement, since the early work of Galton (1880) on individual differences. The authors highlighted the inconsistencies emerging from the literature, and suggested the development of specific imagery tests. More recently, Morris *et al.* (2005) also addressed the question and proposed a classification of imagery-use measures. They notably described the psychological questionnaires used most often in experimental studies. Interestingly, Paivio (1986) reported that individual differences in imagery might result from the interaction between experience and genetic variability. As the second aspect remains difficult to establish, objectively, researchers have been primarily interested in determining whether it was possible to estimate wide individual differences in imagery ability. To do so, many psychological self-report questionnaires have been validated. These explicit measures of motor imagery usually require that participants engage in a motor imagery task, and rate the accuracy of their imagery experience. Usually, the score is given using a Likert-type rating scale to rate the ease or difficulty encountered during motor imagery. Two main kinds of questionnaires should be distinguished: those that measure motor imagery ability and those that evaluate motor imagery use (Hall *et al.* 1998). The questionnaires that assess motor imagery use are usually functional, easy and rapid to complete, and have been extensively proposed in many areas of research and practical applications including motor learning and rehabilitation (for reviews, see Guillot and Collet 2005b; Morris *et al.* 2005). The main question when using such questionnaires is related to subjectivity, as participants report their own representation of motor imagery accuracy. Hence, the use of complementary physiological recordings that correlate with the mental representation of actions has recently been proposed and will be specifically considered in the following sections of this chapter (Guillot and Collet 2005b; Lotze and Halsband 2006; Guillot *et al.* 2008, 2009).

Other measurement tools are post-imagery evaluations, debriefings, and participants' interviews, which are based on detailed manipulations checks. Such interventions usually aim at having explicit descriptions of the imagery content that the participant himself can obtain (through verbal, written, or even sketched form). For instance, it is interesting to know on which key component of the movement the participant focused during his imagery experience (for a review of these qualitative assessments, see Morris *et al.* 2005). Even though the subjectivity of the measure still exists, its use remains beneficial to achieve valid and useful findings.

Finally, a third method consists of requesting the participants to make a decision following the presentation of a stimulus. Though this is not systematic, the participants are understood to be engaged in motor imagery before giving their response, hence involving motor simulation and prospective action judgements. Firstly, the mental rotations tasks are reliable candidate to this type of paradigms. Mental rotation requires cognitive manipulation and spatial transformation of the object to imagine, while the participants are usually required to indicate whether pairs of visual 3-D stimuli, presented from two different angles, are identical or not (Shepard and Metzler 1971; for review, see Zacks 2008). The main findings arising from the literature were that response times increase linearly with the degree of orientation difference between the two stimuli. These conclusions also suggest that participants form a visual image of the object and rotate this image until equivalence with the reference has been reached. Secondly, it is also possible to ask the individuals to make a decision based on the laterality of a body part, or to ask them how they should act to grasp and use an object (e.g., De'Sperati and Stucchi 2000; Johnson 2000; Frak *et al.* 2001; Parsons 2001; Johnson-Frey 2004). In general, the results strongly support the hypothesis that prospective judgements about movement are based on motor simulation and feasibility, in a similar manner to that of actual movements. Their timing is affected by the same influencing factors than actual actions, such as biomechanical constraints and awkwardness of action. These latter measurements are of interest when assessing individual imagery abilities, while they do not evaluate the content of the imagery experience. Hence, conclusions emerging from analyses of responses, and both reaction and discrimination times, should be drawn cautiously, as one cannot be absolutely certain that participants are engaged in motor imagery *per se*.

To conclude, the techniques reviewed above seem to be partially limited, and thus remain restrictive to provide a thorough estimation of the motor imagery quality and ability. As recently suggested by Guillot and Collet (2005b), they should ideally be combined with more 'complementary and objective methods' to investigate the participants' ability to form and manipulate accurate mental images of the movement. Thereby, it appears necessary to assess physiological correlates of motor imagery, to provide a clearer quantification of the imagery content. Understanding the neural correlates of goal-directed action, whether executed or imagined, has been an important domain of cognitive brain research since the advent of functional neuroimaging studies. Such methodological advances have now opened up a space for studying the neural underpinnings of motor imagery in greater details, through a wide range of physiological recordings from both the central and peripheral nervous systems. Moreover, one may now have the opportunity to use biofeedback techniques and control the quality of motor imagery in real-time. Studies showing cases of brain-damaged patients are also likely to provide insight on the preservation or loss of the imagery content. The strengths and weaknesses of each complementary type of recordings will be discussed below, in the following section. Finally, data resulting from mental chronometry paradigms will be briefly reviewed to provide evidence of the crucial role of this measure.

Brain mapping techniques

A large amount of central measures related to the activity of the central nervous system can be recorded during motor imagery. Using these scanning techniques has a specific interest when mapping the anatomy and the physiology of the human brain. These techniques differ in their spatial and temporal resolutions, but are complementary when investigating the neural networks which mediate the imagery experience. Electroencephalography (EEG) is the measurement of the electrical activity of the brain as recorded from electrodes placed on the scalp. Magnetoencephalography (MEG) measures the magnetic fields produced by electrical activity in the brain via extremely sensitive devices. Both techniques have good temporal, but less spatial resolution. In contrast, magnetic resonance imaging (MRI) and positron emission tomography (PET) have good spatial, but poor temporal resolution. Functional MRI (fMRI) is a structural technique, with acceptable temporal resolution, that maps the structures of the brain following excitation of atoms through radio waves. Such methodology is capable of detecting haemodynamic changes throughout the brain through the blood-oxygen dependent level effect. PET is a more invasive method which detects positrons (atomic particles) emitted by radioactive isotopes injected into the blood on a biological active molecule. Finally, transcranial magnetic stimulation (TMS) has more recently been used to stimulate cortical neurons and measure the consequences in terms of motor excitability. Research with TMS has shown that motor imagery may lead to an increase in corticospinal excitability, which is muscle-specific and temporally modulated, and elicits a facilitation of motor-evoked potentials (for review, see Chapter 4 in this book).

We have learned from the relationships between both EEG and MEG recordings and motor imagery in Chapter 5. Generally speaking, the data indicate that similar cerebral structures are involved during both motor imagery and motor performance. Interestingly, Davidson and Schwartz (1977) compared the EEG activity during visual and kinaesthetic imagery, and provided evidence that visual imagery elicited greater activity in the occipital regions than kinaesthetic imagery. Martinez (2000) further reported that kinaesthetic imagery yielded more cortical activity than visual imagery, but failed to clearly identify two distinct neural networks. Also, Neuper et al. (2005) found that the focus of activity was close to the sensorimotor cortex during kinaesthetic imagery, whereas visual imagery did not result in detectable changes.

Typically, the conclusions from neuroimaging studies that compared the neural substrates mediating motor imagery with those involved in the preparation and execution of the motor act, also dovetailed the earlier findings from both behavioural and EEG experiments. For instance, fMRI and PET studies have extensively demonstrated that motor imagery and motor performance shared the same neural networks, including the motor systems, as well as the inferior and superior parietal lobules (Decety et al. 1994; Mellet et al. 1998; Lotze et al. 1999; Gerardin et al. 2000; Guillot et al. 2008). Specifically, the premotor cortex, the supplementary motor area, the precuneus, the putamen, and the cerebellum were found to have a critical role in the formation of the mental images. Even if there are some discrepancies, the primary motor cortex also seems to be activated during motor imagery (for reviews, see Lotze and Halsband 2006; Sharma et al. 2008; see also Chapter 3 in this book). Interestingly, Sharma et al. (2008) recently suggested that this structure may also contribute to the spatial encoding of the movement during imagery. Furthermore, Lafleur *et al.* (2002) and Jackson *et al.* (2003) demonstrated that the cerebral plasticity that occurs following physical practice was reflected during motor imagery, hence strongly supporting the principle of functional equivalence.

A limited number of researchers examined the content of motor imagery, and most specifically whether visual imagery and kinaesthetic imagery may recruit different neural networks. In a first study dealing with this issue, Binkofski *et al.* (2000) showed that the anterior part of the intraparietal sulcus was more active during kinaesthetic imagery of finger movements, while the posterior part was more involved during visual imagery. Also, when bilateral activations were reported during kinaesthetic imagery in the opercular portion of the ventral premotor cortex, a lack of activation in the parietal areas was observed. In two independent groups of participants, Solodkin *et al.* (2004) further investigated the effective connectivity in networks associated with physical execution: visual imagery (group 1) and kinaesthetic imagery (group 2) of hand movements. Even these latter types of imagery were found to share similar neural substrates, including the connection from the superior parietal lobule to the supplementary motor area; the main difference was found in the inputs from the superior parietal lobule and the supplementary motor area to the primary motor cortex, which were opposite to those observed during motor performance. More recently, Guillot *et al.* (2009) examined whether the same group of healthy participants with very good to excellent imagery abilities recruited similar or distinct brain activations during visual imagery and kinaesthetic imagery of hand movements. Visual imagery was found to activate predominantly the occipital regions and the precuneus, whereas kinaesthetic imagery produced more activity in motor-associated structures and the inferior parietal lobule.

Finally, despite accumulated evidence that the benefits of motor imagery are quite dependent upon the individual imagery abilities, there is very few data with respect to the pattern of brain activations involving participants with different motor imagery abilities. A remarkable neuroimaging study that indirectly touched upon this issue (but did not address it directly) comes from Lotze *et al.* (2003). They compared professional musicians and beginners during both imagery and motor performance of a violin concerto; however, their study focused more on highlighting the brain structures related to the effects of the subject's expertise level in music than on their capacity to produce efficient motor imagery. The recent study by Guillot *et al.* (2008) raised this question, and was designed to determine the neural substrates mediating motor imagery in good and poor imagers. Consistent with findings from the motor sequence learning literature (Doyon and Ungerleider 2002; Doyon and Benali 2005), the authors demonstrated that compared to skilled imagers, poor imagers not only needed to recruit the cortico-striatal system, but also to compensate with the cortico-cerebellar system during motor imagery of sequential movements. Interestingly, their findings also suggest that compared to poor imagers, good imagers would have a more efficient recruitment of movement engrams. Although this remains a working hypothesis awaiting further experimental investigation, the authors concluded that the pattern of cerebral activation recorded during motor imagery in poor imagers might improve and evolve close to that observed in the good imagers after imagery training.

In order to confirm this assumption, researchers may now take advantage of the methodological fMRI developments. For instance, such hypothesis could be tested by measuring the dynamic changes in cerebral activity using real-time fMRI. This technique provides a reconstruction of the raw data obtained with the brain scan, while the scan is happening. The participants can therefore receive a feedback of the pattern of brain activation in predetermined regions of interest. This design works even if an average 2–5s lapse time to the signal usually remains necessary, due to the physiological delay of the haemodynamic response (a more simple feedback can also be used, e.g. a score using a Likert-type scale). A significant illustration of the strength of this methodology has been offered by DeCharms *et al.* (2004) during motor imagery of a manual action task. In their study, the participants received feedback information about the level of activation in their somato-motor cortex with a simple virtual reality interface. The results showed that they were able to enhance the fMRI level of activation driven by motor imagery in the somatomotor cortex through the course of training. Moreover, the activation of this region after imagery training was found as robust as that recorded during actual practice. These data strongly support that real-time neuroimaging is a valuable and promising technique to investigate whether participants are able to use a cognitive strategy to control a target brain region in real-time.

Altogether, the results mentioned above clearly indicated that the neuroimaging techniques are highly useful to better understanding the relationships between motor imagery and physiological processes. Furthermore, the data not only provided insight on the neural underpinnings of motor imagery, but also contributed to distinguish among the neural substrates mediating motor imagery in participants with high and poor imagery abilities (Guillot *et al.* 2008). The remarkable research perspectives using real-time fMRI now offer new challenges to the investigators focusing on motor imagery, and more specifically on the cerebral plasticity occurring during mental practice. Also, as the neural networks mediating motor imagery are not identical in good and poor imagers, brain mapping data lead to the conclusion that it is imperative to evaluate the individual imagery ability to determine the optimal training conditions for learning how to use mental practice with motor imagery in neurological rehabilitation. However, since the reliability of these neuroimaging techniques is now well established, their contribution to exploring the foundations of motor imagery is also somewhat limited (Dietrich 2008). First, they cannot be used in the field as they are non-ambulatory methods. Second, the type and the amplitude of movements are limited. Usually, the actual motion must be small enough to avoid head movements. For these reasons, researchers primarily investigate finger, hand, feet, and/or tongue movements. The classical paradigms consist on performing either simple movements (flexion, extension, abduction or adduction, or making a fist), or finger-to-thumb opposition and tapping tasks. Finally, one should keep in mind that brain activations recorded during mental processes remain an inference of brain functioning, which is afterward associated to the content of the mental representation by the experimenter. These limitations must therefore be taken into account to draw cautious conclusions.

Autonomic nervous system activity

We have already learned about the strengths of recording the autonomic nervous system (ANS) activity during imagined actions in the Chapter 7. Here, we would like to primarily focus on the reliability of this methodology, more specially as it offers a possibility to objectively control and analyse the imagery experience in real time. As shown by Hugdahl (1996), higher brain functions can be studied through ANS effectors activity at a peripheral level. Furthermore, ANS parameters can be monitored continuously by non-invasive sensors at the level of the skin. For these reasons, this technique is most particularly adapted to applied research designed to study complex motor skills (Collet *et al.* 2003). In general, literature has provided converging evidence that similar autonomic responses occur during both motor imagery and motor performance. Interestingly, ANS response patterns have also been found to differentiate between good and poor imagers (Roure *et al.* 1999, Guillot *et al.* 2004). Accordingly, ANS responses were recorded after each motor imagery instruction in participants with high imagery ability, thus attesting to mental work during each trial. On the contrary, in individuals with poor imagery ability, ANS recording elicited weaker responses during initial trials which then tended to disappear with mental repetitions, and therefore confirmed that they did not succeed in forming a vivid mental representation of the movement.

Based on the two preliminary studies mentioned above, Guillot *et al.* (2008, 2009) tried to distinguish between subjects who were able to reach a high level of performance from those who were having trouble in using motor imagery. In parallel to imagery questionnaires and mental chronometry data, they recorded the patterns of ANS activity to calculate a global imagery score in order to select good and poor imagers for subsequent fMRI experiments. Specifically, two kinds of measures were provided. The number of ANS responses (phasic activity) was first calculated, and represented on a numeric scale (with reference to the principle that each imagery trial should elicit an autonomic response). In addition, the participant's level of arousal (tonic level) was assessed according to autonomic basal tonic evolution across the imagery session (the participant should remain aroused during the mental rehearsal session). To give equal importance to these two factors, the evolution of the arousal level was graded. The ANS score consisted of the sum of the two preceding measures, and was added (or subtracted) from the other scores (questionnaires and mental chronometry)[1]. Analysing respiratory sinus arrhythmia during the experiment could also be considered and included in this evaluation, as this physiological variable provides evidence of the individual ability to accurately focus attention during motor imagery (Roure et al. 1999). The association of these complementary evaluations has been found to be a valuable procedure to control motor imagery quality, hence guaranteeing the high or poor imagery abilities of the participants (Guillot and Collet 2005b; Lotze and Halsband 2006). Although ANS responses remain an inference of the central nervous system functioning, this thorough procedure is not only a reliable tool to predetermine the individual imagery ability, but may also be used as a potential biofeedback for the participant throughout the imagery training phase per se. For example, ANS recordings may help researchers to adjust in real-time the number of successive imagery trials to be performed when the physiological responses tend to disappear, and/or if the participant strongly decreases its level of arousal.

Peripheral muscular activity and postural data

In Chapter 6 of this book, we extensively described the electromyographic recordings during motor imagery, and we concluded that it is still premature to draw final conclusions, as the literature provided controversial results regarding the use of this physiological measurement to assess individual motor imagery ability. Hence, the electromyographic activity should not be considered a reliable indicator of motor imagery ability, nor of the imagery content, and future investigation is necessary to analyse this physiological activity during various conditions, and explain its origin in greater detail. Similarly, changes in postural control during motor imagery must be interpreted cautiously, due to few experimental investigations and discrepancies in the results. In fact, this topic of research has received limited attention, even though the main results indicated that motor imagery may have contributed to increase the postural control (Rodrigues *et al.* 2003; Guillot and Collet 2005b; Hamel and Lajoie 2005). More recently, Bakker *et al.* (2007, 2008) investigated the motor imagery of gait, as well as its cerebral correlates. They notably demonstrated that a motor imagery protocol might be very useful to explore the neurophysiological correlates of gait, both in healthy subjects and patients with gait disturbances. Altogether, one may assume that the anticipated postural adjustments preceding the action are not inhibited, and contribute to increase the postural control during motor imagery, even though the movement

---

[1] The global imagery score was calculated using this simple formula: (ANS score + imagery questionnaire score + auto-estimation score) – (mental chronometry score). The mental chronometry score was subtracted from the others as a great difference between imagined and actual times did indicate inaccurate motor imagery.

will not be performed. Despite these promising results, however, extreme caution should be exercised before drawing a parallel between the motor imagery-related influence on postural oscillations and the accuracy of the imagery content. At this time, future research is therefore necessary before considering the increase in postural control as a reliable indicator of MI accuracy.

Eye movements

An alternative approach has recently been (re)considered to provide an objective assessment of motor imagery. In fact, early researchers examined oculomotor behaviour during visual imagery, and reported some saccadic eye movements (Jacobson 1931; Totten 1935). Hebb (1968) even suggested that if imagery is the reinstatement of a perceptual process, it should include eye movements. However, other investigators did not find any eye movement during imagery (Shick 1970; Hale 1982), and the substantial results indicating that eye movement provide a window into the mind during imagery have only been obtained within the last decade. More specifically, many experiments have shown that eye movements during visual imagery are not epiphenomenal but should assist the process of image generation. For example, an important study by Laeng and Teodorescu (2002) provided evidence of high correlated patterns of oculomotor activity between perception and imagery. Interestingly, these authors systematically varied the visual stimulation. An absence of eye movement was observed in participants who maintained fixation studying the display, while those who visually explored the pattern made eye movements during imagery. As highlighted by Mast and Kosslyn (2002), it could be hypothesized that the participants used memories of eye movements to help the reconstruction of mental images. Eye movements should thus be stored in memory with the images encoded at each fixation (Kosslyn 1994), which is in line with the results by Spivey and Geng (2000), or Laeng and Teodorescu (2002), who confirmed that eye movements reflect the context of the stimulation, and that scanning eye paths during visual imagery is correlated to those of actual perception.

Similar results were reported during mental rotation tasks, thus supporting the hypothesis that eye movements may be considered a precise marker of the spatiotemporal evolution of the underlying mental processes (De'Sperati *et al.* 2003). In motor imagery *per se*, Rodionov *et al.* (2004) recorded eye movements during mental rotation of the body and showed that they may serve as an objective sign of individual performance. A famous study focusing on the oculomotor behaviours during motor imagery was recently published by Heremans *et al.* (2008). These authors clearly demonstrated that the coupling between neural patterns for eye and hand movements remained intact when hand movements were merely imagined, as opposed to physically being executed. Especially, eye movements during motor imagery with eyes open or closed showed remarkable similarities to those recorded during physical practice. The spatial and temporal coupling between eye and hand control systems may imply that there is a common representation of the target to be reached. Heremans *et al.* (2008) also confirmed that during motor imagery, as well as during actual perception, eyes movement anticipated the position of the hand when it virtually reached peak velocity, leaving sufficient time for correction processes to take place. In addition, and although Johansson *et al.* (2005) suggested that environmental visual features are used as visual indexes of mental image spatial location, the fact that Heremans *et al.* (2008) recorded eye movements during motor imagery with closed eyes demonstrates that they are inherent to the imagery process itself, instead of being triggered by visual cues. These authors concluded that eye movements may be used as a real-time indicator attesting that the participant actually performs motor imagery. Finally, Gueugneau *et al.* (2008) recently examined the timing of eye movements either during imagery with eyes free (eyes were free to move during imagined arm movements) or motionless. In other words, they investigated, whether eye movements during imagery were indispensable for the accurate prediction of arm motion, using a mental chronometry paradigm.

Their findings showed that the accuracy of imagined arm movements did not depend on the presence or absence of eye movements, thus restricting the functional role of oculomotor behaviours during imagery, as compared to observation.

Despite some discrepancies, eye movement recording is a promising method to assess objectively the motor imagery content. However, some limitations can still be underlined, and further investigation is needed to ascertain its reliability. First, the fact that all subjects do not exhibit eye movements remains problematic. Furthermore, experimental data is also warranted to check whether eye movement recordings are sensitive enough to distinguish between good and poor imagers, and thus to measure the motor imagery ability *per se*. In other words: Does a greater similarity of oculomotor behaviour during imagined and actual practice indicate either that the participant is performing its imagery experience accurately, or that his ability to form the mental images of the movement is high? Also, to date, few studies have delineated the role of eye movements during the motor imagery experience. Thus, further research is still necessary to test a wide range of perceptual stimuli. For instance, little is known regarding the occurrence of eye movements during imagery of self-generated movements, as well as during movements which are externally cued with a non-auditory way, or even during more complex and non-visual imagery tasks (Heremans *et al.* 2008). Finally, Mast and Kosslyn (2002) highlighted that it would be interesting to know what happens if the perceived stimulus is imagined in a different orientation from the one which is initially encoded.

Brain-damaged patient data

An increasing number of experimental studies have been conducted in brain-damaged patients during the last decade to investigate whether motor imagery may contribute to the recovery of motor functions (for reviews, see Jackson *et al.* 2001; Lotze and Cohen 2006; Sharma *et al.* 2006; De Vries and Mulder 2007). Also, researchers were generally interested to see whether patients were able to form the mental representation of movements following different types of lesions, in order to adjust the rehabilitation programmes in clinical settings. Taken overall, the results of motor imagery impairments in patients provide strong evidence about the important role of specific cerebral structures within the four operations of the nervous system during imagery (generation, inspection, maintenance, and transformation of the image), which were described by Thompson and Kosslyn (2000). Case reports of brain-damaged patients therefore appeared to substantially contribute to the understanding of the motor imagery underpinnings. It is noteworthy, however, to see that some patients may retain good motor imagery accuracy, hence suggesting that cortical lesions are not systematically associated with motor imagery impairments, and thus that caution must be exercised before drawing final conclusions. This general, topic of research will be extensively considered in the third part of this book, and researchers will most especially provide insight on the preservation or loss of the imagery content following a wide range of brain damages.

Mental chronometry

In the previous sections of this chapter, we reviewed the strengths and weaknesses of a wide range of neurophysiological techniques which can be used to provide a reliable measurement of motor imagery ability. None of them, however, can give the researchers an accurate indication of the individual's ability to preserve the temporal characteristics of the movement during its visualization. As we mentioned earlier, this issue is a crucial dimension of motor imagery accuracy, as it has been shown by its impact on the subsequent and unexpected modifications of the actual speed (see Louis *et al.* 2008, Debarnot *et al.* 2009). For this reason, it remains imperative to control the motor imagery speed through a mental chronometry paradigm. A simple and reliable way consists on measuring the temporal congruence between the actual and the imagined times (Guillot and Collet 2005b; Malouin *et al.* 2008). Usually, the participants are required to, respectively, start and stop a timer upon mental initiation of the first body movement, as well as at the end of the sequence. While no data regarding the vividness or the accuracy of the imagery experience is provided, it may easily indicate if comparable times are spent both to imagine and physically execute the same action. For instance, some researchers reported that Fitts's law, which governs the executed movements, also holds motor imagery (e.g., Decety *et al.* 1989; Decety and Jeannerod 1996; Maruff *et al.* 1999). Also, evidence of the individual difficulty to preserve the temporal characteristics of the movement during imagery is often taken as motor imagery impairment in patients (Sirigu *et al.* 1996; Malouin *et al.* 2004).

Altogether, recording the timing of imagined action is imperative. However, one of the main issues is that the total imagery time is not sufficient, as it does not provide information about the successive and different parts of the imagined action. Furthermore, changes in timing, tempo, and rhythm of the action must also be considered, as they are dependent on one another and can thus disrupt each other (Jagacinsky and Greenberg 1997). Hence, recording several intermediate times would be helpful to detect when the participant is going to either under- or overestimate the duration of the action at a certain point in time. Also, the coupling between the imagery duration, the verbal description of the imagery content during the imagery experience, and the video recording of the actual movement may be of particular interest (McIntyre and Moran 2005).

Conclusion

Because of its concealed nature, motor imagery remains difficult to assess objectively. However, the main conclusions driven by this review are that:

1 A wide range of reliable neurophysiological techniques are now available to assess the individual imagery ability and the accuracy of the motor imagery content.

2 These methods should be combined adequately with self-report questionnaires, and psychological and behavioural evaluations. Such reliable and thorough procedures may therefore benefit from complementary assessments to evaluate motor imagery more objectively.

3 Even though they are quite objective, the neurophysiological methods remain an inference which is afterward associated to the content of the mental representation by the experimenter.

4 While some techniques may provide satisfactory assessment of motor imagery ability, others are not suitable enough, due to discrepancies in the results, and/or received limited attention.

Altogether, the methodological advances and developments offer promising perspectives in the investigation of motor imagery ability and accuracy. Strong theoretical and practical implications for both motor learning and neurological rehabilitation can be drawn. For example, identifying the patient populations that could benefit most from the motor imagery therapeutic approach, by investigating their abilities to generate accurate mental images of movement after stroke, is imperative in clinical investigations.

References

Bakker, M., deLange, F.P., Stevens, J.A., Toni, I., and Bloem, B.R. (2007). Motor imagery of gait: a quantitative approach. *Experimental Brain Research*, **179**, 497–504.

Bakker, M., deLange, F.P., Helmich, R.C., Scheeringa, R., Bloem, B.R., and Toni, I. (2008). Cerebral correlates of motor imagery of normal and precision gait. *NeuroImage*, **41**, 998–1010.

Binkofski, F., Amunts, K., Stephan, K.M. *et al.* (2000). Broca's region subserves imagery of motion: a combined cytoarchitectonic and fMRI study. *Human Brain Mapping*, **11**, 273–85.

Calmels, C., Holmes, P., Lopez, E., and Naman, V. (2006). Chronometric comparison of actual and imaged complex movement patterns. *Journal of Motor Behavior*, **38**, 339–48.

Cocude, M., Mellet, E., and Denis, M. (1999). Visual and mental exploration of visuo-spatial configurations: behavioral and neuroimaging approaches. *Psychological Research*, **62**, 93–106.

Collet, C., Guillot, A., Bolliet, O., Delhomme, G., and Dittmar, A. (2003). Neurophysiological correlates of mental processes through non-invasive micro-sensors recording in the field. *Science and Sports*, **18**, 74–85.

Davidson, R.J. and Schwartz, G.E. (1977). Brain mechanisms subserving self-generated imagery: electrophysiological specificity and patterning. *Psychophysiology*, **14**, 598–602.

De Vries, S. and Mulder, T. (2007). Motor imagery and stroke rehabilitation: a critical discussion. *Journal of Rehabilitation in Medicine*, **39**, 5–13.

De'Sperati, C. and Stucchi, N. (2000). Motor imagery and visual event recognition. *Experimental Brain Research*, **133**, 273–8.

De'Sperati, C. (2003). Precise oculomotor correlates of visuospatial mental rotation and circular motion imagery. *Journal of Cognitive Neurosciences*, **15**, 1244–59.

Debarnot, U., Louis, M., Collet, C., and Guillot, A. (2009). Voluntary changes in motor imagery speed: inconsistent and task-related effects on motor performance. *Submitted for publication*.

Decety, J. and Jeannerod, M. (1996). Mentally simulated movements in virtual reality: does Fitts's law hold in motor imagery? *Behavioural Brain Research*, **72**, 127–34.

Decety, J., Jeannerod, M., and Prablanc, C. (1989). The timing of mentally represented actions. *Behavioural Brain Research*, **34**, 35–42.

Decety, J., Perani, D., Jeannerod, M. *et al.* (1994). Mapping motor representations with positron emission tomography. *Nature*, **371**, 600–2.

DeCharms, R.C., Christoff, K., Glover, G.H., Pauly, J.M., Whitfield, S., and Gabrieli, J.D. (2004). Learned regulation of spatially localized brain activation using real-time fMRI. *NeuroImage*, **21**, 436–43.

Denis, M., Chevalier, N., and Eloi, S. (1985). Visual imagery and the use of mental practice in the development of motor skills. *Canadian Journal of Applied Sport Sciences*, **10**, 4S–16S.

Denis, M., Goncalves, M.R., and Memmi, D. (1995). Mental scanning of visual images generated from verbal descriptions: towards a model of image accuracy. *Neuropsychologia*, **33**, 1511–30.

Dietrich, A. (2008). Imaging the imagination: the trouble with motor imagery. *Methods*, **45**, 319–24.

Doyon, J. and Benali, H. (2005). Reorganization and plasticity in the adult brain during learning of motor skills. *Current Opinion in Neurobiology*, **25**, 161–7.

Doyon, J. and Ungerleider, L.G. (2002). Functional anatomy of motor skill learning, in L.R Squire and D.L. Schacter (ed.), *Neuropsychology of Memory*, pp. 225–38. New York: Guilford Press.

Feltz, D.L. and Landers, D.M. (1983). The effects of mental practice on motor skill learning and performance: a meta-analysis. *Journal of Psychology*, **5**, 25–57.

Frak, V., Paulignan, Y., and Jeannerod, M. (2001). Orientation of the opposition axis in mentally simulated grasping. *Experimental Brain Research*, **136**, 120–7.

Galton, F. (1880). Statistics of mental imagery. *Mind*, **5**, 301–318.

Gerardin, E., Sirigu, A., Lehericy, S. *et al.* (2000). Partially overlapping neural networks for real and imagined hand movements. *Cerebral Cortex*, **10**, 1093–104.

Gueugneau, N., Crognier, L., and Papaxhantis, C. (2008). The influence of eye movements on the temporal features of executed and imagined arm movements. *Brain Research*, **1187**, 95–102.

Guillot, A. and Collet, C. (2005a) Duration of mentally simulated movement: a review. *Journal of Motor Behavior*, **37**, 10–9.

Guillot, A. and Collet, C. (2005b). Contribution from neurophysiological and psychological methods to the study of motor imagery. *Brain Research Reviews*, **50**, 387–97.

Guillot, A. and Collet, C. (2008). Construction of the motor imagery integrative model in sport: a review and theoretical investigation of motor imagery use. *International Review of Sport and Exercise Psychology*, **1**, 31–44.

Guillot, A., Collet, C., and Dittmar, A. (2004). Relationship between visual vs kinaesthetic imagery, field dependence-independence and complex motor skills. *Journal of Psychophysiology*, **18**, 190–8.

Guillot, A., Collet, C., Nguyen, V.A., Malouin, F., Richards, C., and Doyon, J. (2008). Functional neuroanatomical networks associated with expertise in motor imagery ability. *NeuroImage*, **41**, 1471–83.

Guillot, A., Collet, C., Nguyen, V.A., Malouin, F., Richards, C., and Doyon, J. (2009). Brain activity during visual vs. kinaesthetic imagery: an fMRI study. *Human Brain Mapping*, **30**, 2157–72.

Hale, B.D. (1982). The effects of internal and external imagery on muscular and ocular concomitants. *Journal of Sport Psychology*, **4**, 379–87.

Hall, C.R., Pongrac, J., and Buckolz, E. (1985). The measurement of imagery ability. *Human Movement Science*, **4**, 107–18.

Hall, C.R., Mack, D.E., Paivio, A., and Hausenblas, H.A. (1998). Imagery use by athletes: development of the sport imagery questionnaire. *International Journal of Sport Psychology*, **29**, 73–89.

Hamel, M.F. and Lajoie, Y. (2005). Mental imagery. Effects on static balance and attentional demands of the elderly. *Aging in Clinical and Experimental Research*, **17**, 223–8.

Hardy, L. and Callow, N. (1999). Efficacy of external and internal visual imagery perspectives for the enhancement of performance on tasks in which form is important. *Journal of Sport and Exercise Psychology*, **21**, 95–112.

Hebb, D.O. (1968). Concerning imagery. *Psychological Review*, **75**, 466–77.

Heremans, E., Helsen, W.H., and Feys, P. (2008). The eye as a mirror of our thoughts: quantification of motor imagery of goal-directed movements through eye-movement registration. *Behavioural Brain Research*, **187**, 351–60.

Hugdahl, K. (1996). Cognitive influences on human autonomic nervous system function. *Current Opinion in Neurobiology*, **6**, 252–8.

Isaac, A.R. and Marks, D.F. (1994). Individual differences in mental imagery experience: developmental changes and specialization. *British Journal of Psychology*, **85**, 479–500.

Jackson, P.L., Lafleur, M.F., Malouin, F., Richards, C., and Doyon, J. (2001). Potential role of mental practice using motor imagery in neurologic rehabilitation. *Archives of Physical Medicine and Rehabilitation*, **82**, 1133–41.

Jackson, P.L., Lafleur, M.F., Malouin, F., Richards, C.L., and Doyon, J. (2003). Functional cerebral reorganization following motor sequence learning through mental practice with motor imagery. *NeuroImage*, **20**, 1171–80.

Jagacinsky, R.J. and Greenberg, N. (1997). 'Tempo, rhythm and aging in golf'. *Journal of Motor Behavior*, **29**, 159–73.

Jacobson, E. (1931). Electrical measurements of neuromuscular states during mental activities. *American Journal of Physiology*, **96**, 122–5.

Johansson, R., Holsanova, J., and Holmqvist, K. (2005). What do eye movements reveal about mental imagery? Evidence from visual and verbal elicitations, in *Proceedings of the 27th Cognitive Science Conference*, p. 1054. Mahwah, NJ: Erlbaum.

Johnson, S.H. (2000). Thinking ahead: the case for motor imagery in prospective judgements of prehension. *Cognition*, **74**, 33–77.

Johnson-Frey, S.H. (2004). Stimulation through simulation? Motor imagery and functional reorganization in hemiplegic stroke patients. *Brain and Cognition*, **55**, 328–31.

Kosslyn, S.M., Ball, T.M., and Reiser, B.J. (1978). Visual images preserve metric spatial information: evidence from studies of image scanning. *Journal of Experimental Psychology: Human Perception and Performance*, **4**, 47–60.

Kosslyn, S.M. (1994). *Image and Brain: The Resolution of the Imagery Debate*. Cambridge, MA: Harvard University Press.

Kosslyn, S.M., Ganis, G., and Thompson, W.L. (2001). Neural foundations of imagery. *Nature Review Neuroscience*, **2**, 635–42.

Laeng, B. and Teodorescu, D.S. (2002). Eye scanpaths during visual imagery reenact those of perception of the same visual scene. *Cognitive Science*, **26**, 207–31.

Lafleur, M.F., Jackson, P.L., Malouin, F., Richards, C.L., Evans, A.C., and Doyon, J. (2002). Motor learning produces parallel dynamic functional changes during the execution and imagination of sequential foot movements. *NeuroImage*, **2**, 142–57.

Lotze, M. and Cohen, M.G. (2006). Volition and imagery in neurorehabilitation. *Cognitive Behavior and Neurology*, **19**, 135–40.

Lotze, L., Montoya, P., Erb, M. *et al.* (1999). Activation of cortical and cerebellar motor areas during executed and imagined hand movements: an fMRI study. *Journal of Cognitive Neuroscience*, **11**, 491–501.

Lotze, M., Scheler, G., Tan, H.R.M., Braun, C., and Birbaumer, N. (2003). The musician's brain: functional imaging of amateurs and professionals during performance and imagery. *NeuroImage*, **20**, 1817–29.

Lotze, M. and Halsband, U. (2006). Motor imagery. *Journal of Physiology (Paris)*, **99**, 386–95.

Louis, M., Guillot, A., Maton, S., Doyon, J., and Collet, C. (2008). Effect of imagined movement speed on subsequent motor performance. *Journal of Motor Behavior*, **40**, 117–32.

Malouin, F., Richards, C.L., Desrosiers, J., and Doyon, J. (2004). Bilateral slowing of mentally simulated actions after stroke. *Neuroreport*, **15**, 1349–53.

Malouin, F., Richards, C.L., Durand, A., and Doyon, J. (2008). Reliability of mental chronometry for assessing motor imagery after stroke. *Archives in Physical Medicine and Rehabilitation*, **89**, 311–9.

Martinez, R.K. (2000). Changes in the frequency power spectrum of the human EEG during visual and kinaesthetic imagery. *Dissertation Abstracts International*, **61**, 545.

Maruff, P., Wilson, P.H., De Fazio, J., Cerritelli, B., Hedt, A., and Currie, J. (1999). Asymmetries between dominant and non-dominant hands in real and imagined motor task performance. *Neuropsychologia*, **37**, 379–84.

Maruff, P. and Velakoulis, D. (2000). The voluntary control of motor imagery. Imagined movements in individuals with feigned impairment and conversion disorder. *Neuropsychologia*, **38**, 1251–60.

Mast, F.W. and Kosslyn, S.M. (2002). Eye movements during visual mental imagery. *Trends in Cognitive Sciences*, **6**, 271–2.

McIntyre, T. and Moran, A.P. (2005). Mental travel experiments with elite gymnastics and canoe-slalom competitors: an attempt to overcome tacit knowledge. *Proceedings of the 'Congrès International des Chercheurs en Activités Physiques et Sportives' (ACAPS)*, 26–28 Octobre, Paris, p. 577.

Mellet, E., Petit, L., Mazoyer, B., Denis, M., and Tzourio, N. (1998). Reopening the mental imagery debate: lessons from functional anatomy. *NeuroImage*, **8**, 129–39.

Moran, A. (1993). Conceptual and methodological issues in the measurement of mental imagery skills in athletes. *Journal of Sport Behavior*, **16**, 156–70.

Morris, T., Spittle, M., and Watt, A.P. (2005). *Imagery in Sport*. Champaign, IL: Human Kinetics.

Murphy, S.M. and Jowdy, D.P. (1992). Imagery and mental practice, in T.S. Horn (ed.), *Advances in Sport Psychology*, pp. 221–250. Champaign, IL: Human Kinetics.

Murphy, S., Nordin, S.M., and Cumming, J. (2008). Imagery in sport, exercise and dance, in T.S. Horn (ed.), *Advances in Sport Psychology*, pp. 306–315. Champagne, IL: Human Kinetics.

Neuper, C., Scherer, R., Reiner, M., and Pfurtscheller, G. (2005). Imagery of motor actions: differential effects of kinaesthetic and visual-motor mode of imagery in single-trial EEG. *Cognitive Brain Research*, **25**, 668–77.

Paivio, A. (1986). *Mental Representations: A Dual Coding Approach*. Oxford: Clarenton Press.

Parsons, L.M. (2001). Integrating cognitive psychology, neurology and neuroimaging. *Acta Psycholica (Amsterdam)*, **107**, 155–81.

Reed, C.L. (2002). Chronometric comparisons of imagery to action: visualizing versus physically performing springboard dives. *Memory and Cognition, 30*, 1169–78.

Richardson, A. (1994). *Individual Differences in Imaging: Their Measurements, Origins and Consequences.* Amytiville, NY: Baywood.

Rodionov, V., Zislin, J., and Elidan, J. (2004). Imagination of body rotation can induce eye movements. *Acta Otolaryngology, 124*, 684–9.

Rodrigues, E.C., Imbiriba, L.A., Leite, G.R., Magahlaes, J., Volchan, E., and Vargas, C.D. (2003). Mental simulation strategy affects postural control. *Revista Brasilian de Psiquiatria, 25*, 33–5.

Roure, R., Collet, C., Deschaumes-Molinaro, C., Delhomme, G., Dittmar, A., and Vernet-Maury, E. (1999). Imagery quality estimated by autonomic response is correlated to sporting performance enhancement. *Physiology and Behavior, 66*, 63–72.

Sharma, M., Pomeroy, V.M., and Baron, J.C. (2006). Motor imagery: a backdoor to the motor system after stroke? *Stroke, 37*, 1941–52.

Sharma, M., Jones, P.S., Carpenter, T.A., and Baron, J.C. (2008). Mapping the involvement of BA 4a and 4p during motor imagery. *Neuroimage, 41*, 92–9.

Shepard, R.N. and Metzler, J. (1971), Mental rotation of three-dimensional objects. *Science, 171*, 701–3.

Shick, J. (1970). Effects of mental practice on selected volleyball skills for college women. *Research Quarterly, 41*, 88–94.

Sirigu, A., Duhamel, J.R., Cohen, L., Pillon, B., Dubois, B., and Agid, Y. (1996). The mental representation of hand movements after parietal cortex damage. *Science, 273*, 1564–8.

Solodkin, A., Hlustik, P., Chen, E.E., and Small, S.L. (2004). Fine modulation in network activation during motor execution and motor imagery. *Cerebral Cortex 14*, 1246–55.

Spivey, M.J., Tyler, M.J., Richardson, D.C., and Young, E.E. (2000). Eye movements during comprehension of spoken scene description, in *Proceedings of the 22nd Annual Conference of the Cognitive Science Society*, pp. 487–92. Mahwah, NJ: Erlbaum.

Thompson, W.L. and Kosslyn, S.M. (2000). Neural systems activated during visual mental imagery: a review and meta-analysis, in A.W. Toga and J.C. Mazziota (ed.), *Brain Mapping II: The Systems.* San Diego: Academic Press.

Totten, E. (1935). Eye movement during visual imagery. *Comparative Psychology Monographs, 2*, 11–46.

Vadocz, E.A., Hall, C.R., and Moritz, S.E., (1997). The relationship between competitive anxiety and imagery use. *Journal of Applied Sport Psychology, 9*, 241–53.

Vealey, R. and Greenleaf, C.A. (1998). Seeing is believing: understanding and using imagery in sport, in: J.M. Williams (3rd ed.), *Applied sport psychology: Personal Growth to Peak Performance*, pp. 247–283. Mountain View, CA: Mayfield.

Wraga, M., Thompson, W.L., Alpert, N.M., and Kosslyn, S.M. (2003). Implicit transfer of motor strategies in mental rotation. *Brain and Cognition, 52*, 135–43.

Zacks, J.M. (2008). Neuroimaging studies of mental rotation: a meta-analysis and review. *Journal of Cognitive Neurosciences, 20*, 1–19.

Motor imagery in rehabilitation

Chapter 9

Motor imagery and the rehabilitation of movement disorders: An overview

Chris H. Dijkerman, Magdalena Ietswaart, and Marie Johnston

Introduction

Movement disorders are a common consequence of neurological disease. They are often associated with reduced levels of functional independence and, as such, it is important to minimize any motor deficit and to maximize functional recovery. Traditionally, physical therapy and related methods have been used for rehabilitation of motor impairments. In recent years, motor imagery has received increasing attention as a tool to aid recovery. Neuroimaging studies investigating the neural basis of mental simulation of movements suggest that they largely engage similar cortical areas to actual performance of movements (Decety *et al.* 1994; De Lange *et al.* 2005; Orr *et al.* 2008). Moreover, recovery of motor function after brain damage often involves a redistribution of activity within the cortical motor control network (Seitz *et al.* 2004; Ward 2006). For example, early stage attempts to move the impaired limb are associated with widespread activation in a bilateral cortical network, but recovery is dependent on increased efficiency within surviving networks (Ward 2006). Therefore, activating the motor network through motor imagery may aid redistribution of neural activity resulting in enhanced recovery. In addition, practical aspects may make motor imagery attractive within motor rehabilitation. The time patients spend in rehabilitation-related activities is often limited by the need for close supervision by occupational or physiotherapists for safety reasons (Tinson 1989). Motor imagery does not involve overt movements and can therefore be safely practiced alone, increasing the time the patient spends in rehabilitation-related activities.[1] It is therefore not surprising that in the last few years, an increasing number of studies have investigated the effect of motor imagery training on reducing movement disorders in neurologically impaired participants.

Here we review the current literature on the use of motor imagery in rehabilitation. Table 9.1 gives an overview of the studies conducted so far on the use of motor imagery as rehabilitation method for motor impairments. It may be clear that the studies vary widely with respect to the motor imagery training methods used, the patients trained, and also regarding the methodological rigour of the evaluation of effectiveness. Some described single-case studies, while others did not include a control group. We have underlined the studies including 10 or more participants and a control group. Several of them reported randomized controlled trials (RCTs), although it should be noted that the largest study still only included 16 patients in the experimental group. Indeed most studies till date evaluating the effectiveness of motor imagery as a rehabilitation tool

---

[1] Of course this requires the ability to perform motor imagery in an effective way, which may depend on several variables, see below.

Table 9.1 An overview of the studies published so far on motor imagery training for rehabilitation of movement deficits. The studies that are underlined and in italic are those that include a patient control group. The studies printed in bold are large sample randomized controlled trials for which the results have not been reported as yet.

Study	Randomized control trial?	N (treatment-control)	Type of and time since injury	Severity	Training methods	Control training	Outcome
Page (2000)	No	8–8	Chronic stroke		Occupational +Motor imagery, 4 weeks	Occupational therapy only, 4 weeks	Improvement on the Fugl-Meyer
Page et al. (2001a)	No	8–5	Stroke 4–52 weeks	Residual function present	Physical therapy 3 times a week, for 6 weeks; + Verbal scripts describing movements (10 minutes)	Physical therapy 3 times a week, for 6 weeks; + Stroke information	Improvement on ARAT + Fugl Meijer
Page et al. (2001b)	No	1	Stroke, 5 months		Auditory scripts twice a week		Improvement on ARAT + Fugl Meijer
Stevens and Stoykov (2003)	No	2	Stroke 14 months–6 years		Wrist movements, grasping object manipulation, using mirror, 3 times x 4 weeks		Improvement on MT, Fugl Meijer, stable over 3 months.
Crosbie et al. (2004)	No	10	Stroke 10–176 days		Imagining reach to grasp movements daily for 2 weeks		Improvement on the motricity index (up till 3 days)
Malouin et al. (2004a)	No	12–14 (healthy controls)	Stroke 2 months–4 years		Single session combined physical mental practice on load on affected leg		Reduced overload on unaffected limb, correlation with working memory
Malouin et al. (2004b)	No	12–6 (healthy controls)	Stroke 20 months		Single session mental practice of standing up and sitting down		Increased load on affect lower limb
Dijkerman et al. (2004)	No	10–10	> 1 year post-stroke	Residual motor function present	Daily practice of grasping movements 4 weeks unsupervised	Visual imagery or physical practice only	Improvement on practiced task only

Reference	Randomized	N		Condition	Intervention		Results
Jackson et al. (2004)	No	1		Stroke 4 months	Mental + physical practice of foot sequence		Retention + some improvement of MT after mental practice
Liu et al. (2004b)	No	2		Stroke	3-week mental imagery		Improvements on rehearsed and non-rehearsed tasks
Dickstein et al. (2004)	No	1		Stroke 3 months	Motor imagery gait practice 6 weeks		Improvement
Liu et al (2004a)	*Yes*	*26–20*	*Residual function present*	*Stroke 2 weeks*	*15 times during 3 weeks mental practice of daily activities intermixed with actual practice*	*15 times during 3 weeks Functional retraining of same daily activities (with assistance*	*Improved performance on trained and untrained tasks. Also present after 1 month and on Color Trail task, more on more complex tasks*
Gaggioli et al. (2006)	No	1		Chronic stroke	Computer aided VR type of training of arm function		Improvement on Fugl-Meyer and ARAT
Dunsky et al. (2006)	No	4		Chronic stroke	3 days a week for 6 weeks, imagery gait practice		Increased gait speed, stride length, cadence
Butler and Page (2006)	No	4		Stroke, 3–4months	Mental practice (see earlier studies)		fMRI, slight improvement on Wolf motor function test imagery questionnaires

(Continued)

Table 9.1 (Continued) An overview of the studies published so far on motor imagery training for rehabilitation of movement deficits. The studies that are underlined and in italic are those that include a patient control group. The studies printed in bold are large sample randomized controlled trials for which the results have not been reported as yet.

Study	Randomized control trial?	N (treatment-control)	Type of and time since injury	Severity	Training methods	Control training	Outcome
Ietswaart et al. (2006)	**Yes**	**45–45–45**	**Stroke, 1–6 months**	**Residual function present OR ARAT score between 3 and 51**	**45 min a day for 4 weeks focused on the upper limb. Visual, kinaesthetic, combined motor imagery. Elementary motor control and ADL function**	**Group 1: Matched for attention of therapist, visual illusion cognitive demands Group 2: Normal care**	**Results not reported as yet, study protocol**
Cramer et al. (2007)	No	10 –10 healthy controls	chronic spinal cord injruy		Mentally rehearse tongue and foot sequences, audio-visually guided twice daily for one week		Significant improvement for nonparalyzed muscles
Tamir et al. (2007)	*No*	*12–11*	*Parkinson, 7 years since onset*		*Mental rehearsal of variety of practiced movements, 2x a week for 12 weeks*	*Physical practice of movements only*	*Faster performance of movement seq. Higher gains on UPDRS, effects on daily living.*
Page et al. (2007)	*Yes*	*16–16 moderate motor impairment*	*Chronic stroke*	*Some flexion of the wrist necessary*	*2/week for 6 weeks auditory guided mental practice of grasping etc. + physical practice*	*Mental relaxation + physical practice*	*Improved performance on ARA and Fugl Meyer for MI group only*
Sutbeyaz et al. (2007)	*Yes*	*17–16*	*Stroke < 12 months*		*30 minutes a day mirror therapy of leg movements in addition to to 2–5 hours conventional stroke rehabilitation program, for 4 weeks*	*Sham therapy in addition to to 2–5 hours conventional stroke rehabilitation program, for 4 weeks*	*More improvement on the FIM and Brunnstrom stages, not on other measures*

Muller et al. (2007)	*Yes*	*6–6–5*	*Stroke, 28 days*	*Some individual finger movements present*	*Mental non-sequential finger opposition, 30 minutes, 5 days every four weeks*	*Physical non-sequential finger opposition, conventional therapy*	*Increase in peak force of pinch grip, better functionality (Jeben test)*
Verbunt et al. (2008)		**80–80**	**First stroke, 2–6 weeks**	**MRC grade 1–3**	**Mental training of upper limb function with 5 levels (depending on the individual's level), based on the Frenchay Activities Index. Video based instructions**	**Conventional treatment + additional bimanual upper extremity techniques based on conservative neurodevelopmental (NDT) principles**	**Results not reported, study protocol**

are small feasibility studies. Based on these studies we aim to discuss both patient and training variables that seem important. This chapter will conclude with some recommendations concerning both the design and implementation of motor imagery training methods and the evaluation of its effectiveness in enhancing recovery of hand function after stroke.

Patient characteristics

Severity of motor impairment

Movement deficits are common after a wide variety of lesions and in different diseases. It may therefore not be surprising that motor imagery has been used as a retraining method in a number of different patient populations. Most studies report on hemiparesis after stroke, but others describe Parkinson's disease (Tamir *et al.* 2007) and spinal cord injuries (Cramer *et al.* 2007), children with development coordination disorder (DCD; Wilson *et al.* 2002), or a 'normal' ageing population (Mulder *et al.* 2007). Irrespective of its cause, there are a number of aspects of the motor impairment that need to be considered when discussing the effectiveness of motor imagery. Perhaps the most obvious is the severity of the deficit. In particular, the question whether some residual motor function should be present is relevant (although this issue may not be applicable to all patient groups, e.g. Parkinson's, DCD). Recovery of motor function after stroke may be predicted by absence of residual motor function shortly after the event (Kwakkel *et al.* 2003). Several studies report an average initial performance on the outcome measure with some variability present, suggesting that at least part of the group showed some residual motor function (Liu *et al.* 2004a, Page *et al.* 2001a) with at least two studies explicitly stating some residual motor function as inclusion criteria (Dijkerman *et al.* 2004; Page *et al.* 2007; see also Muller *et al.* 2007). Few reported on patients with complete motor deficits. Cramer *et al.* (2007) investigated the effects of motor imagery training on tongue and foot movements in para- and tetraplegic spinal cord patients. Although changes in neural activity were observed for both body parts, behavioural effects were observed only for the tongue and not for the paralysed foot.

Thus, the evidence so far does suggest that motor imagery is beneficial when some residual motor abilities are present. Whether this is the case for patients with complete motor impairments after central lesions remains to be determined. However, no behavioural improvements were observed in patients with spinal cord injuries on movements that could not be performed. Furthermore, in healthy individuals, motor imagery training did not improve performance of a movement (toe abduction) of those participants who were unable to perform this movement prior to training (Mulder *et al.* 2004). In contrast, participants who could already make this movement to some extent did improve through mental training. Thus, beneficial effects of motor imagery training may depend on the presence of a central representation of the imagined movement. Even in the group with some residual function, the relation between severity of motor deficit and effect of retraining needs to be explored, with either a positive or a negative relation being possible.

Time since onset of motor impairment

The question about the relation between time since injury and benefit of motor imagery retraining is perhaps associated with the question of severity of impairment. Again the studies varied regarding to this variable. Most studies assessed patients with chronic and stable motor deficits, presumably to limit the effects of spontaneous recovery (Dijkerman *et al.* 2004; Page 2000; Page *et al.* 2007; Stevens and Stoykov 2003). Most observed positive effects suggesting that patients who are in the post-rehabilitation stage can nevertheless benefit from motor imagery training.

Indeed, as such, motor imagery has been coined the 'backdoor' to the motor system (Sharma *et al.* 2006). However, there are also good reasons for applying motor imagery training at a much earlier stage post-injury. The idea of 'guided recovery' (Robertson and Murre 1999) suggests that recovery may be maximized if the intervention occurs early after onset of the brain lesion. Few studies have assessed the effect of motor imagery early after brain damage.[2] Two studies have been reported with early patients and involving control groups. Liu *et al.* (2004a) performed an RCT in which the patients were on average about two weeks post-stroke. Mental imagery involved not only internal rehearsal of specific movements but also more complex daily activities such as folding laundry and going to a park. Compared to the control group that only performed the activities physically, but not mentally, the experimental group improved on the trained and untrained complex tasks, but not on the cognitive and sensorimotor abilities measures. The difference remained significant at one-month follow-up. Muller *et al.* (2007) took a different approach and asked participants (average 28 days post-stroke) to imagine non-sequential finger movements. They compared this with control groups physically practicing the movement sequences or only receiving conventional therapy. The mental imagery group improved as much as the physical therapy group on pinch grip force and more than the group only receiving conventional therapy. Overall, this suggests that motor imagery training can be effective at an early as well as a chronic stage. Whether early intervention is more beneficial, as suggested by Robertson and Murre (1999), remains to be determined by comparing subacute and chronic patients using the same imagery method.

Motor imagery ability

The ability to mentally simulate performing a movement varies in patients as well as in healthy individuals. Cognitive psychology studies used a variety of methods to study and assess motor imagery ability (Guillot and Collet 2005; Jeannerod 1995). These include mental chronometry, hand laterality judgements, physiological recordings of autonomic nervous system activation, and questionnaires. Certain studies specifically investigated individual differences (Hall 1985) and found them to be related to several variables such as perceptuo-motor ability and developmental stage (Isaac and Marks 1994). In addition, specific neurological abnormalities have been reported to affect the ability to perform motor imagery. Cortical lesions affecting the posterior parietal cortex and putamen have been found to reduce motor imagery (Sirigu *et al.* 1996; Li 2000; Sirigu and Duhamel 2001), although others have reported that physical motor impairments are not necessarily reflected in motor imagery ability (Johnson 2000). Surprisingly, as motor imagery has been considered to involve internal forward models (Schwoebel *et al.* 2002; Kasess *et al.* 2008), possible motor imagery impairments in apraxic patients have received little attention. Sirigu (Sirigu *et al.* 1996; Sirigu and Duhamel 2001) reported first-person motor imagery impairments in a patient suffering from ideomotor apraxia. This relation was explored further by Buxbaum *et al.* (2005), who reported particular motor imagery deficits while imagining movement that required planning and were less dependent on online visuomotor control. In contrast, Anezoulaki (2005) found motor imagery ability, assessed through mental chronometry, to be intact both in ideomotor and ideational apraxia. However, it should be noted that evaluating motor imagery ability through mental chronometry alone may be quite limited as it only provides information about the capacity to imagine in real-time, or not. Overall, the detection of motor imagery impairments seems to depend on the patient's clinical characteristics such as lesion location as well as the task used to assess motor imagery.

Other groups for whom motor imagery impairment has been observed include Parkinson's disease, but not Huntington's disease (Yaguez *et al.* 1999; Helmich *et al.* 2007; Frak *et al.* 2004),

---

[2] Of course, the patient should first be medically stable before any cognitive treatment could be started.

DCD (Williams *et al.* 2008), and hemiplegic cerebral palsy (Mutsaarts *et al.* 2007; but see Steenbergen *et al.* 2007 for evidence that motor imagery ability may be intact in hemiplegic cerebral palsy). Although it may be intuitively logical that patients with motor imagery impairments will not benefit from motor imagery training, this issue has so far not been investigated.

Many studies assessing the effectiveness of motor imagery training have included a measure of motor imagery ability as inclusion criteria. Measures that are used to screen for motor imagery ability include self-report questionnaires, such as the Movement Imagery Questionnaire (Page *et al.* 2001a), Kinaesthetic and Visual Imagery Questionnaire (Malouin *et al.* 2004b). Others have used mental chronometry (Dijkerman *et al.* 2004). Both the kinaesthetic and visual imagery questionnaire and mental chronometry method have recently been found to have satisfactory psychometric characteristics when used with a clinical (stroke) population (Malouin *et al.* 2008a,b). Another possibility is to use more implicit measures of motor imagery such as hand laterality judgements (Parsons 1994; Johnson 2000). However, this has so far not been applied in studies assessing motor imagery training in neurological patients (but see Ietswaart *et al.* 2006). Two notes of caution should be made regarding the screening for motor imagery ability. First, although several measures have been used to investigate motor imagery impairments in patients, there are currently no standard screening tests for motor imagery. Motor imagery as such remains difficult to define and an elusive phenomenon, hence developing screening measures is not straightforward. The studies reporting motor imagery impairments in clinical populations have used a variety of measures, including questionnaires and experimental cognitive psychology tasks, and the approach has mainly been correlational. Nevertheless, recent reviews have suggested that a combination of different methods may be the most sensitive approach to determine motor imagery ability (Guillot and Collet 2005; Lotze and Halsband 2006). The authors suggest that combining mental chronometry, psychological questionnaires, and physiological measures from the autonomic nervous system may be the most suitable approach. It would be useful if this could also be implemented in clinical assessment of patients.

Cognitive impairments

A final aspect that is important when considering motor imagery in patients with movement disorders is the cognitive status of the patients. Brain damage often leads to a variety of cognitive impairments and these can be predictive of functional outcome (Nys *et al.* 2005). Moreover, motor imagery itself can be considered to be a top-down process that activates relevant motor areas (Jeannerod 1997). It is therefore not surprising that the cognitive status of the patient is important in the context of motor imagery training. Several studies investigating the effect of motor imagery training on motor deficits have used a screening measure of cognitive function such as the Mini Mental State Examination (MMSE) or Cognistat to exclude patients with important cognitive deficits (Page *et al.* 2001a, 2001b, 2007; Crosbie *et al.* 2004; Liu *et al.* 2004a; Tamir *et al.* 2007). Few studies have assessed the relation between cognitive function and motor imagery in patients in more detail. Malouin *et al.* (2004a) reported a significant relation between effects of motor imagery training on load placed on the affected limb when standing up and working memory measures. Interestingly, improvement correlated higher with visuo-spatial working memory scores than with kinaesthetic memory. This is somewhat in contrast with reports that particularly kinaesthetic motor imagery activates lower levels of the motor system (see Stinear *et al.* 2006; Li *et al.* 2004). Anezoulaki (2005) assessed motor imagery ability and kinaesthetic working memory in a group of eight patients with ideomotor apraxia and did not observe any relation between motor imagery ability, kinaesthetic working memory, and apraxia. Finally, Dijkerman *et al.* (2004) investigated the effect of motor imagery training on attentional control. They observed no significant relation between improvement in motor performance and attentional control.

Another 'cognitive' variable that may be relevant is body schema. Disorders of body representation are often observed after brain injury (Berlucchi and Aglioti 1997; Dijkerman and De Haan 2007; Haggard and Wolpert 2005) and can be linked to motor imagery ability (Funk *et al.* 2005), but no studies so far have assessed whether body representation disorders also affect motor imagery ability in a rehabilitation context. Thus, although studies have controlled for important cognitive impairments, and it seems intuitively logical that cognitive variables such as working memory, sustained attention, planning, language, or bodily perception may be relevant, little empirical evidence can be found. Clearly, this area requires further exploration in future.

Imagery-related variables

In addition to patient-related variables, of course, the motor imagery used in a rehabilitation context is of prime importance. Studies within cognitive psychology and cognitive neuroscience suggest that motor imagery is not a single process, but can vary according to a number of important variables. For example, a movement can be imagined in first person perspective or from a third person viewpoint. They can differ regarding the dominant modality (visual or kinaesthetic), or the way that motor imagery is induced (scripts, verbal instructions, imitation, observation). Some of these variables are relevant within a motor rehabilitation context. Here we discuss the most important variables.

Perspective

Most studies investigating the effect of motor imagery on rehabilitation use a first person perspective imagery (Page 2000; Page *et al.* 2001a, 2007; Crosbie *et al.* 2004; Dijkerman *et al.* 2004; Cramer *et al.* 2007; Muller *et al.* 2007). Indeed, neuropsychological (Sirigu and Duhamel 2001) and neuroimaging studies (Jackson *et al.* 2006) suggest that motor imagery in a first person perspective engages the motor system more than third person perspective. The effects of first person perspective motor imagery training are visible as improved performance on more motor tasks (Page 2000, Page *et al.* 2001a, 2007; Crosbie *et al.* 2004; Dijkerman *et al.* 2004; Muller *et al.* 2007). In contrast, when first person perspective was not explicitly instructed as in the study by Liu *et al.* (2004a), improvements were observed on ADL tasks, but not on basic motor function as measured by subtests of the Fugl-Meyer (De Vries and Mulder 2007). These subtests assessed upper extremity motor function, lower extremity motor function, and sensation (Gladstone *et al.* 2002). Note that this differential effect of perspective is somewhat in contradiction to the idea that action observation can activate similar motor representations as action execution can (Schutz-Bosbach *et al.* 2006; Rizzolatti and Craighero 2004).

Modality

The modality of the imagery can also vary and may be visual (for both first- and third-person perspective) or kinaesthetic (first-person perspective only). Evidence from experimental psychology and sport science suggests that effectiveness of modality-specific motor imagery may depend on the stage of training and on the type of movement (Dickstein and Deutsch 2007). At the early stages, form of the movement is better learned by visual motor imagery, while for timing of the movements and bimanual coordination kinaesthetic imagery may be more efficient (Fery 2003). Studies on expert dancers and mental practice of walking suggest a greater involvement of kinaesthetic imagery in whole body movements (Golomer *et al.* 2008; Sacco *et al.* 2006); however, when environmental cues are important, visual imagery may again play a role (White and Hardy 1995). Furthermore, functional imaging shows that visual and kinaesthetic motor imagery activate different, albeit overlapping networks (Guillot *et al.* 2009). While visual motor imagery activated occipital and superior parietal regions, kinaesthetic imagery was associated with motor-related areas and the inferior parietal lobule. Furthermore, imagery of hand and finger movements also may benefit particularly from kinaesthetic imagery. Corticospinal activation was found during kinaesthetic, but not visual imagery of thumb movements (Stinear *et al.* 2006). In patients, modality used in motor imagery has received little attention. One of the few studies focusing on this issue showed that kinaesthetic, but not visual motor imagery, affected the CNV (contingent negative variation, an ERP measure associated with anticipation and motor preparation) in Parkinson's suggesting a more direct link between kinaesthetic imagery and motor ability in these patients (Lim *et al.* 2006).

The motor imagery intervention: content, intensity, and duration

In recent years there has been a major move to enhance the reporting of interventions. For example, Davidson *et al.* (2003) provided a checklist of items, based on the CONSORT-statement (www.consort-statement.org) that should be included in reports about RCTs. They particularly named eight items that minimally should be described including: content, provider, recipient, setting, format, intensity, duration, and fidelity checks. Here we will review the motor imagery interventions reported, based on these guidelines. Particularly, we focused on the content, intensity, duration, and setting, as other aspects have already been described (recipient), which did not vary much (provider, format) or received little attention (fidelity checks).

The studies that investigated the effect of motor imagery training on motor recovery varied widely regarding content, intensity, duration, and setting. Two early studies by Page *et al.* (2001a,b) used audio tapes that contained about 5–7 minutes of verbal imagery instructions (e.g. 'imagine yourself reaching for a cup on the table'; 'feel your arm and fingers extending as you reach for the cup', Page *et al.* 2001a, p. 236), preceded by 2 or 3 minutes of relaxation.[3] Although they described this as visual imagery, the instructions suggest that kinaesthetic imagery was also encouraged. The scripts focused on various aspects of upper arm function and different scripts were used in different weeks to maintain interest. All the studies by Page and colleagues reported positive effects of imagery on clinical outcome measures such as the Action Research Arm Test (ARAT) (a measure of upper extremity functional limitation, with a total of 19 items assessing gross motor control, grasp, grip, and pinch. The scores for each item vary from 0-no movement to 3-normal movement) and Fugl-Meyer. In a later double blind RCT, again audio-taped instructions were used, but the sessions lasted longer, and more importantly, focused on creating polysensory images of movements practiced earlier that day during physical therapy (Page *et al.* 2007). Moreover, the patients were discouraged from mentally practicing at home in between the 2 times a week imagery sessions. One week after the six weeks of imagery training had ended, the motor imagery group showed improved performance on both outcome measures (ARAT and Fugl-Meyer), in contrast to a control group who received mental relaxation at a similar rate.

Crosbie *et al.* (2004) used video during the first two days to instruct patients about the movement that had to be imagined ('grasping a cup'). Day 2–14 the patient imagined the movement during therapy, as well as outside, and reported back about it during the therapy session. Improved performance on the motor index was observed 3 days after termination of the mental practice

---

[3] However, sport studies have shown that a relaxed state may not be optimal for inducing motor imagery as participants should have to recall the state they encountered during actual practice (Guillot and Collet 2008).

(note that no control group was involved). Dijkerman *et al.* (2004) instructed participants to imagine grasping a row of tokens and moving them to the opposite side of a board. A single instruction session was used after which patients were required to practice, unsupervised, daily for four weeks. In addition to mental practice, all patients including control groups (who performed visual non-motor imagery or no imagery at all) also practiced the task physically. Participants were required to use a logbook to record when they practiced. After four weeks of training, the motor imagery group performed better on the trained task only.

Liu *et al.* (2004a) used a protocol of nine standardized steps that involved more complex task such as doing the laundry or going to a cafeteria. The steps involved analysis of the movement sequence, identification of patients' problems within motor task, mental (visual) rehearsal of correct performance, and video-based evaluation. Compared to the control group who only performed the activities physically, but not mentally, the experimental group improved on the trained and untrained complex tasks, but not on the cognitive and sensorimotor abilities measures. The difference remained significant at one-month follow-up. Tamir *et al.* (2007) reported combined imagery and physical training in Parkinson's patients (see also Chapter 12, this book). Imagery training was integrated in physical training and focused on the same movement (sitting without support, walking, etc.). Patients received training twice a week for twelve weeks. Compared to the control group (who only received physical training) the combined training resulted in faster performance of movement sequences and improved scores on the Unified Parkinson's Disease Rating Scale (UPDRS) and cognitive tests such as the Stroop. Finally, Muller *et al.* (2007) also used video instruction to train non-sequential finger movements with the affected hand. These instructions were repeated at the beginning of each training session. Training was performed for four weeks (daily 30 minutes) preceded by two weeks of baseline assessment and one week of follow-up. Patients in the motor imagery training group improved in pinch grip force after physical as well as mental training.

Overall, the studies reported here suggest a certain relation between the motor imagery instructions (and therefore content) and the effect observed on the outcome measures. Most studies show positive effects on outcome measures that are closely related to motor imagery content. Thus mentally rehearsing a specific type of hand and finger movements (Dijkerman *et al.* 2004; Muller *et al.* 2007) improves hand and finger movements, whereas training a complex sequence of activities (Liu *et al.* 2004a) results in improvement at this level. Generalization of the trained effects to other tasks has not always been assessed, but those who do, report conflicting results. Some describe generalization in which the type of arm movement mentally rehearsed was not identical to the one assessed (Page and others). At least one study reported effects of non-motor tests (Tamir *et al.* 2007), while another study shows improvements on the rehearsed task only (Dijkerman *et al.* 2004). This latter finding may be due to the relative specific contents of the motor imagery training and the lack of supervision during the training. Finally, the modality in which the instructions are given does not seem to be relevant, nor can any firm conclusion be drawn regarding the intensity and duration of the training.

Evaluation of effectiveness of training

The studies reported in Table 9.1 describe a range of methods of evaluating effectiveness of training. While some simply report case series, others are full RCTs, albeit with relatively few participants. Some report control groups with a variety of specifications of the control group. As a minimum, the experience of the control group should be described. In a pragmatic trial, one would simply wish to know whether motor imagery training could improve on normal care and therefore suggest potential for clinical improvement. However, in an explanatory trial, it would also be important to ascertain whether motor imagery was effective via the hypothesized mechanisms. Demonstrating that a group receiving motor imagery had better recovery than a 'normal care' control group does not demonstrate that motor imagery achieved the effect: the effect may equally well be due to attention placebo given the time invested by the trainer, or to other non-specific effects, for example due to extra motor rehearsal. In order to test whether effects are due to motor imagery training, a control group receiving all the non-specific effects is necessary. Some studies have included a 'normal care' (Page 2000, Page *et al.* 2001a) or physical-practice-only group (Liu *et al.* 2004a; Tamir *et al.* 2007; Muller *et al.* 2007). Other studies included a control group receiving similar amounts of trainer attention, but not involving imagery (Sutbeyaz *et al.* 2007; Verbunt *et al.* 2008), while others also include an imagery control group that engaged in similar amounts of imagery, but not motor imagery (Dijkerman *et al.* 2004; Ietswaart *et al.* 2006; Page *et al.* 2007). Indeed the trial by Ietswaart *et al.* included both a 'care as usual' and 'non-motor imagery' control group. This trial will be able to attribute any effects on recovery of function to motor imagery training if, and only if, the experimental group achieves greater recovery than *both* control groups.

Trials also vary in the duration of follow-up and the measures of outcome (see Table 9.1). Clearly it is important to establish that an effect can be achieved before investigating persistence of effects, but the latter is important for clinical benefits. Outcomes assessed include performance on the training tasks, performance on related motor tasks, impairment of a limb not involved in training, activity limitations, ADL, etc. As a minimum, one should expect evidence of reduced impairment of the motor function included in the imagery training, but effects on disability in everyday life will be necessary to demonstrate clinical value.

In sum, the variety of methods of evaluating the effectiveness of training makes it difficult to compare studies, and suggests some basic standards for trials and trial reporting which are necessary.

Limitations and recommendations for future studies

It may be clear from this review that during the last decade an increasing number of studies have investigated motor imagery as a tool for rehabilitation of motor disorders. Although the studies vary widely regarding the patients' aetiology, motor imagery characteristics, and methodological rigour, the overall outcome has been positive. This is of course encouraging, but there are some important limitations to the current literature that should also be discussed. Furthermore, as may be clear from the review, many questions remain concerning the role of motor imagery within rehabilitation of movement deficits. Here we discuss some of the limitations and describe the most important remaining issues.

An important issue regarding the current literature is that of a possible publication bias. The published results so far are almost entirely positive and one does wonder whether there may also have been studies in which null findings have been obtained that as a consequence have not been published. This would be unfortunate, as a comparison between effective and ineffective studies may provide important information about which aspects of the imagery training are effective and which group of patients may benefit most. Hopefully a more balanced report of motor imagery outcome is provided in the future.

A second limitation is related to methodological rigour. As mentioned previously, this varied widely between studies, with many papers reporting on a few patients without a control group. Some recent papers fortunately do report RCTs, but even in these studies the number of participants is relatively small. Research on the effectiveness of motor imagery training for reducing movement deficits may therefore benefit greatly from double-blind RCTs with sufficiently large groups, which remain to be reported. The protocols of two such studies have recently been published (Ietswaart *et al.* 2006; Verbunt *et al.* 2008), but the results have not yet been reported.

A third limitation concerns the range of patient and imagery-related variables. Although the large range of patient aetiologies and of motor imagery training methodology used perhaps suggests that motor imagery training is a relatively robust method applicable to a number of patient groups, it does leave many questions open about which method may be most effective and which patient group may benefit most. Therefore an important next step in the motor imagery rehabilitation research, if large double-blind RCTs confirm the results, may be to assess patient and imagery-related variables more systematically. Indeed, this review suggests that for each patient characteristic or imagery variable discussed, important questions remain unanswered. With respect to the patient, the role of motor impairment severity is important and in particular whether patients with complete paralysis may benefit. Furthermore, the role of time since the onset of motor impairment is unclear with both subacute and chronic stroke patients being studied with different paradigms. A direct comparison between groups for whom time since onset differs, remains wanting. A third important variable is the ability of the patients to perform motor imagery. Particularly, the relation between motor imagery ability and effectiveness of motor imagery training should be assessed. So far, it is assumed that participants with little motor imagery ability would not benefit, but little experimental evidence exists to support this. In neurologically intact participants, imagery ability is not always related to the effects of motor imagery training. Associated with this issue, further research should be done on the relation between impairments on the different motor imagery measures.

The role of cognitive function in motor imagery training within a clinical setting also requires attention. So far few studies have investigated whether cognitive deficits may affect motor imagery training, and those that did overall found little relation, except with visuo-spatial working memory (Malouin *et al.* 2004a). To our knowledge no studies have assessed the role of executive function, disturbances in bodily perception, and language function in relation to motor imagery. It may therefore be of particular importance to focus on these aspects.

A final issue that requires attention is the motor imagery itself and how it is reported. A wide range of imagery instructions, contents, etc. have been used. Again, overall positive effects have been reported, but a systematic approach to assess how motor imagery variables affect retraining is still missing. Nevertheless some suggestions can be made. First, different studies suggest that training of motor skills actually benefits most from a first person's perspective. In contrast, more complex ADL skills may be improved more by adopting a third person's perspective approach (Liu *et al.* 2004a). With respect to modality of the motor image, studies in experimental psychology and sport science suggest that visual imagery is more effective at early stages and when spatial requirements are high, for example when environmental cues are important. In contrast, kinaesthetic imagery may be more appropriate when somesthetic cues are essential, for bimanual coordination, finger, hand, and whole body movements. Whether this may also be the case when using motor imagery in rehabilitation setting remains to be determined.

The instructions used for training motor imagery also require further attention. Although the modalities in which the instructions are given (verbal, visual) do not seem to be very relevant, most studies used instructions that are closely linked to the outcome measures. Some studies do report generalization to measures other than those emphasized in the instructions; however, it is not clear which instructions may be most effective and again systematic assessment of various forms of instructions is clearly warranted. Furthermore, it should be noted that motor imagery training was generally combined with physical training. The evaluated motor imagery training focused on images of movements practiced during physical therapy. It remains to be seen whether motor imagery is effective if such close association between motor imagery and physical training does not exist, and motor imagery is trained on its own (but see Ietswaart *et al.* 2006). These are complex interventions and require good reporting for replication and implementation in practice. This will require publication of training procedures as well as report of the evaluation and outcome.

Overall, despite increased attention for motor imagery as a rehabilitation tool in the last few years and the generally positive effects reported, much work remains to be done. Several studies designed to evaluate the effectiveness of motor imagery training show serious methodological limitations (although recent studies are promising) and many questions remain. Future studies should focus on further delineating the precise relation between motor imagery training content and mode of delivery, patient variables and motor improvement, using well-designed evaluation trials.

References

Anezoulaki, D. (2005). Motor imagery and kinaesthesia in ideomotor apraxia. *Unpublished MSc thesis, Neuroscience and Cognition.* Utrecht, Utrecht University.

Berlucchi, G. and Aglioti, S. (1997). The body in the brain: neural bases of corporeal awareness. *Trends in Neuroscience,* **20,** 560–4.

Butler, A.J. and Page, S.J. (2006). Mental practice with motor imagery: evidence for motor recovery and cortical reorganization after stroke. *Archives in Physical Medicine and Rehabilitation,* **87,** S2–11.

Buxbaum, L.J., Johnson-Frey, S.H., and Bartlett-Williams, M. (2005). Deficient internal models for planning hand-object interactions in apraxia. *Neuropsychologia,* **43,** 917–29.

Cramer, S.C., Orr, E. L., Cohen, M.J., and Lacourse, M.G. (2007). Effects of motor imagery training after chronic, complete spinal cord injury. *Experimental Brain Research,* **177,** 233–42.

Crosbie, J.H., Mcdonough, S.M., Gilmore, D.H., and Wiggam, M.I. (2004). The adjunctive role of mental practice in the rehabilitation of the upper limb after hemiplegic stroke: a pilot study. *Clinical Rehabilitation,* **18,** 60–8.

De Lange, F.P., Hagoort, P., and Toni, I. (2005). Neural topography and content of movement representations. *Journal of Cognitive Neuroscience,* **17,** 97–112.

De Vries, S. and Mulder, T. (2007). Motor imagery and stroke rehabilitation: a critical discussion. *Journal of Rehabilitation Medicine,* **39,** 5–13.

Decety, J., Perani, D., Jeannerod, M., Bettinardi, V., Tadary, B., Woods, R., Mazziotta, J. C., and Fazio, F. (1994). Mapping motor representations with positron emission tomography. *Nature,* **371,** 600–602.

Dickstein, R. and Deutsch, J. E. (2007) Motor imagery in physical therapist practice. *Physical Therapy,* **87,** 942–53.

Dickstein, R., Dunsky, A., and Marcovitz, E. (2004). Motor imagery for gait rehabilitation in post-stroke hemiparesis. *Physical Therapy,* **84,** 1167–77.

Dijkerman, H.C. and De Haan, E.H. (2007). Somatosensory processes subserving perception and action. *Behavioural Brain Sciences,* **30,** 189–201.

Dijkerman, H.C., Ietswaart, M., Johnston, M., and Macwalter, R.S. (2004). Does motor imagery training improve hand function in chronic stroke patients? A pilot study. *Clinical Rehabilitation,* **18,** 538–49.

Dunsky, A., Dickstein, R., Ariav, C., Deutsch, J., and Marcovitz, E. (2006). Motor imagery practice in gait rehabilitation of chronic post-stroke hemiparesis: four case studies. *International Journal of Rehabilitation Research,* **29,** 351–6.

Fery, Y.A. (2003). Differentiating visual and kinesthetic imagery in mental practice. *Canadian Journal of Experimental Psychology,* **57,** 1–10.

Frak, V., Cohen, H., and Pourcher, E. (2004). A dissociation between real and simulated movements in Parkinson's disease. *Neuroreport,* **15,** 1489–92.

Funk, M., Shiffrar, M., and Brugger, P. (2005). Hand movement observation by individuals born without hands: phantom limb experience constrains visual limb perception. *Experimental Brain Research,* **164,** 341–6.

Gaggioli, A., Meneghini, A., Morganti, F., Alcaniz, M., and Riva, G. (2006). A strategy for computer-assisted mental practice in stroke rehabilitation. *Neurorehabil Neural Repair,* **20**, 503–7.

Gladstone, D.J., Danells, C.J., and Black, S.E. (2002). The fugl-meyer assessment of motor recovery after stroke: a critical review of its measurement properties. *Neurorehabilitation and Neural Repair,* **16**, 232–40.

Golomer, E., Bouillette, A., Mertz, C., and Keller, J. (2008). Effects of mental imagery styles on shoulder and hip rotations during preparation of pirouettes. *Journal of Motor Behavior,* **40**, 281–90.

Guillot, A. and Collet, C. (2005). Contribution from neurophysiological and psychological methods to the study of motor imagery. *Brain Research Reviews,* **50**, 387–97.

Guillot, A. and Collet, C. (2008). Construction of the motor imagery integrative model in sport: a review and theoretical investigation of motor imagery use. *International Review of Sport and Exercise Psychology,* **1**, 31–44.

Guillot, A., Collet, C., Nguyen, V. A., Malouin, F., Richards, C., and Doyon, J. (2009). Brain activity during visual versus kinesthetic imagery: an fMRI study. *Human Brain Mapping,* **30**, 2157–72.

Haggard, P. and Wolpert, D.M. (2005). Disorders of body scheme, in Freund, H. J., Jeannerod, M., Hallett, M., and Leiguarda, R. (eds), *Higher-Order Motor Disorders,* pp. 261–272. Oxford: Oxford University Press.

Hall, C.R. (1985). Individual differences in the mental practice and imagery of motor skill performance. *Canadian Journal of Applied Sport Science,* **10**, 17S–21S.

Helmich, R.C., De Lange, F.P., Bloem, B.R., and Toni, I. (2007). Cerebral compensation during motor imagery in Parkinson's disease. *Neuropsychologia,* **45**, 2201–15.

Ietswaart, M., Johnston, M., Dijkerman, H. C., Scott, C. L., Joice, S. A., Hamilton, S., and Macwalter, R. S. (2006). Recovery of hand function through mental practice: a study protocol. *BMC Neurology,* **6**, 39.

Isaac, A.R. and Marks, D.F. (1994). Individual differences in mental imagery experience: developmental changes and specialization. *British Journal of Psychology,* **85**(Pt 4), 479–500.

Jackson, P.L., Doyon, J., Richards, C.L., and Malouin, F. (2004). The efficacy of combined physical and mental practice in the learning of a foot-sequence task after stroke: a case report. *Neurorehabilitation and Neural Repair,* **18**, 106–11.

Jackson, P.L., Meltzoff, A.N., and Decety, J. (2006). Neural circuits involved in imitation and perspective-taking. *Neuroimage,* **31**, 429–39.

Jeannerod, M. (1995). Mental imagery in the motor context. **33**, 1419–32.

Jeannerod, M. (1997). *The Cognitive Neuroscience of Action.* Oxford: Blackwell.

Johnson, S.H. (2000). Imagining the impossible: intact motor representations in hemiplegics. *Neuroreport,* **11**, 729–32.

Kasess, C.H., Windischberger, C., Cunnington, R., Lanzenberger, R., Pezawas, L., and Moser, E. (2008). The suppressive influence of SMA on M1 in motor imagery revealed by fMRI and dynamic causal modeling. *Neuroimage,* **40**, 828–37.

Kwakkel, G., Kollen, B.J., Van Der Grond, J., and Prevo, A.J. (2003) Probability of regaining dexterity in the flaccid upper limb: impact of severity of paresis and time since onset in acute stroke. *Stroke,* **34**, 2181–6.

Li, C.R. (2000). Impairment of motor imagery in putamen lesions in humans. *Neuroscience Letters,* **287**, 13–6.

Li, S., Kamper, D.G., Stevens, J.A., and Rymer, W.Z. (2004). The effect of motor imagery on spinal segmental excitability. *Journal of Neuroscience,* **24**, 9674–80.

Lim, V.K., Polych, M.A., Hollander, A., Byblow, W.D., Kirk, I.J., and Hamm, J.P. (2006). Kinesthetic but not visual imagery assists in normalizing the CNV in Parkinson's disease. *Clinical Neurophysiology,* **117**, 2308–14.

Liu, K.P., Chan, C.C., Lee, T.M., and Hui-Chan, C.W. (2004a). Mental imagery for promoting relearning for people after stroke: a randomized controlled trial. *Archives in Physical Medicine and Rehabiliation,* **85**, 1403–8.

Liu, K.P., Chan, C.C., Lee, T.M., and Hui-Chan, C.W. (2004b). Mental imagery for relearning of people after brain injury. *Brain Injury,* **18**, 1163–72.

Lotze, M. and Halsband, U. (2006). Motor imagery. *Journal of Physiology Paris,* **99**, 386–95.

Malouin, F., Belleville, S., Richards, C.L., Desrosiers, J., and Doyon, J. (2004a). Working memory and mental practice outcomes after stroke. *Archives in Physical Medicine and Rehabilitation,* **85**, 177–83.

Malouin, F., Richards, C., Durand, A., and Doyon, J. (2008a). Clinical assessment of motor imagery after stroke. *Neurorehabilitation and Neural Repair,* **22**, 330–40.

Malouin, F., Richards, C.L., Doyon, J., Desrosiers, J., and Belleville, S. (2004b). Training mobility tasks after stroke with combined mental and physical practice: a feasibility study. *Neurorehabilitation and Neural Repair,* **18**, 66–75.

Malouin, F., Richards, C.L., Durand, A., and Doyon, J. (2008b). Reliability of mental chronometry for assessing motor imagery ability after stroke. *Archives in Physical Medicine and Rehabilitation,* **89**, 311–9.

Mulder, T., Hochstenbach, J.B., Van Heuvelen, M.J., and Den Otter, A.R. (2007). Motor imagery: the relation between age and imagery capacity. *Human Movement Science,* **26**, 203–11.

Mulder, T., Zijlstra, S., Zijlstra, W., and Hochstenbach, J. (2004). The role of motor imagery in learning a totally novel movement. *Experimental Brain Research,* **154**, 211–7.

Muller, K., Butefisch, C.M., Seitz, R.J., and Homberg, V. (2007). Mental practice improves hand function after hemiparetic stroke. *Restorative Neurology Neuroscience,* **25**, 501–11.

Mutsaarts, M., Steenbergen, B., and Bekkering, H. (2007). Impaired motor imagery in right hemiparetic cerebral palsy. *Neuropsychologia,* **45**, 853–9.

Nys, G.M., Van Zandvoort, M.J., De Kort, P.L., Van Der Worp, H.B., Jansen, B.P., Algra, A., De Haan, E.H., and Kappelle, L.J. (2005). The prognostic value of domain-specific cognitive abilities in acute first-ever stroke. *Neurology,* **64**, 821–7.

Orr, E.L., Lacourse, M.G., Cohen, M.J., and Cramer, S.C. (2008). Cortical activation during executed, imagined, and observed foot movements. *Neuroreport,* **19**, 625–30.

Page, S.J. (2000). Imagery improves upper extremity motor function in chronic stroke patients: a pilot study. *The Occupational Therapy Journal of Research,* **20**, 200–215.

Page, S.J., Levine, P., and Leonard, A. (2007). Mental practice in chronic stroke: results of a randomized, placebo-controlled trial. *Stroke,* **38**, 1293–7.

Page, S.J., Levine, P., Sisto, S., and Johnston, M.V. (2001a). A randomized efficacy and feasibility study of imagery in acute stroke. *Clinical Rehabilitation,* **15**, 233–40.

Page, S.J., Levine, P., Sisto, S.A., and Johnston, M.V. (2001b). Mental practice combined with physical practice for upper-limb motor deficit in subacute stroke. *Physical Therapy,* **81**, 1455–62.

Parsons, L.M. (1994). Temporal and kinematic properties of motor behavior reflected in mentally simulated action. *Journal of Experimental Psychology, Human Perception and Performance,* **20**, 709–30.

Rizzolatti, G. and Craighero, L. (2004) The mirror-neuron system. *Annual Review of Neuroscience,* **27**, 169–92.

Robertson, I.H. and Murre, J.M. (1999). Rehabilitation of brain damage: brain plasticity and principles of guided recovery. *Psychological Bulletin,* **125**, 544–75.

Sacco, K., Cauda, F., Cerliani, L., Mate, D., Duca, S., and Geminiani, G.C. (2006). Motor imagery of walking following training in locomotor attention. The effect of 'the tango lesson'. *Neuroimage,* **32**, 1441–9.

Schutz-Bosbach, S., Mancini, B., Aglioti, S.M., and Haggard, P. (2006). Self and other in the human motor system. *Current Biology,* **16**, 1830–4.

Schwoebel, J., Boronat, C.B., and Branch Coslett, H. (2002). The man who executed 'imagined' movements: evidence for dissociable components of the body schema. *Brain and Cognition,* **50**, 1–16.

Seitz, R.J., Butefisch, C.M., Kleiser, R., and Homberg, V. (2004). Reorganisation of cerebral circuits in human ischemic brain disease. *Restorative Neurology Neuroscience,* **22**, 207–29.

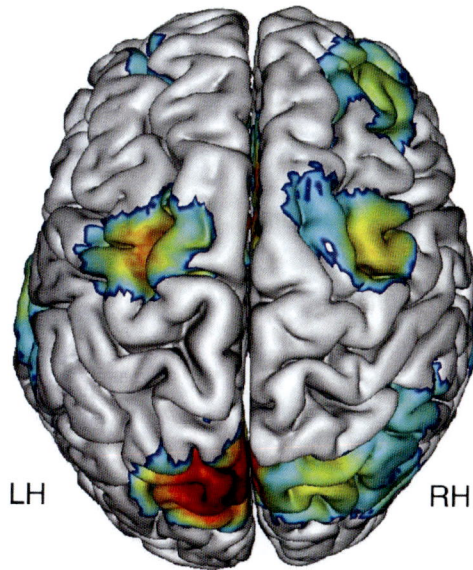

Fig. 2.1 3-D rendering of areas activated during a mental navigation task in environments learned from different modalities (actual navigation learning, map learning, and text learning, see Mellet *et al.*, 2000a, 2002). This conjunction analysis revealed the basic parieto-frontal network involved as soon as subjects use a spatial mental representation ($P_{uncorr} < 0.001$, LH: left hemisphere, RH: right hemisphere). See p.19.

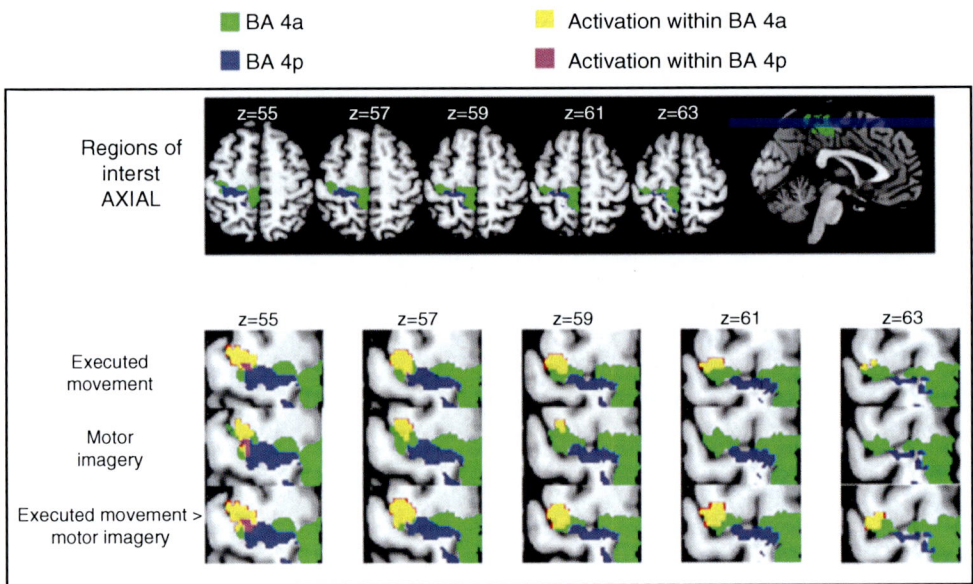

Fig. 3.1 Contribution of primary motor cortex during a finger opposition sequence. Activation clusters are shown in cytoarchitectural masks (indicated in green and blue) of highest probability for Brodmann's area 4a (yellow) and 4p (pink). The figure is printed with permission from Sharma, Carpenter, and Baron, NeuroImage 2008. See p. 34.

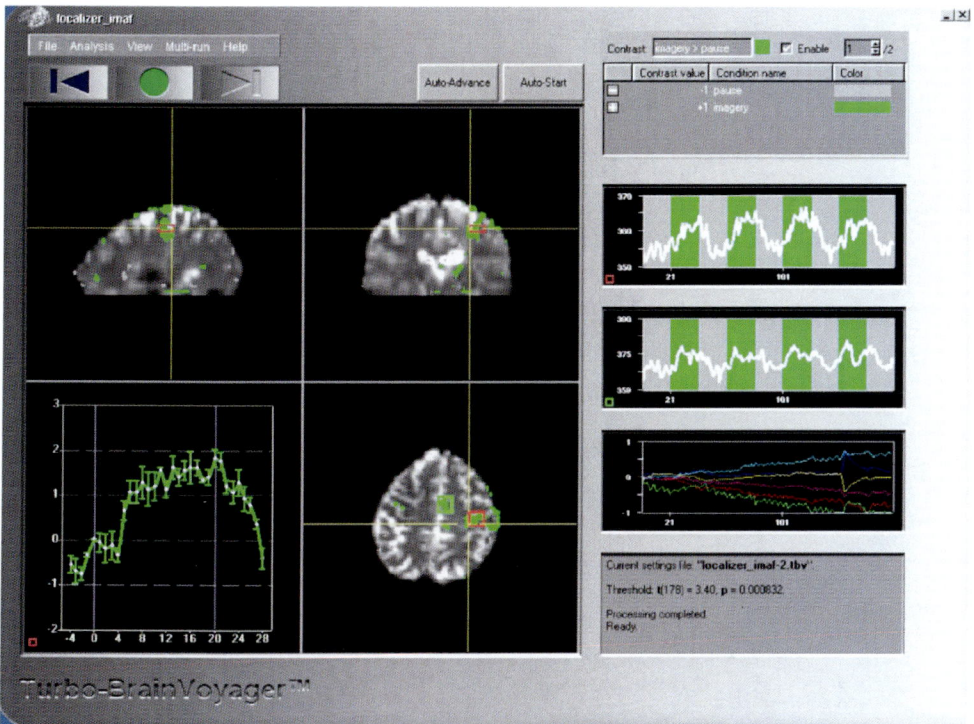

Fig. 3.2 Blood-oxygenation level-dependent (BOLD)-feedback training session of a patient suffering from motor impairment of the left hand due to a stroke in the internal capsule 3.5 years before fMRI. This is a screen shot of a Turbo Brain Voyager session of a left-hand imagery training session. Online visual inspection of the hand in the scanner was used to exclude execution. Left: The red rectangle in the three echo planar images indicates the Region-of-Interest (ROI) for M1c; the green, the reference area in the medial SMA. The bottom left panel shows the averaged BOLD plot of activation (%) over time (28 s) for one block. On the right, the top graph shows the BOLD time course for the ROI (cM1); the middle one, that for the reference area (SMA). The bottom graph indicates movement of the head in mm and rotations in degrees (each for 3 directions). This partici-pant showed considerable problems with imagery intensity during training without fMRI (vividness score: 2 from a maximum of 6), but he was perfectly able to increase BOLD magnitude by fMRI visual feedback with an average temporal delay of 5 s. See p. 40.

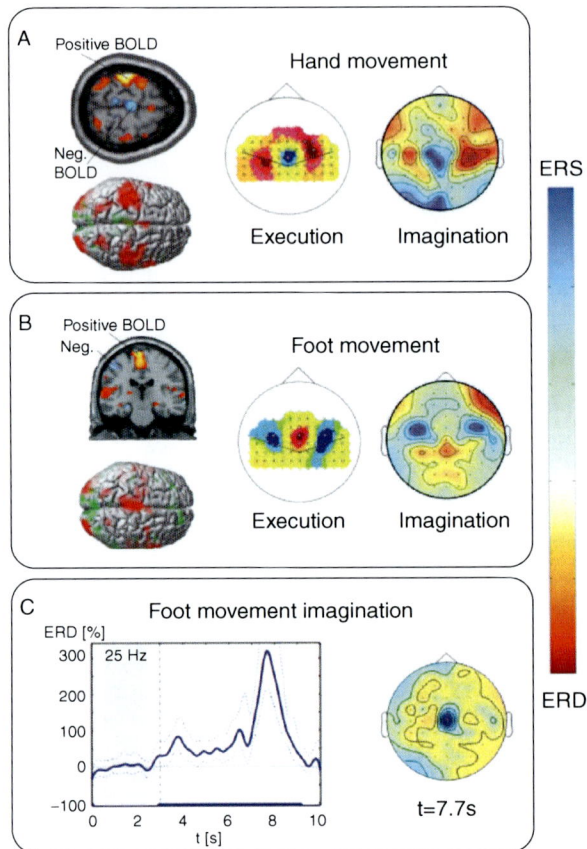

Fig. 5.1 Examples of activation patterns obtained with functional magnetic resonance imaging (fMRI) and EEG (ERD/ERS) during execution and imagination of hand (A) and foot movements (B). Note the correspondence between the focus of the positive BOLD signal and ERD, and between the negative BOLD signal and ERS, respectively. C: Topoplot and time course of the beta rebound in the foot motor imagery task for a representative subject (illustrating a group effect). The dominant frequency of the beta rebound (25 Hz) and the latency of its maximum (7.7 s) are indicated. The subject started imagery at second 3 and stopped it at second 7. See p. 69.

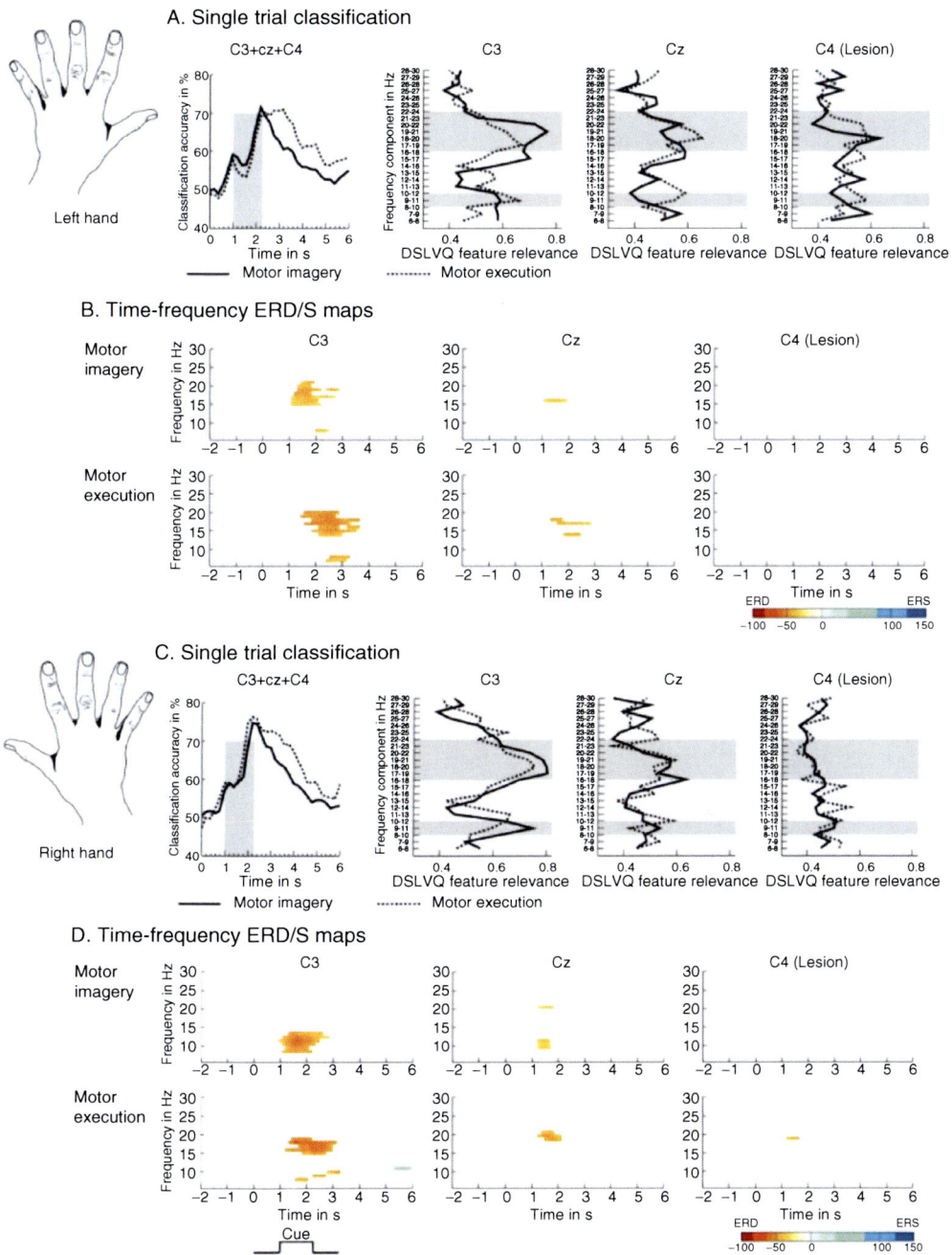

Fig. 5.3 Results of single trial classification, depicted in the form of time curves of DSLVQ classification accuracies for the combination of channels C3, Cz, and C4 and diagrams representing the corresponding feature relevance values of overlapping frequency bands for the 3 channels, separately for left-hand (A) and right-hand (C) motor tasks. Grand-average time-frequency ERD/S maps (confidence level α=0.05) for electrode locations C3 (undamaged), Cz and C4 (damaged hemisphere) are shown for left (affected)-hand (B) and right (unaffected)-hand motor imagery and execution (D). Modified from Scherer et al. (2007). See p. 75.

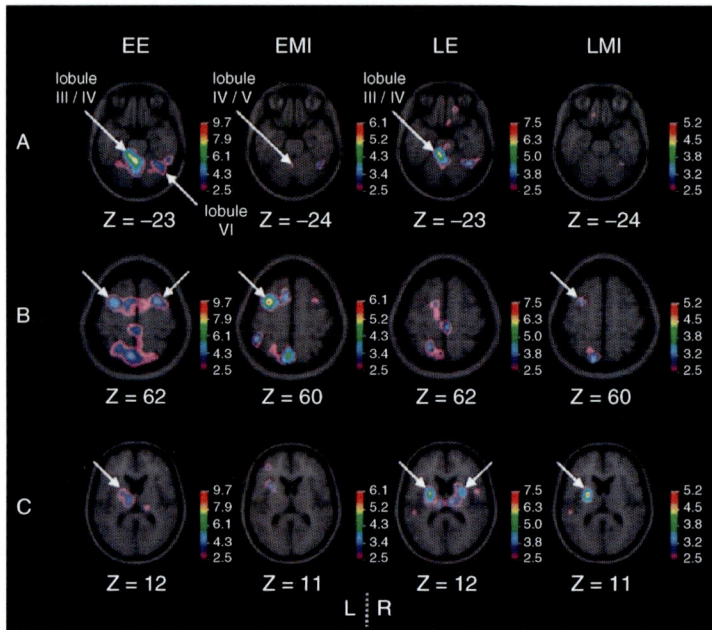

Fig. 10.1 Merged PET-MRI sections illustrating increases of regional cerebral blood flow (rCBF) associated with the execution and MI conditions, both before and after training on the foot-sequence task. The images were averaged over the nine subjects and represent the four different experimental conditions (EE, early execution; EMI, early motor imagery; LE, late execution; LMI, late motor imagery) minus the perceptual control condition. Each subtraction yielded focal changes in blood flow shown as t statistic images; the range is coded by the colour scale (L, left; R, right). Areas of activation in the (A) cerebellar lobules, (B) dorsal premotor cortex, and (C) striatum. (reprinted with permission from Elsevier, Jackson et al. 2003). See p. 152.

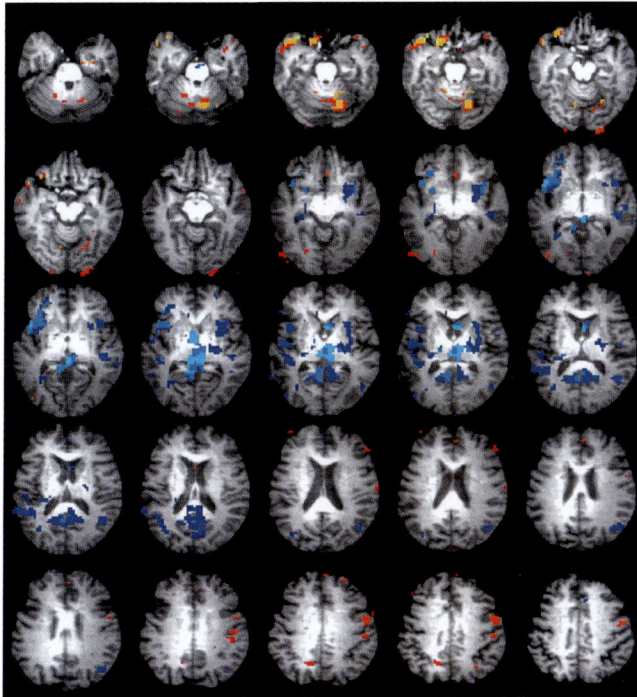

Fig. 10.2 Group fMRI activation patterns after a 10-week programme of MI targeting the affected arm. Orange depicts areas of increased cortical activation; blue depicts areas of decreased activation. In this particular study, subjects became more adept at using the affected arm; it is likely that the large decreases in activation suggest a more efficient brain pattern and/or consolidation of the activations, both commiserate with subjects' increased motor abilities. This figure is authors', taken from his previously unpublished material. See p. 154.

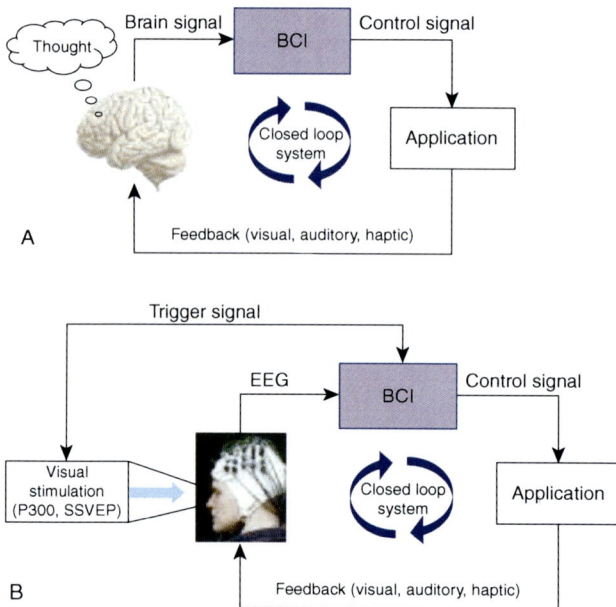

Fig. 14.1 A. Principal schemes of BCIs operated with motor imagery. B. visual- or gaze-directed attention to visual stimulation. See p. 204.

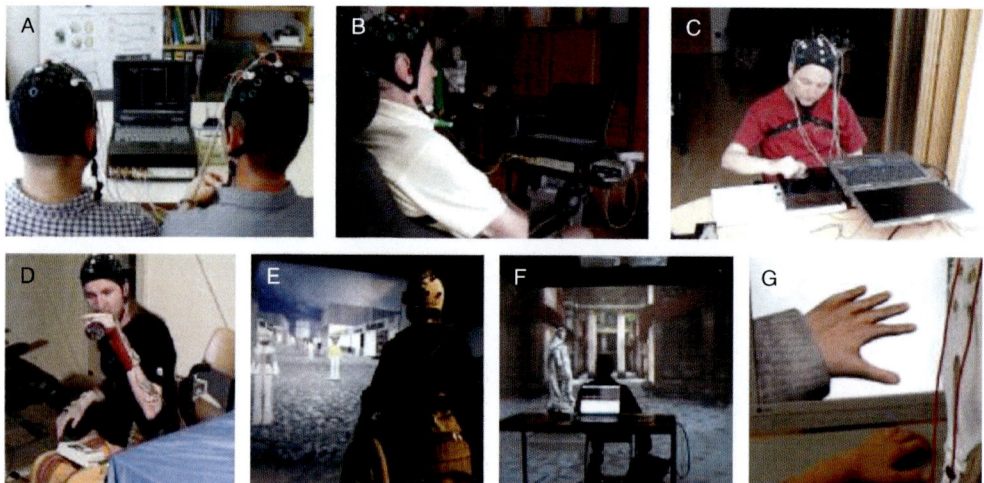

Fig. 14.2 A Two students playing table tennis; B. ALS patient operating a spelling system at home; C. thought-based control of a neuroprosthesis through implanted functional electrical stimulation (FES) of hand muscles; D. thought-based control of a neuroprosthesis through FES of hand muscles using surface electrodes; E. 'wheel chair movement' in a virtual environment; F. navigation through thought in a virtual library; G. and opening/closing of a virtual hand through hand motor imagery. See p. 209.

Sharma, N., Pomeroy, V.M., and Baron, J.C. (2006). Motor imagery: a backdoor to the motor system after stroke? *Stroke*, **37**, 1941–52.

Sirigu, A. and Duhamel, J.R. (2001). Motor and visual imagery as two complementary but neurally dissociable mental processes. *Journal of Cognitive Neuroscience*, **13**, 910–9.

Sirigu, A., Duhamel, J.R., Cohen, L., Pillon, B., Dubois, B., and Agid, Y. (1996). The mental representation of hand movements after parietal cortex damage. *Science*, **273**, 1564–8.

Steenbergen, B., Van Nimwegen, M., and Craje, C. (2007). Solving a mental rotation task in congenital hemiparesis: motor imagery versus visual imagery. *Neuropsychologia*, **45**, 3324–8.

Stevens, J.A. and Stoykov, M.E. (2003). Using motor imagery in the rehabilitation of hemiparesis. *Archives in Physical Medicine and Rehabilitation*, **84**, 1090–2.

Stinear, C.M., Byblow, W.D., Steyvers, M., Levin, O., and Swinnen, S.P. (2006). Kinesthetic, but not visual, motor imagery modulates corticomotor excitability. *Experimental Brain Research*, **168**, 157–64.

Sutbeyaz, S., Yavuzer, G., Sezer, N., and Koseoglu, B.F. (2007). Mirror therapy enhances lower-extremity motor recovery and motor functioning after stroke: a randomized controlled trial. *Archives in Physical Medicine and Rehabilitation*, **88**, 555–9.

Tamir, R., Dickstein, R., and Huberman, M. (2007). Integration of motor imagery and physical practice in group treatment applied to subjects with Parkinson's disease. *Neurorehabilitation and Neural Repair*, **21**, 68–75.

Tinson, D.J. (1989). How stroke patients spend their days. An observational study of the treatment regime offered to patients in hospital with movement disorders following stroke. *International Disabilities Studies*, **11**, 45–9.

Verbunt, J.A., Seelen, H.A., Ramos, F.P., Michielsen, B.H., Wetzelaer, W.L., and Moennekens, M. (2008). Mental practice-based rehabilitation training to improve arm function and daily activity performance in stroke patients: a randomized clinical trial. *BMC Neurology*, **8**, 7.

Ward, N.S. (2006). The neural substrates of motor recovery after focal damage to the central nervous system. *Archives in Physical and Medicine Rehabilitation*, **87**, S30–5.

White, A. and Hardy, L. (1995). Use of different imagery perspectives on the learning and performance of different motor skills. *British Journal of Psychology*, **86**(Pt 2), 169–80.

Williams, J., Thomas, P.R., Maruff, P., and Wilson, P.H. (2008). The link between motor impairment level and motor imagery ability in children with developmental coordination disorder. *Human Movement Science*, **27**, 270–85.

Wilson, P.H., Thomas, P.R., and Maruff, P. (2002). Motor imagery training ameliorates motor clumsiness in children. *Journal of Child Neurology*, **17**, 491–8.

Yaguez, L., Canavan, A., Lange, H., and Homberg, V. (1999). Motor learning by imagery is differentially affected in Parkinson's and Huntington's diseases. *Behavioural Brain Research*, **102**, 115–27.

Chapter 10

An overview of the effectiveness of motor imagery after stroke: A neuroimaging approach

Stephen J. Page

Stroke remains the leading cause of long-term disability in the United States (U.S.) (American Heart Association, 2008). The prevalence of stroke in the U.S. is estimated to be 5.5 million, with approximately 700,000 additional strokes occurring annually (Kissela *et al.* 2004; Kleindorfer *et al.* 2006). Data also show that stroke incidence is not changing (Kleindorfer *et al.* 2006). Thus, the human and financial burden of stroke in the U.S. will only increase over time, especially as the U.S. population ages and becomes more obese (for a review, see Rundek and Sacco 2008). Similar stroke incidence and prevalence trends are also being observed internationally, making stroke truly an international concern.

Hemiparesis (i.e., weakness on one side of the body) is one of the most common and, perhaps, the most disabling, of all stroke sequelae. This is because hemiparesis frequently undermines fundamental abilities such as eating, driving, writing, and ambulation, causing increased reliance on the healthcare system and on others. For example, in the Framingham Stroke Study, 50% of patients had some degree of hemiparesis at 6 months after stroke (Kelly-Hayes *et al.* 2003), and 30–70% of patients were unable to use their more affected arms functionally following discharge (Gresham *et al.* 1975). Similarly, the majority of stroke patients exhibit insufficient leg function to simply ambulate outside of their homes or function effectively within their communities (Corr and Bayer 1992; Goldie *et al.* 1996; Hill *et al.* 1997). Gait velocity is also affected: a velocity of .58 ±.38m/s was reported for a diverse group of subjects with hemiplegia in the chronic stage of recovery (Titianova *et al.* 2003); in contrast, velocity for healthy adults is approximately 1.49 m/s (Chen *et al.* 2005).

Given its devastating impact, and the rapidly increasing number of stroke survivors, effective hemiparesis treatments are needed. Recently, the use of motor imagery (MI) has been shown to reduce hemiparesis and improve function. 'Plasticity,' which appears to be a critical factor underlying MI efficacy, refers to the capability of the central nervous system to alter function and structure in response to use and motor learning (Donoghue *et al.* 1991; Kaas 1991). This chapter examines the co-occurrence of plasticity with provision of MI, as measured by neuroimaging. This discussion will briefly highlight basic principles of plasticity, followed by the promise of MI for hemiparesis recovery, the neural and physical events observed during MI, and how plasticity, measured by neuroimaging, may be an important mechanism mediating MI efficacy for stroke-induced hemiparesis.

Importantly, MI may also hold promise for other stroke-induced impairments. However, given the high prevalence and impact of hemiparesis, this chapter primarily focuses on the neuroimaging experiments of MI, and their functional relation to hemiparesis, while the Chapter 9 reviewed MI behavioural and kinematic studies in greater detail.

Plasticity

Emboldened (and, some would argue, initiated) by Broca's work (Broca 1861) the neurosciences had been dominated by localizationist concepts for decades. Central to this paradigm was the belief that specific brain regions primarily controlled specific functions. Yet, it was also known that, although particular cells serve specific functions, there is considerable sharing and overlap among cells in the functional representation of motor control. For example, motor representations can vary from moment to moment at a particular site, as first shown by Leyton and Sherrington (Leyton *et al.* 1917). Similarly, many have demonstrated that individual neurons subserve a myriad of functions (Hebb 1949; Bach y Rita 1964).

Given their versatility, it is, perhaps, unsurprising that *groups* of cells adapt very quickly to behaviour. 'Neuroplasticity' refers to the capability of cells or groups of cells to alter function and/ or structure according to repetition and demand. In humans, brain-mapping techniques that measure neuroplasticity-mediated brain function during rehabilitation include regional cerebral blood flow (rCBF), regional metabolic rate of glucose (rCMRglc) PET or SPECT, functional magnetic resonance imaging (fMRI), near infrared spectroscopy (NIRS), electroencephalography (EEG), magnetoencephalography (MEG), and transcranial magnetic stimulation (TMS). The word 'function', as used here, implies either the manipulation of a person's behaviour in order to influence signal amplitude or the measurement of regional blood flow or metabolism in the absence of behavioural manipulations. In either case, the signal is assumed to relate to the ability of nearby neurons to process information, i.e., to function.

The way in which brain function is assessed depends upon the technique in question. For fMRI, function is assessed by measuring changes in blood flow that vary with the changing metabolic demands of neurons nearby. PET can measure not only blood flow but also oxygen and sugar metabolism directly. TMS can be used to determine the electrical excitability of brain tissue by measuring the muscular response to stimulation. EEG and MEG measure an electrical or magnetic signature of cortical pyramidal neuron excitation. Roughly speaking, fMRI, PET, and NIRS measure blood flow related signals, while EEG and MEG record brain-electrical activity, and TMS directly induces brain-electrical activity.

Examples of neuroplasticity abound in both animal and human studies. Specifically, in animals, repetitive training on a task requiring manual skill results in enlargement of the digit and wrist representations in the motor cortex, and decreases in proximal areas, each correlating with learning of a novel motor skill (Nudo *et al.* 1996). In humans, Jenkins and colleagues (Jenkins *et al.* 1990) similarly showed that repeated tapping training with the 2nd, 3rd, and 4th, fingers caused expansion in the cortical representations corresponding to these areas, and correlative motor improvements. Karni and colleagues (Karni *et al.* 1995) similarly reported enlargement in human primary motor cortices engaging in daily practice of several motor tasks, while Classen and colleagues (Classen *et al.* 1998) showed that even simple thumb movements repeated over a short period of time induce lasting cortical representational changes. Others have repeated this finding, using a number of practice scenarios (Elbert *et al.* 1995; Sterr *et al.* 1998; Liepert *et al.* 1999). From these data, it is clear that individual cells, and groups of cells, can reconfigure quickly in response to motor behaviour.

After stroke, a reduction in motor cortex excitability and a decrease in the size of the cortical representations of paretic muscles occur (Cicinelli *et al.* 1997; Liepert *et al.* 1998). These cortical changes are likely attributable to reductions in affected limb use. However, when repetitive, task specific, affected limb practice (RTP) is provided to hemiparetic stroke patients, the same effects are seen as those reported above in animals and humans; the size of the cortical areas representing that limb increase, and correlative functional changes can be seen (Dean and Shephard 1997;

Smith *et al.* 1999; Galea *et al.* 2001). This cortical plasticity is brought about only when motor learning and repetitive affected limb use occur; plasticity is not typically observed when non-functional limb use and/or strength training are undertaken (for a recent review, see Nudo 2006). This use dependent, motor learning-induced, plasticity has been shown to be a mechanism underlying motor function changes following a number of efficacious stroke rehabilitative therapies (Schaecter *et al.* 2002; Luft *et al.* 2004; Szaflarski *et al.* 2006) (including MI as discussed later), and is believed to be a prerequisite for motor function changes to occur. For more information on this phenomenon, see Chapter 11 in this book.

Motor imagery: a promising treatment for stroke hemiparesis

Conventional rehabilitative strategies have typically focused on compensation with the unaffected limb, and/or non-functional exercises involving the affected limb. However, a number of newer programmes have taken advantage of the above neurophysiologic findings. Specifically, they have emphasized repetitive, task specific, RTP to produce motor changes, even years after stroke.

The most notable example has been constraint-induced movement therapy (CIT) (Taub *et al.* 1993; Miltner *et al.* 1999; van der Lee *et al.* 1999), which emphasizes affected arm RTP by: (1) restricting participants' less affected upper limbs during 90% of waking hours of a 2-week period; and (2) requiring subjects to engage in 6-hour activity sessions using their more affected limbs on the 10 weekdays of the same 2-week period. Shaping (see Taub 1977 for a description) is also applied during the 6-hour therapy sessions, in which the subject is verbally encouraged to perform progressively more difficult components of the movement. Although CIT efficacy was shown in a recently completed multicenter trial (Wolf *et al.* 2006) its feasibility has been questioned (Siegert *et al.* 2004) as its intensive parameters may be difficult to clinically implement and/or may encounter resistance, low adherence, and be fatiguing (Kaplon *et al.* 2007) for some subjects. Shorter CIT versions have been developed with comparable efficacy (Sterr *et al.* 2002; Pierce *et al.* 2003; Page *et al.* 2004) yet issues of intensive home and/or clinical practice still linger.

To provide RTP, yet assuage CIT contact time concerns, a variety of researchers have developed robotic (see Volpe and colleagues 2005, for a review) or other mechanized approaches to administering affected arm RTP (Whitall *et al.* 2000; Taub *et al.* 2005; Merians *et al.* 2006). Still others are attempting to augment or facilitate RTP with implanted devices (Chae and Hart 2003; Baker *et al.* 2007; Northstar Neuroscience 2003–2007) or other machinery. Despite this explosion in the diversity of efficacious RTP approaches, the above regimens often require particular equipment to administer, can be intensive and/or taxing for the patient and therapist, and/or can be invasive. Many of the strategies and devices inherent in the above approaches are also costly for individual clinics or hospitals, and are not reimbursed by insurance plans, making them also implausible for individual patient purchase. Thus, there has remained a need for easily implemented, inexpensive, non-invasive RTP approaches for affected arm hemiparesis.

Motor imagery for affected arm retraining after stroke

MI is a non-invasive, cost-effective, easily implemented technique in which physical skills are cognitively rehearsed in the absence of overt, physical movements. Since the 1890s studies have reported improved motor function when MI is combined with physical practice (Bachman 1990; Yaguez *et al.* 1998). As we will discuss later, the same neural and muscular areas are activated during MI as during physical practice of the same skill. Thus, MI provides the user with the opportunity to non-invasively, safely gain additional practice on a variety of motor skills, by repetitively activating similar neural and muscular regions as during physical practice. This MI facet is especially advantageous in rehabilitative settings, where certain skills may be difficult and/or unsafe to physically practice (e.g., walking). Consistently, MI has been widely shown to increase relearning of motor skills in rehabilitative settings (Fansler *et al.* 1985; Linden *et al.* 1989; Williams *et al.* 2004; Maring 1990; Sidaway and Trzaska 2005).

Given the above evidence, as well as decades of evidence showing MI efficacy in sport/exercise settings, our team was the first to examine MI use as an adjunctive strategy to affected arm RTP in stroke (Page 2000). Since some of our studies have been among the first and most comprehensive MI studies performed to date for the stroke-affected arm, below we present some of these studies as exemplars of the possible impact of MI when combined with RTP.

1 **Motor imagery reduces affected arm impairment: a pilot study** (Page 2000). We initially provided eight chronic stroke patients with right-arm hemiparesis a 4-week programme combining MI and RTP (Group 1), while eight controls received exposure to stroke information + RTP (Group 2). At the pretesting period (PRE), mean scores of Group 1 and Group 2 on the upper extremity section of the Fugl-Meyer Assessment (FM), a stroke-specific impairment measure were nearly identical (i.e., subjects in the two groups exhibited comparable levels of impairment in their affected arms). The FM is a stroke-specific measure of arm movement that examines the patient's ability to perform isolated, active movements at each joint (e.g., elbow extension; wrist flexion; pincer grasp). The patient is rated either 0, 1, or 2, depending on how well he/she performs each movement.

However, after treatment (POST), scores indicated that MI + RTP patients exhibited significantly greater reductions in impairment than patients in Group 2 (F [1, 14] = 14.71; $P < .05$). This study was small and pilot in nature, and, thus, suffered from limitations associated with studies of this size. However, this was the first study in the literature examining the relationships among MI and function in any brain-injured population. Later in this section we provide additional discussion of positive findings in this population: both by our group and by other groups.

2 **Motor imagery improves reaching kinematics** (Hewett *et al.* 2007). We also showed that MI + RTP use improves the kinematics with which the affected arm performs a reaching task. In other words, not only did MI improve function, but the quality and efficiency with which patients performed a functional activity also improved.

Before and after MI + RTP, five chronic stroke patients (3 males; mean age = 52.6 ± 15.4 years, age range 38–76 years; mean time since stroke = 51.2 months, range 13 – 126 months) were instrumented with 15 retro-reflective markers placed bilaterally. Subjects were seated at an adjustable chair and feet positioned flat. They then randomly performed two different reaching tasks: reach out and reach up. Both tasks consisted of reaching a plastic cylinder (5-cm diameter; 17-cm high) positioned in line with the olecranon and at a height of either the olecranon (reach out) or the acromioclavicular joint (reach up). Before MI + RTP, mean horizontal reaching distance was 8.3 ± 1.7 cm and 10.9 ± 2.2 cm for the reach up and reach out tasks, respectively. After intervention, ability to reach up significantly improved to 9.9 ± 1.6 cm ($P < 0.001$); horizontal reach distance improved insignificantly during the reach out task (11.7 ± 2.2 cm, $P = 0.366$). Subjects exhibited marked, non-significant increases in linear hand velocity (<u>reach out</u>: pre 20.5 ± 3.4 cm/s, post 27.3 ± 4.8 cm/s, $P = 0.068$; <u>reach up</u>: pre 19.3 ± 3.9 cm/s, post 26.1 ± 3.8 cm/s, $P = 0.072$) by 7 cm/s (approximately 35%). As we noted in the article, while subjects did not exhibit significant kinematic changes in all planes, their motor changes translated to improved (and, in some cases, new) ability to reach for and grasp objects (e.g., comb, toothbrush), as well as new supination/pronation during activities, such as pouring from a cup. Thus, the changes were still sufficiently robust to be clinically meaningful.

3 **Motor imagery increases affected arm use and reduces functional limitation: a pilot study** (Page *et al.* 2005). In 2005, we reported that, in addition to functional changes, MI + RTP increases community-based affected arm use as measured by the Motor Activity Log. Eleven chronic stroke patients were administered the same RTP programme discussed above. Six of the subjects also received the MI intervention, while five received a relaxation tape with the same duration and frequency as the MI intervention. Outcome measures, administered once before and once after intervention, were the Action Research Arm Test (ARAT), and the Motor Activity Log (MAL). The former is a test of functional limitation that mostly examines the ability to actively perform fine movements with the distal areas of the arm. Items include pinching, grasping, and gripping small objects between fingers (e.g., a marble between the thumb and each of the four digits), as well as larger items (e.g., grasping a block). The MAL is a self-report instrument in which the patient rates the quality and amount with he/she performs each of 30 valued activities (e.g., turning on a light with a switch; turning a key in a lock) all with the affected hand. Increased scores are indicative of increased use and/or function in the affected hand.

Affected limb use as rated by MI + RTP patients and their caregivers increased (1.55, 1.66, respectively), as did patient and caregiver ratings of quality of movement (2.33, 2.15, respectively) and ARAT scores (10.7). In contrast, the controls showed nominal MAL changes. A Wilcoxon test on the ARAT scores revealed significantly ($P < .004$) greater changes in the MI + RTP group's scores.

4 **A randomized, placebo-controlled study of MI in chronic stroke** (Page *et al.* 2007). The above studies culminated in a recently completed, clinical trial. Using a multiple baseline design, all subjects (n = 32) were administered the FM and ARAT on two occasions. Patients were then randomly assigned to an MI + RTP or relaxation tape + RTP. No pre-existing group differences were found on any demographic variable or movement scale. Subjects receiving MI + RTP showed significant reductions in affected arm impairment and functional limitation (both at the $P < 0.0001$ level). Functionally patients receiving MI + RTP were able to perform valued activities that they had not performed in years, such as writing, and using a computer keyboard with the affected hand.

5 **Other relevant MI studies.** Other relevant MI work includes the following:

♦ Page *et al.* 2001 compared the arm impairment and functional restriction levels of a patient with a sub-acute stroke MI combined with RTP versus those of a patient with sub-acute stroke received only RTP. Patient 'A' received RTP for the affected side 3 times per week for 6 weeks. In addition, 2 times per week, he listened to a 10-minute audiotape containing stroke information. Patient 'B' was an age-matched male who received identical amounts and types of RTP for the affected side from the same therapist as Patient A. However, 2 times per week, Patient B listened to an audiotape in which he imaged himself functionally using the affected limb as well as listening to the tape at home 2 times per week. PRE and POST measures were the upper extremity scale of the FM and ARAT. At POST, Patient B, who received MI, exhibited a higher score on the FM and considerable improvements in fine motor skill, as measured by the ARAT while Patient A's scores remained stable between PRE and POST.

♦ Expanding the work in subacute stroke, Page *et al.* 2001 conducted a study examining MI + RTP efficacy in reducing impairment levels and improving functional outcomes of sub-acute stroke patients. Upper extremity impairment, as measured by the upper extremity component of the FM, remained stable for all subjects during pre-testing. Specifically, subjects in the control group averaged 35.00 on the FM after the first pretesting session (PRE-1), and 37.00 on the FM during the second pretesting session (PRE-2). Subjects in the experimental group scored FM averages of 19.4 and 19.75 during PRE-1 and PRE-2, respectively. At POST, scores of subjects in the control group remained stable at 37.00. However, subjects in the experimental group exhibited tremendous improvement, scoring a mean of 35.5.

In all of our above work, the therapy and MI components have remained fairly consistent. The therapy has typically consisted of repetitive, task specific practice (RTP), and is usually administered 2–3 days per week in one and half hour increments. During these sessions, emphasis is placed on breaking down tasks that patients want to relearn into their smallest components, and working on the most deficient components repetitively until mastery is achieved.

MI is most effective when the skills being mentally rehearsed are also physically practiced. This is because the physical practice component is believed to create a motor plan or 'schema' that MI then augments or emboldens. Thus, the MI programme provides MI + RTP subjects with RTP, plus additional practice of the five aforementioned physical skills via MI. Specifically, directly after their half hour RTP sessions, subjects receive a 60 minute, recorded MI intervention. The tape typically consists of 6–8 opening minutes of relaxation, asking patients to imagine themselves in a warm, relaxing place (e.g., a beach), and asking them to contract and relax their muscles (i.e., progressive relaxation). This portion of the tapes is typically followed by suggestions for internal, cognitive polysensory (i.e., using both kinaesthetic and visual cues) images (Paivio, 1985) related to using the affected arm in one of functional tasks, which are also practiced during RTP sessions. The final minutes allow patients to refocus into the room.

Using the above format, other research groups have corroborated the finding that MI reduces affected arm impairment and increases movement in stroke patients (Dijkerman *et al.* 2004)

♦ Crosbie and colleagues (2004) administered MI as part of a therapy programme to 10 men and women between 10 and 176 days post stroke. The study design incorporated a single case design in which each patient acted as his/her own control. Specifically, each patient with two weeks baseline, two weeks intervention, and one week withdrawal. The intervention consisted of structured daily MI sessions of a reach and grasp task, in addition to their usual therapy. Using the Motricity Index as their primary outcome measure, the authors showed that 9 of the 10 subjects exhibited motor changes that were attributable to the MI intervention.

♦ During that same year, Dijkerman and colleagues (2004) showed the same effect on a group of 20 patients with long-term motor impairments (mean two years post-stroke). All subjects assessed before and after four weeks of MI training using measures of motor function (training task, pegboard, and dynamometer), perceived locus of control, attention control, and ADL independence. Ten patients mentally rehearsed movements with their affected arm. Their recovery was compared with patients who performed non-MI ($n = 5$), or who were not engaged in mental rehearsal ($n = 5$). The authors reported that all patient groups improved on all motor tasks except the dynamometer. Improvement was greater for the MI group on the training task (average of 14% versus 6%).

Motor imagery use for affected leg retraining after stroke

As mentioned above, MI is especially useful in situations where physical practice may be difficult or unsafe. For example, walking is, perhaps, the primary goal after stroke. Indeed, Lord *et al.*

(2004) found that the ability to 'get out and about' in the community was considered to be either essential or very important by 75% of stroke patients. Yet, practicing walking in one's hospital room or one's home is unwise for most patients, especially if they lack substantive care partner support. In such situations, MI may be a viable, safe method of practicing walking, since skills are cognitively rehearsed without actual, physical practice.

Spurred by the above findings, MI has been tested in small pilot studies targeting the stroke-affected leg. These studies included: (a) A case series (Dunsky et al. 2006) in which four chronic stroke subjects were administered MI in combination with exercises addressing gait impairments, and some gait training, all occurring three days per week for six weeks. Subjects exhibited increased gait velocity, stride length, and cadence, and a decrease in double support time. (b) A single case (Dickstein et al. 2004) who also received the above intervention. He also showed a 23% increase in gait velocity, and reduced double support time. One other study (Jackson et al. 2004) has shown that MI participation increases serial response time to a task performed with the affected leg, while another (Yoo and Chung 2006) showed that subjects who incorporated MI with visual feedback exhibited better responses to a symmetrical weight bearing training programme compared to those who used visual feedback only. (c) Finally, a group (Jackson et al. 2003) has suggested that M1 and the orbitofrontal cortex are implicated in motor skill relearning of the affected leg following mental practice. The latter data are discussed in greater detail later in this chapter.

Mechanisms during MI

Although individuals do not always physically move during MI, decades of research show that widespread muscular activations occur during MI as if the activity is being physically performed (see Chapter 6 of this book, for greater discussion). Indeed, in one group's words, MI produces 'an identical, minute innervation in localised muscles activated during the same overt movement (Hale, 1982).

Evidence for this finding first came from Jacobsen (1931) who reported activations in the biceps brachii of participants who were asked to visualize bending their right arms. More recent studies have confirmed Jacobsen's findings using electromyography (EMG; Bakker et al. 1996). Moreover, the EMG force characteristics observed during MI are proportional to the force characteristics of the task imaged (Hale 1982), and vegetative responses (e.g., heart rate, oxygen consumption) during MI covary with degrees of imagined effort on a particular task (Decety et al. 1991). In other words, an imagined task that is physically more strenuous elicits greater physiologic responses than one that is less strenuous. A number of studies have also reported correlative neural activity during MI. Indeed, motor evoked potentials, EEG activity, and increased cerebral blood flow to cortical areas that used during physical performance of a particular task, are all observed during MI (Izumi et al. 1995; Salford et al. 1995).

Although beyond the scope of this review, it is interesting to note that the time needed to mentally execute actions is nearly identical to the time needed to physically execute them (Decety et al. 1989; Louis et al. 2008). This evidence has led researchers (Decety 1996) to further conclude that imagined actions rely on same neuromuscular substrates as actual, voluntary physical movements.

Neural changes during MI

As discussed previously, mapping techniques that measure brain function during or after rehabilitation include rCBF, rCMRglc PET or SPECT, fMRI, and TMS, among others. During use of

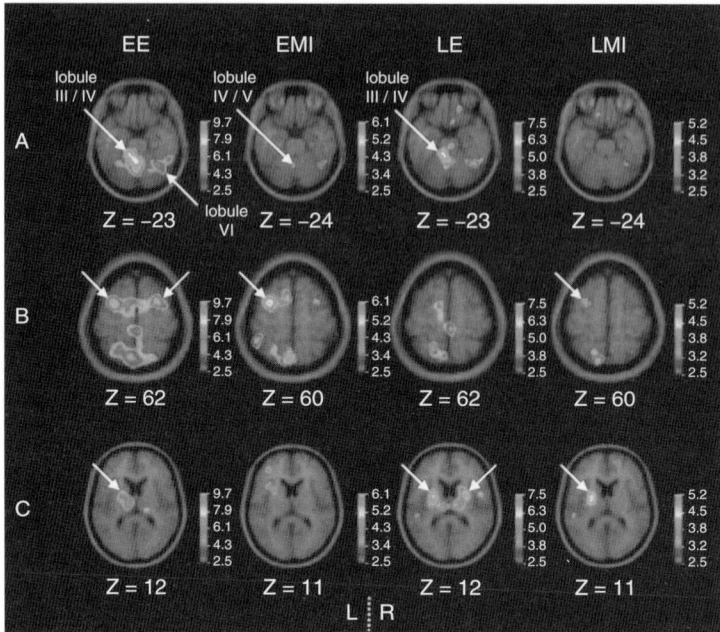

Fig. 10.1 Merged PET-MRI sections illustrating increases of regional cerebral blood flow (rCBF) associated with the execution and MI conditions, both before and after training on the foot-sequence task. The images were averaged over the nine subjects and represent the four different experimental conditions (EE, early execution; EMI, early motor imagery; LE, late execution; LMI, late motor imagery) minus the perceptual control condition. Each subtraction yielded focal changes in blood flow shown as t statistic images; the range is coded by the colour scale (L, left; R, right). Areas of activation in the (A) cerebellar lobules, (B) dorsal premotor cortex, and (C) striatum. (reprinted with permission from Elsevier, Jackson et al. 2003). See colour plate section.

these techniques, a subject's behaviour (e.g., affected limb movement) is manipulated. This movement is of course, initiated by the brain. The above techniques measure changes in signal amplitude, regional blood flow, and/or metabolism during the behaviour. If changes are present in particular brain regions, they are believed to be illustrative of the brain area controlling that behaviour. For example, if a stroke subject moves his/her affected arm, blood flow to the cortical area controlling the affected arm should increase. During fMRI, one measures regional blood flow changes that vary with the changing metabolic demands of neurons nearby.

Using the above techniques, several studies have compared the neural events that co-occur with MI versus those that occur during physical performance of the same task. The genesis of new and improved brain-imaging techniques has revealed that the same neural structures subserve both physical and imagined movements (Figure 10.1) (Lafleur *et al.* 2002; Lacourse *et al.* 2004). For example, Lacourse and colleagues (Lacourse *et al.* 2005) required subjects to mentally and physically practice an intensive button pushing sequence. Using fMRI, they recorded cortical activity during each condition, both before subjects learned the task ('Novel') and after subjects learned the task ('Skilled'). As the subjects became more skilled at the task, the fMRI patterns during mental practice became more congruent with those observed during physical practice. Other fMRI studies (Lotze *et al.* 1999) have similarly shown that the same neural networks are activated during mental and physical performance of the same task.

MI use produces cortical reorganizations/cortical plasticity after stroke

As discussed above, during MI, similar musculature and neural networks are activated as if the imagined activity was being physically performed. Over time, the repetitive activations brought about by MI likely cause cortical plasticity in the same fashion as RTP does. This cortical plasticity may be a primary mechanism underlying the functional changes observed after MI. Restated, if the same processes are occurring during MI and physical practice, repetitive MI should facilitate cortical reorganization and correlative reacquisition of function in the same way as massed physical performance (Carr and Shepherd 1998).

While the body of evidence showing cortical activations *during* MI is quite large, only a handful of studies have examined whether cortical organizations occur *as a result of* MI participation. Below, we discuss the two largest studies showing these changes.

1 Jackson and colleagues (2003) administered a specific ankle dorsiflexion/plantar flexion task to nine subjects with stroke. Subjects were presented with two different auditory signals, and either executed or imagined a dorsiflexion in response to a high-pitched sound (2000 Hz), or a plantar flexion in response to a low-pitched sound (100 Hz). During conditions involving the imagination of movements, subjects imagined that their foot reached the target position following each sound using the first-person perspective.

   The subjects also participated in two scanning sessions (Session 1: Early Learning; Session 2: Late Learning) using positron emission tomography (PET). Before scanning began in Session 1, subjects completed one block of 20 random trials, in both physical and MI conditions, in order to become familiar with the task. Subsequently, a 10-element sequence of dorsiflexion (D) and plantar flexion (P) movements (sequence = D-D-P-D-P-P-D-P-D-P) was explicitly taught to the subjects until they were able to reproduce it correctly three times in a row, thus demonstrating declarative knowledge of the sequence.

   Subjects exhibited a decreased movement response time, which was deduced to be indicative of learning. Parallel to this finding, subjects exhibited a significant decrease in the time taken to imagine the foot movement sequence, and increased rCBF in the right medial orbitofrontal cortex. Direct comparisons of the cerebral blood flow before and after MI showed that this frontal region was significantly more activated during both the execution and imagination of the sequence after practice. This study provides a well-controlled examination of dorsiflexion and plantar flexion, and the impact of learning via MI and physical practice on these processes. This is an important information given that dorsiflexion is a critical component of the gait cycle (Dobkin 2003). However, this study neither examined the influence of MI on actual ambulation outcomes (e.g., gait velocity), nor the impact of MI depicting 'real world' ambulation activities on cortical changes.

2 A recent study by our group (Page *et al.* in press) administered a battery of affected arm functional activities (e.g., reacing for and grasping a cup) to 10 chronic stroke patients (mean time post stroke = 36.7 months). Under occupational therapist supervision, subjects physically practiced these activities during half hour therapy sessions, occurring three days per week over a 10-week period. Directly after therapy sessions, subjects mentally rehearsed the same activities that they had just physically rehearsed.

   Subjects had exhibited no motor changes in months (and in some cases, years), and initially exhibited minimal ability to move their affected wrists. However, after participating in the above-described regimen, subjects displayed new movements in their affected wrists and fingers. These new isolated movements enabled subjects to perform valued activities (e.g., striking a computer key) that they had not performed in months. Using fMRI,

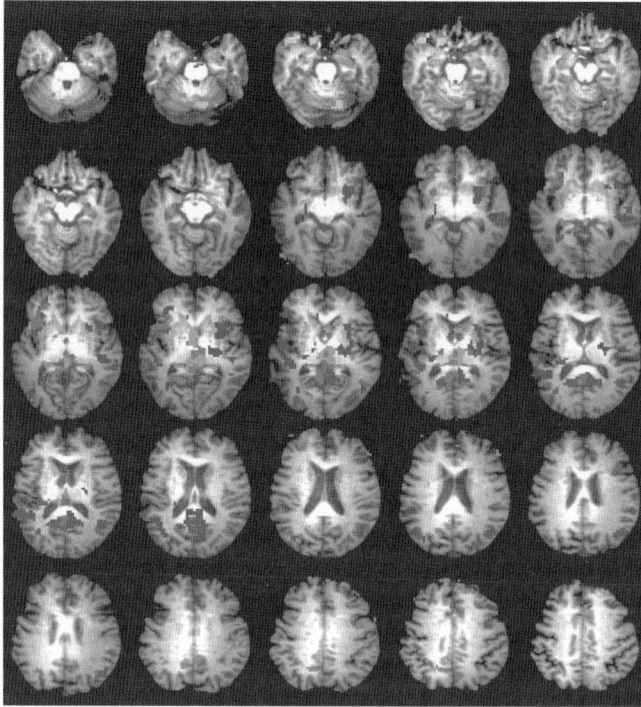

Fig. 10.2 Group fMRI activation patterns after a 10-week programme of MI targeting the affected arm. Orange depicts areas of increased cortical activation; blue depicts areas of decreased activation. In this particular study, subjects became more adept at using the affected arm; it is likely that the large decreases in activation suggest a more efficient brain pattern and/or consolidation of the activations, both commiserate with subjects' increased motor abilities. This figure is authors', taken from his previously unpublished material. See colour plate section.

we showed that 'plastic' changes coincided with the above motor changes. Since subjects had not exhibited motor changes in months, and they were not receiving any other rehabilitative regimens, we concluded that the intervention was most likely responsible for the motor and neural changes observed.

Across our MI studies for the affected arm, fMRI data have shown initial activation in contralateral primary motor cortex, SMA, and superior parietal lobule, with small clusters in the ipsilateral primary motor cortex. A small number of subjects have shown no detectable activation before intervention. Post-treatment, subjects have shown reductions in the extent of contralateral primary motor and parietal activation, and significantly increased activation in ipsilateral primary motor and premotor regions, and increased activation in the ipsilesional SMA. Activation increases included both an expansion of activation and an increase in activation magnitude.

Figure 10.2 provides a group depiction of subjects' activation patterns thus far, at pre and post MI intervention. These subjects were several years post stroke and, thus, were medically and neurologically stable, and receiving no rehabilitative therapies. Their clinicians had reported that these individuals had 'plateau', meaning that no additional motor responses were elicited when these subjects were administered rehabilitative therapies.

As shown in Figure 10.2, after being administered MI in combination with RTP for a period of 10 weeks, and using the format described previously, significant cortical activation changes were observed. In the figure, orange-coloured regions are areas where activation increased after MI treatment, while blue regions are cortical regions that decreased with MI treatment. Notice the orange regions in ipsilateral motor cortex, bottom row, and ipsilateral cerebellum that increase with treatment. While the same reorganization patterns have been seen regardless of side of injury, to make review easier, all patients in the figure are right-hand affected.

With its ease of use and low cost, it is likely that more groups will examine the mechanisms underlying MI efficacy in the future.

Conclusion

MI offers similar benefits to physical practice, including activating the same neural and muscular structures as physical practice. Yet, unlike existing physical rehabilitation modalities for stroke, MI is non-invasive, does not require extensive set-up or equipment, and is neither cost nor personnel intensive. Several studies suggest MI efficacy, even years after stroke, and MI appears to produce the same neuroplastic changes as physical modalities. Although more work is needed to optimize its dosing and confirm its neural effects, these facets make MI a viable treatment strategy in stroke.

References

American Heart Association (2008). Heart disease and stroke statistics – 2008 update. *American Heart Association, Inc.*

Bachman, K. (1990). Using mental imagery to practice a specific psychomotor skill. *Journal of Continuing Education in Nursing*, **21**, 125–8.

Bach y Rita, P. (1964). Convergent and long latency unit responses in the reticular formation of the cat. *Experimental Neurology*. **9**, 327–44.

Baker, L.L., Eberly, V., Rakoski, D., *et al.* (2007). Preliminary experience with implanted microstimulators for management of post-stroke impairments. *Journal of Neurologic Physical Therapy*, **30**, 209–22.

Bakker, F.C., Boschker, M., and Chung, J. (1996). Changes in muscular activity while imagining weight lifting using stimulus response propositions. *Journal of Sport and Exercise Psychology*, **18**, 313–24.

Broca, P. (1861). Remarques sur le siege de la faculte du language articule; suivies d'une observation d'a phemie. *Bulletin of the Society of Anatomy of Paris*, **6**, 330–57.

Carr, J. and Shepherd, R. (1998). *Neurological Rehabilitation: Optimizing Motor Performance*. Oxford: Butterworth-Heineman.

Chae, J. and Hart, R. (2003). Intramuscular hand neuroprosthesis for chronic stroke survivors. *Neurorehabilitation and Neural Repair*, **17**, 109–17.

Chen, G., Patten, C., Kothari, D.H., and Zajac, F.E. (2005). Gait differences between individuals with post-stroke hemiparesis and non-disabled controls at matched speeds, *Gait and Posture*, **22**, 51–6.

Cicinelli, P., Traversa, R., and Rossini, P.M. (1997). Post-stroke reorganization of brain motor output of the hand: a 2–4 month follow-up with focal magnetic transcranial stimulation. *Electroencephalography and Clinical Neurophysiology*, **105**, 438–50.

Classen, J., Liepert, J., Wise, S.P., Hallett, M., and Cohen, L.G. (1998). Rapid plasticity of human cortical movement representation induced by practice. *Journal of Neurophysiology*, **79**, 1117–23.

Corr, S. and Bayer, A. (1992). Poor functional status of stroke patients after hospital discharge: scope for intervention. *British Journal of Occupational Therapy*, **55**, 383–5.

Crosbie, J., McDonough, S.M., Gilmore, D.H., and Wiggam, M.I. (2004). The adjunctive role of mental practice in the rehabilitation of the upper limb after hemiplegic stroke: a pilot study. *Clinical Rehabilitation*, **18**, 60–8.

Dean, C.M., and Shepherd, R.B. (1997). Task-related training improves performance of seated reaching tasks after stroke. A randomized controlled trial. *Stroke*, **28**, 722–28.

Decety, J. (1996). Do imagined and executed actions share the same neural substrate? *Cognitive Brain Research*, **3**, 87–93.

Decety, J., Jeannerod, M., Germain, M., and Pastene, J. (1991). Vegetative response during imagined movement is proportional to mental effort. *Behavioral Brain Research*, **42**, 1–5.

Decety, J., Jeannerod, M., and Prablanc, C. (1989). The timing of mentally represented actions. *Behavioral Brain Research*, **34**, 35–42.

Dickstein, R., Dunsky, A., and Marcovitz, E. (2004). Motor imagery for gait rehabilitation in post-stroke hemiparesis. *Physical Therapy*, **84**, 1167–77.

Dijkerman, H.C., Letswaart, M., Johnston, M., and MacWalter, R.S. (2004). Does motor imagery training improve hand function in chronic stroke patients? A pilot study. *Clinical Rehabilitation*, **18**, 538–49.

Dobkin, B.H. (2003). *The Clinical Science of Neurologic Rehabilitation.* New York: Oxford University Press.

Donoghue, J.P., Hess, G., and Sanes, J.N. (1991). Motor cortical substrates and mechanisms for learning, in: J.R. Bloedel, T.J. Ebner, S.P. Wise (eds), *Acquisition of Motor Behavior in Vertebrates*, pp. 363–86. Cambridge MA: MIT Press.

Dunsky, A., Dickstein, R., Ariav, C., Deutsch, J., and Marcovitz, E. (2006). Motor imagery practice in gait rehabilitation of chronic post-stroke hemiparesis: four case studies. *International Journal of Rehabilitation Research*, **29**, 351–6.

Elbert, T., Pantev, C., Wienbruch, C., Rockstroh, B., and Taub, E. (1995). Increased cortical representation of the fingers of the left hand in string players. *Science*, **270**, 305–7.

Fansler, C.L., Poff, C.L., and Shepard, K.F. (1985). Effects of motor imagery on balance in elderly women. *Physical Therapy*, **65**, 1332–7.

Galea, M.P., Miller, K.J., and Kilbreath, S.L. (2001). Early task-related training enhances upper limb function following stroke. Poster presented at the annual meeting of the Society for Neural Control of Movement, Sevilla, Spain.

Goldie, P.A., Matyas, T.A., and Evans, O.M. (1996). Deficit and change in gait velocity during rehabilitation after stroke. *Archives of Physical Medicine and Rehabilitation*, **77**, 1074–82.

Gresham, G., Fitzpatrick, T., Wolf, P., McNamara, P., Kannel, W., and Dawber, T. (1975). Residual disability in survivors of stroke – the framingham study. *New England Journal of Medicine*, **293**, 954–6.

Hale, B.D. (1982). The effects of internal and external imagery on muscular and oular concomitants. *Journal of Sport Psychology*, **4**, 379–87.

Hebb, D.O. (1949). *The Organization of Behavior.* New York: Wiley.

Hewett, T.E., Ford, K.R., Levine, P., and Page, S.J. (2007). Reaching kinematics to measure motor changes after mental practice in stroke. *Top Stroke Rehabil.* Jul-Aug;**14**, 23–9.

Hill, K., Ellis, P., Bernhardt, J., Maggs, P., and Hull, S. (1997). Balance and mobility outcomes for stroke patients: a comprehensive review. *Australian Journal of Physiotherapy*, **43**, 173–80.

Izumi, S., Findley, T., Ikai, T., *et al.* (1995). Facilitatory effect of thinking about movement on motor evoked potentials to transcranial magnetic stimulation of the brain. *American Journal of Physical Medicine and Rehabilitation*, **74**, 207–13.

Jackson, P.L., Doyon, J., Richards, C.L., and Malouin, F. (2004). The efficacy of combined physical and mental practice in the learning of a foot-sequence task after stroke: a case report. *Neurorehabilitation and Neural Repair,* **18**, 106–11.

Jackson, P.L., Lafleur, M.F., Malouin, F., Richards, C.L., and Doyon, J. (2003). Functional cerebral reorganization following motor sequence learning through mental practice with motor imagery. *Neuroimage*, **20**, 1171–80.

Jacobsen, E. (1931). Electrical measurement of neuromuscular states during mental activities: a note on mental activities concerning an amputated limb. *American Journal of Physiology*, **43**, 122–5.

Jenkins, W.M., Merzenich, M.M., Ochs, M.T., *et al.* (1990). Functional reorganization of primary somatosensory cortex in adult owl squirrel monkeys after behaviorally controlled tactile stimulation. *Journal of Physiology,* **63**, 82–104.

Kaas, J. H. (1991). Plasticity of sensory and motor maps in adult mammals. *Annual Review of Neuroscience*, **14**, 137–67.

Kaplon, R.T., Prettyman, M.G., Kushi, C.L., and Winstein, C.J. (2007). Six hours in the laboratory: a quantification of practice time during constraint-induced therapy (CIT). *Clinical Rehabilitation*, **21**, 950–8.

Karni, A., Meyer, G., Jezzard, P., Adams, M.M., Turner, R., and Ungerleider, L.G. (1995). Functional MRI evidence for adult motor cortex plasticity during motor skill learning. *Nature*, **377**, 155–8.

Kelly-Hayes, M., Beiser, A., Kase, C.S., Scaramucci, A., D'Agostino, R.B., and Wolf, P.A. (2003). The influence of gender and age on disability following ischemic stroke: the Framingham study. *Journal of Stroke and Cerebrovascular Disease*, **12**, 119–26.

Kissela, B., Schneider, A., Kleindorfer, D., *et al.* (2004). Stroke in a biracial population: the excess burden of stroke among blacks. *Stroke*, **35**, 426–31.

Kleindorfer, D., Broderick, J., Khoury, J., *et al.* (2006). The unchanging incidence and case-fatality of stroke in the 1990s: a population-based study. *Stroke*, **37**, 2473–8.

Lacourse, M.G., Orr, E.L., Cramer, S.C., and Cohen, M.J. (2005). Brain activation during execution and motor imagery of novel and skilled sequential hand movements. *Neuroimage*, **27**, 505–19.

Lacourse, M.G., Turner, J.A., Randolph-Orr, E., Schandler, S.L., and Cohen, M.J. (2004). Cerebral and cerebellar sensorimotor plasticity following motor imagery-based mental practice of a sequential movement. *Journal of Rehabilitation Research and Development*, **41**, 505–24.

Lafleur, M.F., Jackson, P.L., Richards, C., Malouin, F., and Doyon, J. (2002). Motor learning produces parallel dynamic functional changes during the execution and the imagination of sequential foot movements. *NeuroImage*, **16**, 142–57.

Leyton, A.S., and Sherrington, C.S. (1917). Observations on the excitable cortex of the chimpanzee, orangutan, and gorilla. *Quarterly Journal of Experimental Psychology*, **11**, 135–222.

Liepert, J., Bauder, H., Sommer, M., *et al.* (1998). Motor cortex plasticity during constraint-induced movement therapy in chronic stroke patients. *Neuroscience Letters*, **250**, 5–8.

Liepert, J., Terborg, C., and Weiller, C. (1999). Motor plasticity induced by synchronized thumb and foot movements. *Experimental Brain Research*, **125**, 435–9.

Linden, C.A., Uhley, J.E., Smith, D., and Bush, M.A. (1989). The effects of motor imagery on walking balance in an elderly population. *Occupational Therapy Journal of Research*, **9**, 155–69.

Livesay, J.R., and Samras, M.R. (1998). Covert neuromuscular activity of the dominant forearm during visualization of a motor task. *Perceptual and Motor Skills*, **86**, 371–4.

Lord, S.E., McPherson, K., McNaughton, H.K., Rochester, L., and Weatherall, M. (2004). Community ambulation after stroke: how important and obtainable is it and what measures appear predictive? *Archives of Physical Medicine and Rehabilitation*, **85**, 234–9.

Louis, M., Guillot, A., Maton, S., Doyon, J., and Collet, C. (2008). Effect of imagined movement speed on subsequent motor performance. *Journal of Motor Behavior*, **40**, 117–32.

Lotze, M., Montoya, P., Erb, M., *et al.* (1999). Activation of cortical and cerebellar motor areas during executed and imagined hand movements: an fMRI study. *Journal of Cognitive Neuroscience*, **11**, 491–501.

Luft, A.R., McCombe-Waller, S., *et al.* (2004). Repetitive bilateral arm training and motor cortex activation in chronic stroke: a randomized controlled trial. *Journal of the American Medical Association*, **292**, 1853–61.

Maring, J.R. (1990). Effects of motor imagery on rate of skill acquisition. *Physical Therapy*, **70**, 165–72.

Merians, A.S., Poizner, H., Boian, R., Burdea, G., and Adamovich, S. (2006). Sensorimotor training in a virtual reality environment: does it improve functional recovery poststroke? *Neurorehabilitation and Neural Repair*, **20**, 252–67.

Miltner, W., Bauder, H., Sommer, M., Dettmers, C., and Taub, E. (1999). Effects of constraint-induced movement therapy on patients with chronic motor deficits after stroke: a replication. *Stroke*, **30**, 586–92.

Northstar Neuroscience, Inc. Safety and effectiveness of cortical stimulation in hemiparetic stroke patients. Northstar study code 'Everest'; study # VO267

Nudo, R.J. (2006). Plasticity. *NeuroRx*, **3**, 420–7.

Nudo, R.J., Milliken, G. W., Jenkins, W. M., and Merzenich, M. M. (1996). Use-dependent alterations of movement representations in primary motor cortex of adult squirrel monkeys. *Journal of Neuroscience*, **16**, 785–807.

Page, S.J. (2000). Imagery improves motor function in chronic stroke patients with hemiplegia: a pilot study. *Occupational Therapy Journal of Research*, **20**, 200–15.

Page, S.J., Levine, P., and Leonard, A.C. (2005). Effects of motor imagery on affected limb use and function in chronic stroke. *Archives of Physical Medicine and Rehabilitation*, **86**, 399–402.

Page, S.J., Levine, P., and Leonard, A. (2007). Motor imagery in chronic stroke: results of a randomized, placebo controlled trial. *Stroke*, **38**, 1293–7.

Page, S.J, Levine, P., Sisto, S., and Johnston, M. (2001). Imagery combined with physical practice for upper limb motor deficit in sub-acute stroke: a case report. *Physical Therapy*, **81**, 1455–62.

Page, S.J., Sisto, S., Levine, P., and McGrath, R. (2004). Efficacy of modified constraint-induced therapy in chronic stroke: a single blinded randomized controlled trial. *Archives of Physical Medicine and Rehabilitation*, **85**, 14–18.

Page, S.J., Szaflarski, J.P., Eliassen, J., Pan, H., and Cramer, S.C. (in press). Cortical Plasticity Following Motor Skill Learning During Mental Practice in Stroke. Neurorehabilitation and Neural Repair.

Paivio, A. (1985). Cognitive and motivational functions of imagery in human performance. *Journal of Applied Sport Science*, **10**, 22–28.

Pierce, S.R., Gallagher, K.G., Schaumburg, S.W., Gershkoff, A.M., Gaughan, J.P., and Shutter, L. (2003). Home forced use in an outpatient rehabilitation program for adults with hemiplegia: a pilot study. *Neurorehabilitation and Neural Repair*, **17**, 214–19.

Rundek, T. and Sacco, R.L. (2008). Risk factor management to prevent first stroke. *Neurology Clinical*, **26**, 1007–45.

Salford, E., Ryding, E., Rosen, I., *et al.* (1995). Motor performance and motor ideation of arm movements after stroke: a SPECT rCBF study. In Proceedings if the World Confederation of Physical Therapy Congress: Washington, D.C. p. 793.

Schaechter, J.D., Kraft, E., Hilliard, T.S. *et al.* (2002). Motor recovery and cortical reorganization after constraint-induced movement therapy in stroke patients: a preliminary study. *Neurorehabilitation and Neural Repair*, **16**, 326–38.

Sidaway, B. and Trzaska, A.R. (2005). Can motor imagery increase ankle dorsiflexor torque? *Physical Therapy*, **85**, 1053–60.

Siegert, R.J., Lord, S., and Porter, K. (2004). Constraint-induced movement therapy: time for a little restraint? *Clinical Rehabilitation*, **18**, 110–14.

Smith, G.V., Silver, K.H., Goldberg, A.P., and Macko, R.F. (1999). 'Task-oriented' exercise improves hamstring strength and spastic reflexes in chronic stroke patients. *Stroke*, **30**, 2112–8.

Sterr, A., Müller, M.M., Elbert, T., Rockstroh, B., Pantev, C., and Taub, E. (1998). Changed perceptions in Braille readers. *Nature*, **391**, 134–5.

Sterr, A., Elbert, T., Berthold, I., Kolbel, S., Rockstroh, B., and Taub, E. (2002). Longer versus shorter daily constraint-induced movement therapy of chronic hemiparesis: an exploratory study. *Archives of Physical Medicine and Rehabilitation*, **83**, 1374–7.

Szaflarski, J.P., Page, S.J., Kissela, B.M., Lee, J.H., Levine, P. and Strakowski, S.M. (2006). Cortical reorganization following modified constraint-induced movement therapy: a study of 4 patients with chronic stroke. *Archives of Physical Medicine and Rehabilitation*, **87**, 1052–8.

Taub, E. (1977). Movement in nonhuman primates deprived of somatosensory feedback, in: *Exercise and Sports Science Reviews* pp. 335–74. Santa Barbara: Journal Publishing Affiliates.

Taub, E., Lum, P.S., Hardin, P., Mark, V.W., and Uswatte, G. (2005). Automated delivery of CI therapy with reduced effort by therapists. *Stroke*, **36**, 1301–4.

Taub, E., Miller, N. E., Novack, T. A., *et al.* (1993). Technique to improve chronic motor deficit after stroke. *Archives of Physical Medicine and Rehabilitation*, **74**, 347–54.

Titianova, E.B., Pitkanen, K., Paakkonen, A., Sivenius, J., and Tarkka, I.M. (2003). Gait characteristics and functional ambulation profile in patients with chronic unilateral stroke. *American Journal of Physical Medicine and Rehabilitation*, **82**, pp. 778–86.

van der Lee, J.H., Wagenaar, R.C., Lankhorst, G.J., Vogelaar, T.W., Deville, W.L., and Bouter, L.M. (1999). Forced use of the upper extremity in chronic stroke patients: results from a single-blind randomized clinical trial. *Stroke*, **30**, 2369–75.

Volpe, B.T., Ferraro, M., Lynch, D., *et al.* (2005). Robotics and other devices in the treatment of patients recovering from stroke. *Current Neurology and Neuroscience Reports*, **5**, 465–70.

Whitall, J., McCombe-Waller, S., Silver, K.H., and Macko, R.F. (2000). Repetitive bilateral arm training with rhythmic auditory cueing improves motor function in chronic hemiparetic stroke. *Stroke*, **31**, 2390–5.

Williams, J.G., Odley, J.L., and Callaghan, M. (2004). Motor imagery boosts proprioceptive neuromuscular facilitation in attainment and retention of range of motion at the hip joint. *Journal of Sports Science and Medicine*, **3**, 160–6.

Wolf, S.L., Winstein, C.J., Miller, J.P., *et al.* (2006). Effect of constraint-induced movement therapy on upper extremity function 3 to 9 months after stroke: the EXCITE randomized clinical trial. *Journal of the American Medical Association*, **296**, 2095–104.

Yaguez, L., Nagel, D., Hoffman, H., Canavan, A.G., Wist, E., and Homberg, V. (1998). A mental route to motor learning: improving trajectorial kinematics through imagery training. *Behavioral and Brain Research*, **90**, 95–106.

Yoo, E.Y. and Chung, B.I. (2006). The effect of visual feedback plus mental practice on symmetrical weight-bearing training in people with hemiparesis. *Clinical Rehabilitation*, **20**, 388–97.

Chapter 11

Motor imagery for optimizing the reacquisition of locomotor skills after cerebral damage

Francine Malouin, Carol L. Richards, Philip L. Jackson, and Julien Doyon

Introduction

Mental practice through motor imagery (MI) has been proposed for retraining motor function after cerebral lesions. To date, most of the clinical studies in neurorehabilitation have focused on the retraining of upper limb function (Braun *et al.* 2006). The present chapter will address the potential use of mental practice through MI for retraining locomotor skills after stroke. First, the rationale and evidence for using mental practice through MI for the retraining of locomotor-related tasks will be reviewed. The second part will examine whether MI ability is preserved after stroke. In the third part, findings from clinical studies using MI to retrain locomotor-related tasks following stroke will be reported, and finally, training strategies to optimize the relearning of locomotor skills with MI will be discussed.

Rationale for using motor imagery for the retraining of locomotor-related tasks

Motor imagery is an active process during which the representation of an action is internally reproduced within working memory without any overt output (Decety and Grèzes 1999). Over the past 25 years, an increasing number of studies investigating the psychophysical and physiological correlates of MI have provided evidence that support the benefit of using mental practice through MI for retraining locomotor-related skills. A first confirmation of functional similarity between executed and imagined movements comes from autonomic studies that have demonstrated an increase in the heart and respiration rates of subjects engaged in the MI of walking (Decety *et al.* 1991; Wuyam *et al.* 1995; Fusi *et al.* 2005; see Guillot and Collet 2005b for a review). Imagining walking on a treadmill at different speeds produces speed-related increases in ventilation which amounts to about 20–50% of that observed during real walking in normal subjects (Decety *et al.* 1991; Wuyam *et al.* 1995; Fusi *et al.* 2005). These responses are likely to be of central origin because nuclear magnetic resonance spectroscopy did not find evidence for changes in muscle metabolic activity during imagined exercise (Decety *et al.* 1993). However, because a large fraction of the increased ventilation occurs at the onset of exercise (real and imagined) the vegetative response is thought to be due to the effects of motor preparation (Decety *et al.* 1991, 1993; Jeannerod 1995). Based on such findings, it has been proposed that during imagined activities, a significant portion of the observed increase in autonomic response is of central origin as though the mind deludes the body into believing that some movements are being executed (Decety 1996).

Another example of the correlation between imagined and executed locomotor movements comes from chronometric studies showing that the timing of walking, either performed physically or imagined, is subject to common laws and principles (Decety *et al.* 1989; Decety and Jeannerod 1996; Guillot and Collet 2005a; Bakker *et al.* 2007a). Indeed, temporal congruence between imagined and executed walking times has been observed in subjects instructed to walk towards targets placed at different distances (Decety *et al.* 1989; Decety and Boisson 1990; Decety and Jeannerod 1996; Courtine *et al.* 2004; Bakker *et al.* 2007a). In addition, when the walking task was made more difficult by having subjects walk or imagine themselves walking on narrow beams (Decety *et al.* 1989), through gates (Decety and Jeannerod 1996) or along paths of different widths (Bakker *et al.* 2007a), uphill or downhill (Courtine *et al.* 2004), and at different speeds (Courtine *et al.* 2004), the actual and imagined walking times increased as a function of the difficulty of the task. This effect of task difficulty in both actual and imagined movement times indicates that Fitts' law (Fitts 1954), which states that more difficult movements take more time to produce physically than easier ones, applies also to MI of walking.

Additional confirmation of functional similarity between executed and imagined movements originates from the results of brain imaging studies examining functional neuroanatomical correlates of MI of walking. Using near infrared spectroscopy (NIRS), which enables a direct comparison of cortical activity evoked during actual gait and the imagination of gait, Miyai and colleagues (2001) found that both walking conditions (actual and simulated) increased brain activity bilaterally in the medial primary sensorimotor cortices and the SMA. In addition, cortical activations found during actual walking with NIRS were comparable to activations revealed with functional magnetic resonance imaging (fMRI) during the imagination of walking (Miyai *et al.* 2001). Subsequent positron emission tomography (PET) and fMRI studies used MI to study brain activation patterns of several locomotor-related tasks such as standing (Ouchi *et al.* 1999; Malouin *et al.* 2003), initiating gait (Malouin *et al.* 2003; Wagner *et al.* 2008), normal walking (Malouin *et al.* 2003; Bakker *et al.* 2008a; Iseki *et al.* 2008), walking with obstacles (Malouin *et al.* 2003), precision gait (Bakker *et al.* 2008a), walking along a curved path (Wagner *et al.* 2008) running (Jahn *et al.* 2004; Szameitat *et al.* 2007), as well as other complex movements (Szameitat *et al.* 2007) involving the whole body (e.g. swimming, dancing, lifting a heavy box). These studies have shown that the simulation of locomotor-related activities and complex whole body tasks results in the activation of cortical networks similar to those found during MI of simple movements, hence suggesting that the overlapping between neural substrates during real and imagined movements also applies to complex body movements (Szameitat *et al.* 2007). In addition, when the task is made more difficult by asking subjects to imagine themselves walking around obstacles, increased activity is observed in additional brain areas (e.g. parahippocampal gyrus, SMA, precuneus, the parietal inferior cortex) suggesting that higher brain centres become progressively engaged when demands of locomotor tasks require increasing cognitive and sensory information processing (Malouin *et al.* 2003). Likewise, imagery of precision gait along narrow paths led to increased cerebral activity and effective connectivity within a network involving the superior parietal lobule, the dorsal precentral gyri, and the right middle occipital gyrus, suggesting that MI is sensitive to the constraints imposed by a narrow walking path (Bakker *et al.* 2008a). These results emphasize the role of cortical structures outside primary motor regions in imagining locomotor movements when accurate foot positioning and increased postural control is required.

In summary, the above findings indicate that mentally simulated and physically executed locomotor tasks rely on similar motor representation, temporal organization and activate neural networks that greatly overlap suggesting that both conditions share similar mechanisms. These findings are in accordance with the suggestion that mental practice through MI is effective because it activates a cerebral network comparable to that of physical practice (Jackson *et al.* 2001; Szameitat *et al.* 2007).

Motor imagery ability after stroke

While MI is defined as an active process during which the representation of an action is internally reproduced within working memory without any overt output (Decety and Grèzes 1999), mental practice through MI is the repetition or rehearsing of imagined motor acts with the intention of improving their physical execution. Therefore, the ability to form internal representations of motor acts is a prerequisite for training with mental practice. Obviously, one can ask whether the ability to imagine movements is affected following a stroke. This question has been investigated through different approaches such as mental rotation (Johnson 2000; Johnson *et al.* 2002), mental chronometry (Decety and Boisson 1990; Sirigu *et al.* 1995, 1996; Malouin *et al.* 2004c, 2007b, 2008b; Sabate *et al.* 2007; Stinear *et al.* 2007), and an MI questionnaire (Malouin *et al.* 2007a, 2008a). Findings suggest that, except in a few cases with focalized lesions in the superior region of the parietal cortex or the frontal cortex (Johnson 2000; Sirigu *et al.* 1996), MI ability is preserved (Malouin *et al.* 2008a; Sirigu *et al.* 1995) even in chronic and severely motor impaired subjects (Johnson *et al.* 2002). The general level of MI vividness after stroke, as measured by the Kinesthetic and Visual Imagery Questionnaire (KVIQ), has been found to be similar to that of age-matched persons and was not affected by the side of the brain lesion (Malouin *et al.* 2008a). However, patients had higher imagery scores when imagining movements with the unaffected side than with the affected side (Malouin *et al.* 2008a). Such side difference was not found in healthy individuals. Modulation in MI vividness has also been reported after lesion to the peripheral nervous system. Indeed, the ability to generate vivid images of movements was specifically weakened by the loss of a limb (amputation) or disuse following the immobilization of the non-dominant lower limb (Malouin *et al.* 2009). Altogether these findings suggest that the ability to generate vivid images of movements is a dynamic process that can be modulated by changes in sensorimotor inputs.

Because of its mental nature, however, MI is difficult to assess (for a review see Guillot and Collet 2005a,b and Chapter 8). As a clinical assessment procedure for MI, it has recently been proposed (Malouin *et al.* 2008a) to combine standardized tests such as the Time Dependent Motor Imagery (TDMI) screening test (Malouin *et al.* 2008b) and the KVIQ (Malouin *et al.* 2007a, b). The TDMI is a chronometric screening test wherein the examiner records the number of movements imagined over three time periods (15s, 25s, 45s); it assumes that subjects who display an increase in the number of movements imagined with increasing time are able to simulate movements and likely engage in MI. The test–retest reliability of the TDMI screening test has been confirmed in a group of 20 persons who had recovered from stroke with intraclass correlation coefficients ranging from .88 to .93 (Malouin *et al.* 2008b). Results have shown that the number of imagined stepping movements increased significantly with longer time periods in persons with stroke, and that the increase was comparable to that of age-matched healthy subjects, hence suggesting that persons following stroke maintain their ability to simulate stepping movements (Malouin *et al.* 2004a, 2008b).

Additional evidence confirming the maintenance of MI abilities following stroke comes from a study examining MI vividness with the KVIQ (Malouin *et al.* 2008a). The KVIQ is a standardized MI questionnaire with recognized psychometric properties that is adapted for persons with physical disabilities (Malouin *et al.* 2007a). This MI questionnaire assesses the clarity of images (visual imagery) and intensity of sensations (kinaesthetic imagery) of 10 body movements (including the head, trunk, shoulders, upper, and lower limbs) on a 5-point ordinal scale

(5 = highest imagery). Using the KVIQ, the MI vividness of a group of 32 persons post-stroke was compared to that of age-matched healthy subjects. Between-group comparisons of imagery scores showed that the vividness of MI was preserved, and that there were good and bad imagers in both groups. As mentioned above, comparisons of imagery scores between sides for movements involving the upper and lower limbs, however, showed that post-stroke MI vividness was better when imagining movements of the unaffected than the affected side, hence indicating an overestimation possibly related to a hemispheric imbalance or to a recalibration of MI perception (Malouin *et al.* 2008a).

As mentioned in the first section, movement times during the imagination and during the execution of a given movement are generally very similar; this has been referred to as temporal coupling or functional equivalence effect. However, functional equivalence does not always hold as several external factors (e.g. complexity of movement, level of experience, etc.) can result in an over- or underestimation of movement times (Guillot and Collet 2005a). Nevertheless, impaired temporal coupling has been reported after stroke for simple movements such as stepping, arm pointing, and fingers movements that normally show a functional equivalence (Jackson *et al.* 2004; Malouin *et al.* 2004c, 2007b; Sabate *et al.* 2007; Stinear *et al.* 2007). In the latter studies, comparisons between real and simulated movements revealed longer imagination times after stroke.

Furthermore, the slowing during the imagination condition appears to be linked to the side of the lesion. For instance, studies comparing movement times during the imagination and execution of a stepping task (Malouin *et al.* 2004c, 2007b) and of hand movements (Stinear *et al.* 2007) have shown that contrary to patients with a left stroke, those with a right-hemispheric lesion had longer imagination times than execution times. It was suggested that right hemispheric strokes may affect higher order aspects of movement planning, as the right parietal cortex is involved in spatial processing and attention (Stinear *et al.* 2007). While these results suggest that much of the temporal features during MI depend on spatio-temporal processes, it does not necessarily exclude the contribution of other sources.

The temporal organization of gait and locomotor-related tasks after stroke is not well known. Recently, we investigated whether the temporal congruence and the temporal structure of the timed-up-and-go (TUG) task were retained following stroke. The TUG is a complex locomotor task divided into the following four subtasks: rising from a chair, walking forward, turning around, walking back to the chair, and sitting down. Our study involved 21 persons recovering from a right ($n=7$) or a left ($n=14$) cerebral vascular accident (CVA) in cortical or subcortical regions with a mean age of 62.6 years (SD: 8.8; range: 45–75) and 21 age-matched with a mean: 65.3 years (SD: 7.3; range 46–77) healthy persons (CTL). The time to imagine (I) and execute physically (E) the total TUG task and each of the four subtasks was recorded. The duration of each subtask was normalized in per cent of the total TUG time. ANOVAs with repeated measures were used for group comparisons (CTL–CVA) of movement times during both conditions (I and E). Imagination/Execution (I/E) time ratios of total TUG and of each subtask were computed to quantify the temporal coupling. I/E time ratios were expected to be near 1 if the temporal congruence was preserved. Results from the ANOVAs revealed that in both groups there was no difference between the time to imagine and execute the total TUG (Figure 11.1: upper left). I/E time ratios were close to 1 in both groups: CVA: .98; CTL: 1.09 (Figure 11.1: upper right). Note that in each group some subjects had longer or shorter imagination than execution times indicating a similar variability across groups (Figures 11.1 lower graphs). Likewise, there was no difference between the imagination and execution times for the four subtasks and the relative time dedicated to each subtask was similar in both groups (Figures 11.2: upper graphs). Again, corresponding I/E time ratios were close to 1 in both groups: CVA: .90–1.02; CTL: .97–1.15

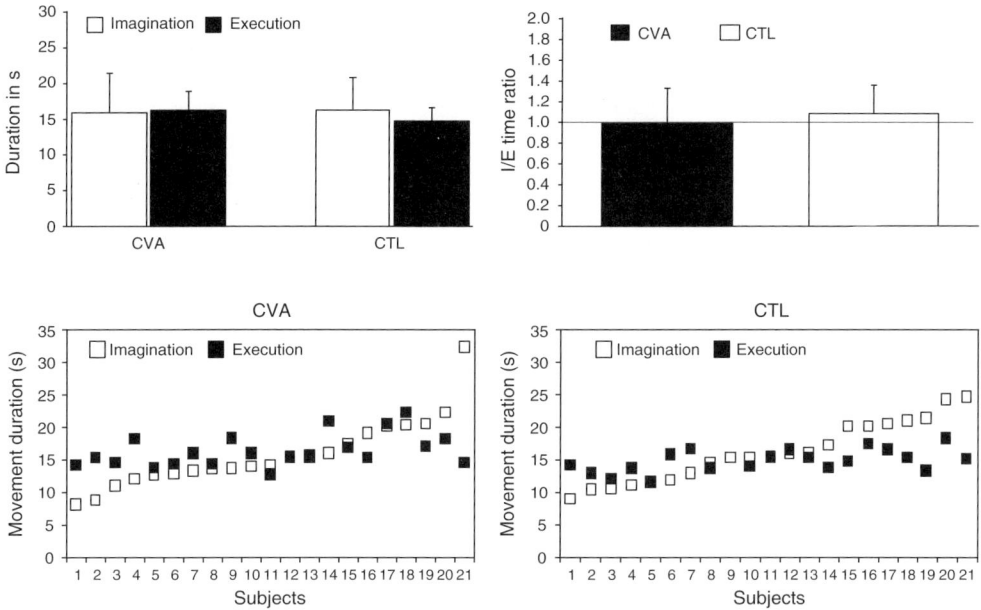

Fig. 11.1 Upper graphs: mean (SD) movement times during the imagination and execution of the timed-up-and-go-task (upper left) and corresponding mean (SD). Imagination/Execution (I/E) time ratios (upper right) in a group of persons with stroke (CVA: n=21) and a group of age-matched healthy subjects (CTL: n=21).

Lower graphs illustrate individual imagination and execution times in the CVA (lower left) and the CTL (lower right) groups, respectively.

(Figures 11.2: lower graphs). Altogether these results suggest that both the temporal coupling and the temporal structure of the TUG are retained after stroke and that the patients had a good spatio-temporal representation of each subset of the TUG. These results are important because they indicate that following stroke patients remain capable of rehearsing mentally complex motor tasks, which is a prerequisite for mental practice.

Clinical outcomes of mental practice

Mental practice with MI offers the possibility of enhancing gait performance through safe, intensive, and self-paced locomotor training in persons with severe disability that makes walking practice difficult and limited in time, especially in the early phase of rehabilitation (Jackson *et al.* 2001; Dickstein *et al.* 2004). However, to date, the few randomized clinical trials that have investigated the effects of mental practice on functional recovery have focused on upper limb function (see Braun *et al.* 2006 for a review). Yet, the potential use of mental practice for optimizing locomotor-related function such as walking (Dickstein *et al.* 2004; Dunsky *et al.* 2008), rising from a chair and sitting (Malouin *et al.* 2004a,b), as well as sequential foot movements (Jackson *et al.* 2004) has been examined in exploratory studies and case reports.

In a first report of a 69-year-old man with a left hemiparesis, improvement in gait spatiotemporal parameters was found after a six-week training programme with mental practice (Dickstein *et al.* 2004). Fifteen-minute sessions of imagery practice were held three times a week for six consecutive weeks. No physical intervention was applied during the six-week programme. Both internal and external perspectives of MI were used. The main goals were to

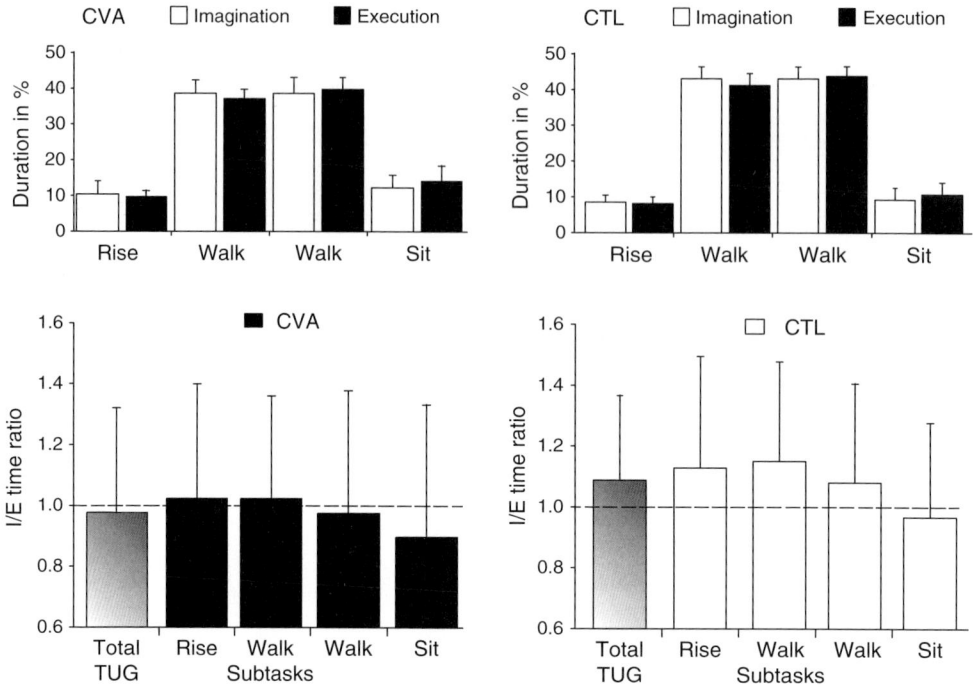

Fig. 11.2 Upper graphs: mean (SD) duration in percent of total TUG for each subtask during the imagination and execution conditions in the CVA group (upper left) and in the CTL group (upper right). Corresponding mean (SD) Imagination/Execution (I/E) time ratios are illustrated for the total TUG and each subtask for the CVA (lower left) and CTL groups (lower right).

facilitate movements and posture of the affected lower limb by focusing on the patient's specific impairments (e.g. forefoot initial contact, push-off) and to enhance functional walking in his own environment). Results indicated that most of the 20–23% increases in gait speed, stride length, and double limb support were retained at follow-up, three weeks after the end of the intervention.

Using a similar training approach, the feasibility of a home programme for enhancing gait through mental practice was investigated in 17 persons post-stroke (Dunsky *et al.* 2008). Mental practice training was provided at home by a visiting therapist three times a week for six weeks. Most patients increased their gait speed with gains ranging from about 10% to 80% for a mean increase of 15 cm/s (baseline: 38 cm/s ±17cm/s; post-training: 53 cm/s ±25cm/s). The effect size for gait speed was .64, which corresponds to a moderate treatment effect. Most interestingly, these gains in gait speed were retained at follow-up (52 cm/s ± 24cm/s) as were gains in stride length, step length, and double-limb support. Although the study did not include a control group, the mean gain in gait speed (15 cm/s) represents twice the amount of the mean gain (7 cm/s) measured in the control group of a randomized controlled study of a home-based exercise programme (including balance and walking activities) in patients with chronic stroke (Duncan *et al.* 1998). Moreover, gains after MI correspond to 60% of the mean gain (25cm/s) found in the experimental group after an eight-week physical training programme (Duncan *et al.* 1998). These results are of great interest because they support the idea that walking skills can be enhanced by MI training. However, as there was no monitoring of the amount of real walking during the home programme, one cannot exclude that part of the gains could also be attributed to an increase in walking time as a result of the home programme.

Although there is no evidence yet that MI of walking after stroke can induce brain reorganization, findings from one fMRI study in healthy adults suggest that focusing attention on walking motor schemes can modify sensorimotor activations of the brain. Indeed, after MI training of a specific sequence of leg movements through tango lessons, an expansion of the bilateral motor areas and a reduction of the visuospatial activation in the posterior cortex were found suggesting that focusing a subject's attention on the movements involved in dancing decreases the role of visual imagery processes in favour of motor-kinaesthetic ones (Sacco *et al.* 2006). In addition, deactivations observed after training in the anterior and posterior cerebellum are also in line with decreases in cerebellar activations following mental practice of a foot movement sequence during five days (Jackson *et al.* 2003).

Beneficial effects of mental practice in 12 persons with chronic stroke have also been reported in another feasibility study that examined the potential of mental practice in combination with a small amount of physical practice (7 series of 1 physical repetition for 5 mental repetitions: 1P/5M ratio) to improve limb loading on the affected leg during rising from a chair and sitting down (Malouin *et al.* 2004a,b). Changes in motor strategies, immediately after one training session and 24 hours later, were assessed by recording vertical forces under each foot. After training, the loading on the affected leg had significantly improved by 17.9% when rising from the chair and by 16.2% while sitting down. Gains were still significant 24 hours later during rising (12.8%) and sitting down (11.2%), hence indicating a learning effect. In contrast, the duration of the subjects' performance did not change with training, suggesting that in the early stage of learning, changes in motor strategies (increase in weight bearing on the affected leg) predominate over changes in speed of execution. This further suggests that, at this stage, changes in vertical forces (limb loading) represent a more sensitive measure of performance than movement time. Moreover, it was reported that patients with deficits in at least two domains of working memory had a smaller improvement (27% vs 72%) and showed no retention at follow-up, thus suggesting that the learning effect is strongly related to working memory abilities of the participants and especially in the visuospatial domain (Malouin *et al.* 2004a). Although, this study did not tease out the specific effects of mental practice, the gains which took place with a relatively small amount of physical practice (7 physical repetitions and 35 mental repetitions) had a magnitude similar to those measured after three weeks of regular physical training (Engardt *et al.* 1993). It has been proposed that the reason for improvement with such little physical practice is the combination of physical with mental practice that requires the person to mentally and explicitly rehearse the sequence of movements associated with the mobility task. Such rehearsal makes the subjects focus each time on the preparation and planning of the proper strategy, hence increasing their awareness of the required movements. Such an interpretation is in line with the results of Pascual-Leone and colleagues (1995) who, using transcranial magnetic stimulation (TMS), have demonstrated that mental practice has preparatory effects and increases the efficiency of subsequent physical training. Likewise, using PET, Jackson and colleagues (2003) found that, after five days of intensive mental practice, changes in brain activity were found in the medial aspect of the orbitofrontal cortex (increase) and cerebellum (decrease) supporting the idea that mental practice through MI initially improves performance by acting on motor preparation and planning.

Further support to the priming effects of MI comes from the findings of a controlled pilot study (Malouin *et al.* in press) that showed that a small amount of physical repetitions alone (total of 120, over a 4-week period) did not enhance the motor performance (limb loading of the affected leg during rising up and sitting down tasks), whereas, when these relatively few physical repetitions were combined with a large number of mental repetitions (total of 1100), the loading on the affected leg was significantly increased and was retained three weeks after training. Thus, the latter findings confirm the added effects of mental rehearsal on motor performance when patients rehearse the tasks mentally 10 times after each physical execution (for a ratio of 1:10).

As for the findings in the feasibility study (Malouin *et al.* 2004a,b), the improved performance immediately after one training session did not necessarily imply learning. The retention of the improved motor performance one day later, however, indicated that learning had occurred. Such retention of performance one day later could be related to the added effect of combining mental and physical repetitions, and also to sleep-related effects of MI on motor performance (Debarnot *et al.* 2009).

Another example pertaining to the retention of the lower limb function is a case study investigating the effect of mental practice on the learning of a foot-sequence task in a 38-year-old man who suffered a left hemorrhagic subcortical stroke four months prior to the study (Jackson *et al.* 2004). The patient practiced a serial response time task with the lower limb in three distinct training phases over a period of five weeks: two weeks of physical practice, one week of combined physical and mental practice, and then two weeks of mental practice alone at home. Performance on the task was measured through response times. The patient's average response time improved significantly during the first five days of physical practice (26%), but then failed to show further improvement (plateau) during the following week of physical practice. The combination of mental and physical practice during the third week yielded additional improvement (10.3%), while the following two weeks of mental practice resulted in a marginal increase in performance (2.2%). The latter findings indicate that the addition of mental practice when the performance has reached a plateau can further improve the performance of a sequential motor skill in a person who had a stroke. Moreover, the retention of the motor skill with cessation of physical practice when MI is practiced at home suggests that mental practice could play a role in the retention of newly acquired abilities. Although foot movements seem remote from the more complex movements involved during walking, a recent TMS study demonstrated a close relationship in the control of the TA muscle during MI of simple foot dorsiflexion and gait (Bakker *et al.* 2008b). Indeed, it was found that corticospinal effects of a simple MI task (foot dorsiflexion) can predict corticospinal effects of a more complex MI task involving the same muscle.

In summary, although results from clinical studies suggest that mental practice can be beneficial to improve locomotor-related tasks, randomized clinical trials with larger samples are needed to confirm and generalize findings about the effects reported so far in a small number of subjects. Yet, despite limitations related to their design, case reports, feasibility, and exploratory studies have provided interesting information about the patients' ability to comply with various training approaches, the sensitivity of outcome measures and the amount of training required to obtain significant gains. The knowledge gained is useful as it provides critical information for the planning of future randomized clinical trials.

Training strategies to optimize the relearning of locomotor skills

The use of MI training in rehabilitation is still relatively new. Several questions need to be answered to improve our understanding of how MI can be used to promote the relearning of functional activities such as walking. In this section, findings from behavioural, psychophysical and brain imaging studies in healthy subjects will be examined to extract guiding principles for the development of training strategies in rehabilitation. More specifically, questions about (1) the imagery perspective; (2) the influence of posture; (3) combining mental and physical practice: optimal ratios, order and timing and serial and block training, will be discussed.

Motor imagery perspective

Several issues arise when planning interventions with MI. The first concerns the selection of the perspective: should one use an internal or external perspective? For example, the patient can be instructed to imagine another person walking as if he/she was a spectator; this is referred to as an external, third person perspective. On the other hand, the patient can be asked to imagine him/herself walking from the inside and be the actor; this corresponds to an internal, first-person perspective (Jackson *et al.* 2001; Solodkin *et al.* 2004; Bakker *et al.* 2007b, 2008a). Each perspective has different properties. While the external perspective implies, primarily, a visual representation of the motor task, the internal perspective entails, in addition to the visual representation, the kinaesthetic sensations associated with the simulated movements, and thus both visual and kinaesthetic inputs.

Behavioural, neurophysiological, and brain-imaging studies have shown that, compared to third-person perspective (external imagery), first-person perspective (internal imagery) shares more physiological characteristics with those observed during the execution of movement, and thus, that movement imagery in the first-person perspective is closest to the real execution of movement (Naito *et al.* 2002; Solodokin *et al.* 2004; Vargas *et al.* 2004; de Lange *et al.* 2006; Fourkas *et al.* 2006a; Stinear *et al.* 2006; Bakker *et al.* 2007b, 2008a;). Likewise, recent findings from fMRI studies, during MI in the first-person perspective (Guillot *et al.*, 2008, 2009), indicated that although both visual and kinaesthetic representations yielded activation of primary sensori-motor areas, the motor systems were more strongly involved during kinaesthetic representation. Based on these findings, the challenge with MI is to ascertain that the persons are really imagining the task in the first-person perspective and focus their attention on both visual and kinaesthetic cues to promote activation of neural networks associated with MI of gait. Recently, Bakker and colleagues (2007a,b) have described an experimental protocol to quantify MI of gait by distinguishing it from visual processes, and by comparing its temporal correspondence with actual gait. In this paradigm, the duration of actual walking is compared to external representation and internal representation of walking. During internal imagery, the subjects are asked to imagine walking along a path (image displayed on a monitor); while, during external imagery, they have to imagine seeing a disc moving along a similar path. Finally during actual walking they are required to physically walk along the same trajectory. Findings revealed that movement times increased with increasing path length and decreasing path width in all three tasks, further confirming the generalization of Fitt's law to locomotor tasks. However, the effects of path width on movement times was significantly stronger during internal imagery and the actual walking conditions than during external imagery, suggesting that MI in the first-person perspective taps into similar cerebral resources as those used during actual gait. In a subsequent fMRI study using this novel experimental protocol, the same research group (Bakker *et al.* 2008a) examined the cerebral correlates of MI during precision gait (subjects walking along a narrow path). They found that imagery times were longer for the narrow path during internal imagery, but not during external imagery. In addition, only the internal representation of precise gait increased cerebral activity and effective connectivity within a network involving the superior parietal lobule, the dorsal precentral gyrus, and the middle right occipital gyrus, further suggesting that internal imagery was sensitive to the constraints imposed by a narrow walking path. The latter findings corroborate those for hand movements (Solodkin *et al.* 2004).

The above findings underline the functional similarities between actual walking and MI in the first person perspective and support its use in MI training (Solodkin *et al.* 2004; Bakker *et al.* 2007b, 2008a). Therefore, instructions should direct the person or patient to focus on both visual and kinaesthetic components seen and felt from inside. Thus, the patients should envision walking within an environment (e.g. imagine the path's width, the size, and position of the obstacles), the displacement of the limbs (e.g. see the top of the feet, the inside of the swinging arms), and recreate the sensations associated with the task (e.g. feeling the push-off, the effort to increase the step height or length). Moreover, the therapist should ask questions about what subjects see and feel during the imagination phase to ascertain that they are engaged in first-person MI. An additional way to verify whether the person is imagining the walking task in the first-person perspective would be to compare their movement times while imagining walking along a wide path versus a narrow path. If the person adopts a first-person perspective, movement times while imagining walking are expected to be shorter for a wide path than a narrow path.

Influence of posture on MI

Another aspect to be taken into consideration during MI training is the subject's posture. Indeed, mentally representing a movement implies a motor plan based on a body-centered frame of reference which depends on visuo-kinaesthetic inputs (Imbiriba *et al.* 2006). Results from fMRI and TMS studies during MI of hand movements have shown that hand postures influence imagery. For instance, higher levels of cortical facilitation and brain activations have been reported when the position of the imagined hand is congruent with the actual hand position suggesting that MI generates motor plans that depend on the current configuration of the limbs (Vargas *et al.* 2004; de Lange *et al.* 2006; Fourkas *et al.* 2006b). Consequently, during MI of locomotor-related activities, care should be taken to place the subject in a similar position or a position close to that usually taken during the actual execution of the motor task. If these findings for the upper limbs can be generalized to lower extremity functions (Imbiriba *et al.* 2006), they would argue for positioning the patients closest to the position that they adopt during the execution of the task. For instance, during MI of rising from a chair and sitting down, training MI with the subjects in a seated position rather than lying down should promote a better representation of the body spatial orientation and of the limb and body movements, hence facilitating brain activations. While a standing position could be too demanding during MI of walking, training the subject in sitting rather than lying down on his back could be more suitable as it would promote vertical body orientation and assist in the representation of visuospatial cues (Imbiriba *et al.* 2006).

Combining physical and mental repetitions

Another question that needs to be answered concerns the optimal conditions for the use of MI. First, it is recognized that mental practice represents only an adjunct to habitual therapy and that mental rehearsal of a task does not replace physical practice of the same task (Jackson *et al.* 2001). To date, only a few clinical studies (Jackson *et al.* 2004; Malouin *et al.* 2004a; Malouin *et al.* in press) have controlled the amount of physical practice during mental practice training. Second, although mental rehearsal alone can promote brain reorganization and have a priming effect on subsequent physical training (Pascual-Leone *et al.* 1995; Jackson *et al.* 2003), it remains to be shown how to better combine physical and mental repetitions to reach the best learning conditions.

This type of question has been addressed in a recent study that examined in young healthy adults how many mental repetitions of a complex manipulative task (in which subjects were required to grasp a small object and to insert it into a support with different orientations) were needed before observing significant reduction in the movement time of the first physical execution of the same task (Allami *et al.* 2008). These authors reported that 60 trials of MI (within a single training session) were not enough to induce a learning effect for this precision task. However, mental rehearsal of 120 trials or more led to a significant improvement. Their results suggest that subjects need to rehearse mentally for a relatively large number of trials for learning to occur especially for the more complex manual skills. More importantly, this study shows that mental rehearsal alone (120 trials) is sufficient to reach the same level of performance as that reached after 240 trials of physical practice, and thus are in line with the priming effects reported by Pascual-Leone and colleagues (1995). While the number of sessions and repetitions required to observe motor improvement may depend on the type and complexity of the task (Louis *et al.* 2008) and cannot be generalized to the learning of walking skills, they raise interesting possibilities especially for patients who cannot walk or who can walk for a very short time. For instance, patients who mentally rehearse walking prior to actual walking could show improvement faster than those who do not. More research, however, is needed to determine whether these findings can be generalized to both gait and rehabilitation.

When combining both physical and mental executions of a task, does the order and timing of the actual and imagined performance affect the imagery? This question was tackled in young healthy adults (Papaxanthis *et al.* 2002). Two groups of subjects were asked to actually execute or imagine a walking task. The first group executed ten trials of the actual walking task and then imagined the same task at different intervals of 25, 50, and 75 minutes afterwards. In contrast, the second group was requested to imagine and then execute physically the same task. They found that the duration of the imagined walking conditions was very similar to those of actual walking regardless of whether the interval elapsed from the actual task (first group), or the order of performance (second group). Thus, the results show that the temporal correspondence between imagination and actual walking movements remains unchanged regardless of the order of performance and the time elapsed from the actual task. Since the temporal correspondence between real and imagination conditions were preserved in subjects imagining the walking task, one could predict that patients unable to walk would still have a good spatiotemporal representation of walking.

Another important finding from Papaxanthis and colleagues (2002) is that, whether the imagined condition precedes or follows an actual walking condition, the variability in the mean duration across trials for blocks of imagined walking is greater than for blocks of actual walking. These observations could suggest that the greater temporal inter-trial variability during mental rehearsal is due to the absence of the peripheral feedback generated during actual walking. The latter hypothesis was examined in a subsequent study. In fact, they found that when subjects alternate between imagination and execution conditions (e.g. each imagination trial is separated by one execution trial: serial training), the variability in the mean duration of mental walking is smaller compared to subjects who performed in blocks (e.g. all the trials of one condition are followed by all the trials of the other condition) (Courtine *et al.* 2004). Their findings show that timing variability during imagined walking decreases when actual movements precede mental rehearsal, hence suggesting that afferent information stored in working memory can thus be used for the consistent reproduction of the next imagined movement. Therefore, if a smaller inter-trial variability during walking imagery translates into better performance then their findings suggest a facilitating effect of motor memory when execution and imagination trials are mixed in a serial fashion.

To date, in the clinical setting, good compliance and learning effects have been reported with training paradigms combining physical execution trials (P) and mental rehearsal trial (M) in proportions from 1 P for 5 M to 1 P for 10 M for retraining rising and sitting down in persons following stroke (Malouin *et al.* 2004a,b; Malouin *et al.* in press). The reason for including the physical execution of the motor task between series of mental trials is to refresh the memory of the sensations associated with the motor task, while minimizing the number of physical executions. Such kinaesthetic inputs likely assist in developing and maintaining the motor representation of the task and in promoting MI in a first-person perspective (Malouin *et al.* 2004a,b).

Conclusions

In this chapter, an overview of studies pertaining to the application of MI for the retraining of human locomotor activities has been presented. Although several lines of evidence suggest that mental practice can be applied to locomotion, to date only case reports and feasibility studies have investigated its use in persons following stroke (Dickstein *et al.* 2004; Dunsky *et al.* 2008). However, the beneficial effects of MI training reported so far warrant future randomized clinical trials with larger samples to confirm and generalize the positive findings reported.

Although the ability to engage in MI can be assessed reliably through mental chronometry and imagery questionnaires, complementary objective tools for measuring MI capability, such as eye movement recordings (Heremans *et al.* 2008) and electrodermic responses (Guillot and Collet 2005b; Guillot *et al.* 2008, 2009) need to be examined for their potential use in clinical settings. Similar to what is reported in normal populations, good and bad imagers coexist after stroke (Malouin *et al.* 2008a), hence the need in some cases to improve MI ability before introducing MI training. For instance, being able to rehearse mentally even complex movements (such as in the TUG) is a good indicator that MI can be used to retrain more complex locomotor tasks. Moreover, based on recent findings that the mental representation of actions is highly modulated by imagery practice (Malouin *et al.* 2009), patients who initially demonstrate difficulty in generating mental representation of movements may eventually improve their MI ability with repeated exposures. Virtual environments (Fung *et al.* 2004) and observation of gait (Iseki *et al.* 2008) could provide the visual reinforcements necessary to promote the generation of proper mental images in persons who have difficulty to engage in MI of walking or who cannot yet walk. In addition to free walking, MI training protocols should also comprise a variety of walking conditions that resemble those usually met daily: stairs, ramps, fixed, or moving obstacles to assist in developing strategies required for dealing with real life situations. Finally, there is a need to look at principles guiding training procedures in neurorehabilitation; attention should be directed to issues regarding modes of delivery of mental practice through MI. For instance, should the patients be lying down and relaxing prior to listening to pre-recorded instruction tapes? Or, in contrast, should they be more actively engaged in their training? Should they learn to self-monitor their training and solve problems along the way (Liu *et al.* 2004; Malouin *et al.* 2004a,b; Malouin *et al.* in press; Braun *et al.* 2008) so that MI can be eventually practiced alone (Jackson *et al.* 2004), or at home without supervision (Braun *et al.* 2008)? Given the increasing interest towards mental practice through MI in neurorehabilitation over the recent years, it is expected that some answers to issues raised in this chapter will soon be provided.

Acknowledgements

This work was supported by the Quebec Provincial Research network REPAR, the CIHR, and the FRSQ. The authors thank Anne Durand, PhD, P.T. for data collection and data analysis as well as Daniel Tardif, BSc, for preparing the figures.

References

Allami, N., Paulignan, Y., Brovelli, A., and Boussaoud, D. (2008). Visuo-motor learning with combination of different rates of motor imagery and physical practice. *Experimental Brain Research*, **184**, 105–13.

Bakker, M., de Lange, F.P., and Stevens, J.A. (2007a). Motor imagery of gait: a quantitative approach. *Experimental Brain Research*, **179**, 497–504.

Bakker, M., Verstappen, C.C.P., Bloem, B.R., and Toni, I. (2007b). Recent advances in functional neuroimaging of gait. *Journal of Neural Transmission*, **114**, 1323–31.

Bakker, M., De Lange, F.P., Helmich, R.C., Scheeringa, R., Bloem, B.R., and Toni, I. (2008a). Cerebral correlates of motor imagery of normal and precision gait. *Neuroimage*, **41**, 998–1010.

Bakker, M., Overeem, S., Snijders, A.H., *et al.* (2008b). Motor imagery of foot dorsiflexion and gait: effects on corticospinal excitability. *Clinical Neurophysiology*, **119**, 2519–27.

Braun, S.M., Beurskens, A.J., Borm, P.J., Schack, T., and Wade, D.T. (2006). The effects of mental practice in stroke rehabilitation. *Archives of Physical Medicine and Rehabilitation*, **87**, 842–52.

Braun, S., Kleynen, M., Schols, J., Schack, T., Beurskens, A., and Wade, D. (2008). Using mental practice in stroke rehabilitation: a framework. *Clinical Rehabilitation*, **22**, 579–91.

Courtine, G., Papaxanthis, C., Gentili, R., and Pozzo, T. (2004). Gait-dependent motor memory facilitation in covert movement execution. *Cognitive Brain Research*, **22**, 67–75.

Debarnot, U., Creveaux, T., Collet, C., Gemignani, A., Massarelli, R., and Doyon, J., Guillot, A. (2009). Sleep-related improvements in motor learning following mental practice. *Brain Cognition*, **69**, 398–405.

Decety, J. (1996). The neurophysiological basis of motor imagery. *Behavioural Brain Research*, **77**, 45–52.

Decety, J. and Boisson, D. (1990). Effect of brain and spinal cord injuries on motor imagery. *European Archives of Psychiatry and Clinical Sciences*, **240**, 39–43.

Decety, J. and Grèzes, J. (1999). Neural mechanisms subserving the perception of human actions. *Trends in Cognitive Science*, **3**, 172–8.

Decety, J. and Jeannerod, M. (1996). Mentally simulated movements in virtual reality: does Fitts' law hold in motor imagery? *Behavioral Brain Research*, **72**, 127–34.

Decety, J., Jeannerod, M., and Prablanc, C. (1989). The timing of mentally represented action. *Behavioral Brain Research*, **34**, 35–42.

Decety, J., Jeannerod, M., Germain, M., and Pastene, J. (1991). Vegetative responses during imagined movement is proportional to mental effort. *Behavioural Brain Research*, **42**, 1–5.

Decety, J., Jeannerod, M., Durozard, D., and Baverel, G. (1993). Central activation of autonomic effectors during mental simulation of motor actions in man. *Journal of Physiology*, **461**, 549–63.

de Lange, F.P., Helmich, R.C., and Toni, I. (2006). Posture influences motor imagery: an fMRI study. *Neuroimage*, **33**, 609–17.

Dickstein, R., Dunsky, A., Marcovitz, E. (2004). Motor imagery for gait rehabilitation in post-stroke hemiparesis. *Physical Therapy*, **84**, 1167–77.

Duncan, P., Richards, L., Wallace, D., *et al.* (1998). A randomized, controlled pilot study of a home-based exercise program for individuals with mild and moderate stroke. *Stroke,* **29**, 2055–60.

Dunsky, A., Dickstein, R., Marcovitz, E., Levy, S., and Deutsch, J. (2008). Home-based motor imagery training for gait rehabilitation of people with chronic poststroke hemiparesis. *Archives of Physical Medicine and Rehabilitation*, **89**, 1580–8.

Engardt, M., Ribbe, T., and Olsson, E. (1993). Vertical ground reaction force feedback to enhance stroke patients' symmetrical body-weight distribution while rising/sitting down. *Scandinavian Journal of Rehabilitation and Medicine*, **25**, 41–8.

Fitts P.M. (1954). The information capacity of the human motor system in controlling the amplitude of movement. *Journal of Experimental Psychology*, **47**, 381–91.

Fung, J., Malouin, F., McFadyen, B.J., *et al.* (2004). Locomotor rehabilitation in a complex virtual environment. Conf. Poceed, IEEE Eng Biol Soc, **7**, 4859–61.

Fourkas, A.D., Avenanti, A., Urgesi, C., and Aglioti, S.M. (2006a). Corticospinal facilitation during first and third person imagery. *Experimental Brain Research*, **168**, 143–51.

Fourkas, A.D., Ionta, S., and Aglioti, S.M. (2006b). Influence of imagined posture and imagery modality on corticospinal excitability. *Behavioral Brain Research*, **168**, 190–6.

Fusi, S., Cutuli, D., Valente, M.R., Bergonzi, P., Porro, C.A., and Di Prampero, P.E. (2005). Cardioventilatory responses during real or imagined walking at low speed. *Archives Italiennes de Biologie*, **143**, 223–8.

Guillot, A. and Collet, C. (2005a). Duration of mentally simulated movement: a review. *Journal of Motor Behavior*, **37**, 10–20.

Guillot, A. and Collet, C. (2005b). Contribution from neurophysiological and psychological methods to the study of motor imagery. *Brain Research Review*, **15**, 287–97.

Guillot, A., Collet, C., Nguyen, V.A., Malouin, F., Richards, C., and Doyon, J. (2008). Functional neuroanatomical networks associated with expertise in motor imagery. *Neuroimage*, **41**, 1471–83.

Guillot, A., Collet, C., Nguyen, V.A., Malouin, F., Richards, C.L., and Doyon, J. (2009). Brain activity during visual versus kinesthetic imagery: an fMRI study. Human Brain Mapping, **30**, 2157–72.

Heremans, E., Helsen, W.F., and Feys, P. (2008). The eyes as a mirror of our thoughts: quantification of motor imagery of goal-directed movements through eye movement registration. *Behavioural Brain Research*, **187**, 351–60.

Imbiriba, L.A, Rodrigues, E.C., Magalhães, J., and Vargas, C.D. (2006). Motor imagery in blind subjects: the influence of the previous visual experience. *Neuroscience Letters*, **400**, 181–5.

Iseki, K., Hanakawa, T., Shinozaki, J., Nankaku, M., and Fukuyama, H. (2008). Neural mechanisms involved in mental imagery and observation of gait. *Neuroimage*, **41**, 1021–31.

Jackson, P.L., Lafleur, M.F., Malouin, F., Richards, C.L., and Doyon, J. (2001). Potential role of mental practice using motor imagery in neurological rehabilitation. *Archives of Physical Medicine and Rehabilitation*, **82**, 1133–41.

Jackson, P.L., Lafleur, M.F., Malouin, F., Richards, C.L., and Doyon, J. (2003). Functional cerebral reorganization following motor sequence learning through mental practice with motor imagery. *Neuroimage*, **20**, 1171–80.

Jackson, P.L., Doyon, J., Richards, C.L., and Malouin, F. (2004). The efficacy of combined physical and mental practice in learning of a foot-sequence task after stroke: a case study. *Neurorehabilitation and Neural Repair*, **18**, 106–11.

Jahn, K., Deutschländer, A., Stephan, T., Strupp, M., Wiesmann, M., and Brandt, T. (2004). Brain activation patterns during imagined stance and locomotion in functional magnetic resonance imaging. *Neuroimage*, **22**, 1722–31.

Jeannerod, M. (1995). Mental imagery in the motor context. *Neuropsychologia*. **33**, 1419–32.

Johnson, S.H. (2000). Imagining the impossible: intact motor representations in hemiplegics. *Neuroreport*, **11**, 729–32.

Johnson, S.H., Sprehn, G., and Saykin, A.J. (2002). Intact motor imagery in chronic upper limb hemiplegics: evidence for activity-independent action representations. *Journal of Cognition and Neuroscience*, **14**, 841–52.

Liu, K.P., Chan, C.C., Lee, T.M., and Hui-Chan, C.W. (2004). Mental imagery for promoting relearning for people after stroke: a randomized controlled trial. *Archives of Physical Medicine and Rehabilitation*, **85**, 1403–8.

Louis, M., Guillot, A., Maton, S., Doyon, J., and Collet, C. (2008). Effect of imagined movement speed on subsequent motor performance. *Journal of Motor Behavior*, **40**, 117–32.

Malouin, F., Richards, C.L., Jackson, P.L., Dumas, F., and Doyon, J. (2003). Brain activations during motor imagery of locomotor-related tasks: a PET study. *Human Brain Mapping*, **19**, 47–62.

Malouin, F., Belleville, S., Desrosiers, J., Doyon, J., and Richards, C.L. (2004a). Working memory and mental practice after stroke. *Archives of Physical Medicine and Rehabilitation*, **85**, 177–83.

Malouin. F., Richards, C.L., Belleville, S., Desrosiers, J., and Doyon, J. (2004b). Training mobility tasks after stroke with combined mental and physical practice: a feasibility study. *Neurorehabilitation and Neural Repair*, **18**, 66–75.

Malouin, F., Richards, C.L., Desrosiers, J., and Doyon, J. (2004c). Bilateral slowing of mentally simulated actions after stroke. *Neuroreport*, **7**, 1349–53.

Malouin, F., Richards, C.L., Jackson, P.L., Lafleur, M.F., Durand, A., and Doyon, J. (2007a). The Kinesthetic and Visual Imagery Questionnaire (KVIQ) for assessing motor imagery in persons with physical disabilities: a reliability and construct validity study. *Journal of Neurologic Physical Therapy*, **31**, 20–9.

Malouin, F., Doyon, J., Durand, A., and Richards, C.L. (2007b). Slowing of motor imagery after stroke. (2007b). *Proceedings of the World Confederation of Physical Therapy*, Abstract **1852**, Vancouver, June 2–6, 2007.

Malouin, F., Richards, C., Durand, A., and Doyon, J. (2008a).Clinical assessment of motor imagery after stroke. *Neurorehabilitation and Neural Repair*, **22**, 330–40.

Malouin, F., Richards, C.L., Durand, A., and Doyon, J. (2008b). Reliability of mental chronometry for assessing motor imagery ability after stroke. *Archives of Physical Medicine and Rehabilitation*, **89**, 311–9.

Malouin, F., Richards, C.L., Durand, A.J., *et al.* (2009). Effects of practice, visual loss, limb amputation and disuse on motor imagery vividness. *Neurorehabilitation and Neural Repair*, **23**, 449–63.

Malouin, F., Richards, C.L., Durand, A., and Doyon, J. (In press). Added value of mental practice combined with a small amount of physical practice on the relearning of rising and sitting post-stroke: a pilot study. *Journal of Neurologic Physical Therapy*.

Miyai, I., Tanabe, H.C., Sase, I., *et al.* (2001). Cortical mapping of gait in humans: a near-infrared spectroscopic topography study. *Neuroimage*, **14**, 1186–92.

Naito, E., Kochiyama, T., Kitada, R., *et al.* (2002). Internally simulated movement sensations during motor imagery activate cortical motor areas and the cerebellum. *Journal of Neuroscience*, **22**, 3683–91.

Ouchi, Y., Okada, H., Yoshikawa, E., Nobezawa, S., and Fatatsubashi, M. (1999). Brain activation during maintenance of standing postures in humans. *Brain*, **122**, 329–38.

Pascual-Leone, A., Nguyet, D., Cohen, L.G., Brasil-Neto, J.P., Cammarota, A., and Hallett, M. (1995). Modulation of muscle responses evoked by transcranial magnetic stimulation during the acquisition of new fine motor skills. *Journal of Neurophysiology*, **74**, 1037–45.

Papaxanthis, C., Pozzo, T., Skoura, X., and Schieppati, M. (2002). Does order and timing in performance of imagined and actual movements affect the motor imagery process? The duration of walking and writing task. *Behavioural Brain Research*, **134**, 209–15.

Sabate, M., Gonzalez, B., and Rodriguez, M. (2007). Adapting movement planning to motor impairments: the motor-scanning system. *Neuropsychologia*, **45**, 378–86.

Sacco, K., Cauda, F., Cerliani, L., Mate, D., Duca, S., and Geminiani, G.C. (2006). Motor imagery of walking following training in locomotor attention. The effect of "the tango lesson". *Neuroimage*, **32**, 1441–9.

Sirigu, A., Cohen, L., Duhamel, J.R. *et al.* (1995). Congruent unilateral impairments for real and imagined hand movements. *Neuroreport*, **6**, 997–1001.

Sirigu, A., Duhamel, J.R., Cohen, L. *et al.* (1996). The mental representation of hand movements after parietal cortex damage. *Science*, **273**, 1564–8.

Solodkin, A., Hlustik, P., Chen, E.E., and Small, S.I. (2004). Fine modulation in network activation during motor execution and motor imagery. *Cerebral Cortex*, **14**, 1246–55.

Stinear, C.M., Byblow, W.D., Steyvers, M., Levin, O., and Swinnen, S.P. (2006). Kinesthetic, but not visual, motor imagery modulates corticomotor excitability. *Experimental Brain Research*, **168**, 157–64.

Stinear, C.M., Fleming, M.K., Barber, P.A., and Byblow, W.D. (2007). Lateralization of motor imagery following stroke. *Clinical Neurophysiology*, **118**, 1794–1801.

Szameitat, A.J., Shen, S., and Sterr, A. (2007). Motor imagery of complex everyday movements. An fMRI study. *Neuroimage*, **34**, 702–13.

Vargas, C.D., Olivier, E., Craighero, L., Fadiga, L., Duhamel, J.R., and Sirigu. A. (2004). The influence of hand posture on corticospinal excitability during motor imagery: a transcranial magnetic stimulation study. *Cerebral Cortex*, **14**, 1200–6.

Wagner, J., Stephan, T., Kalla, R., *et al.* (2008). Mind the bend: cerebral activations associated with mental imagery of walking along a curved path. Experimental Brain Research, [Epub ahead of print] PMID: 18696057 [PubMed – as supplied by publisher]

Wuyam, B., Moosavi, S.H., Decety, J., Adams, L., Lansing, R.W., and Guz, A. (1995). Imagination of dynamic exercise produced ventilatory responses which were more apparent in competitive sportsmen. *Journal of Physiology*, **482**, 713–24.

Chapter 12

Motor imagery practice in individuals with Parkinson's disease

Ruth Dickstein and Ruth Tamir

Motor Imagery (MI) and its practice is a complex self-generated cognitive operation that involves the activation of several motor-related neuronal circuits (Kosslyn *et al.* 2001; Hanakawa *et al.* 2003; Michelon *et al.* 2006; Guillot *et al.* 2008; Hanakawa *et al.* 2008). The employment of motor imagery is accomplished by high-order sensory and perceptual processes that enable the reactivation of specific motor actions in working memory without motor output (Annett 1995; Kosslyn *et al.* 2001; Malouin *et al.* 2004a). Working memory has been described as a process of retention of representations of active information, with these representations being employed in mental processes such as imagery. It entails activity in a network of brain structures, rather than a single unit activity, with domain-specific areas as part of this network (Zimmer 2008 for a recent review).

The generation and rehearsal (practice) of motor imagery context involve activity in neuronal networks of the cortical and subcortical brain areas that play roles in motor planning and execution. Of specific relevance to the current subject are the neuronal networks shared by the basal ganglia and the striato-thalamo-cortico-striatal pathways, which are activated during both real and imagined movements (Gerardin *et al.* 2000; Frak *et al.* 2004; Oullier *et al.* 2005; Szameitat *et al.* 2007; Munzert *et al.* 2008). As the input of the basal ganglia is critical for normal cortical function, diseases of the basal ganglia could affect the ability to become engaged in motor imagery and to practice motor acts via imagery. Particularly noteworthy is the fact that the basal ganglia influence wide areas of the cortex, including the pre-supplementary, supplementary and premotor area, the dorsal prefrontal cortex, and the orbitofrontal cortex. As a result, motor, cognitive and emotional faculties could be affected by malfunction of the basal ganglia (Braak and Del Tredici 2008).

Parkinson's disease (PD) is the second most common progressive neurodegenerative disease, affecting about 1% of individuals over the age of 65 (Tanner and Goldman 1996). The disorder is manifested by a loss of dopaminergic input from the substantia nigra pars compacta to the striatum, which disrupts the basal ganglia-cortical circuitry, particularly the frontal-striatal networks (Stephens *et al.* 2005). As a result, individuals present with various levels of motor (tremor, rigidity, bradykinesia, postural instability), cognitive, and emotional impairments (Rowe *et al.* 2008). At the same time, deficits are also expected to be manifested in the so-called 'internal states' and transition between them (Dominey *et al.* 1995), namely, in the neuronal processes that encode sequential and non-sequential movements in working memory and precede motor output; movement planning and preparation and motor imagery belong to these processes (Holmes 2007).

The nature of the disorder in PD raises several questions regarding the ability of individuals with PD to generate motor imagery and to apply it for the practice of motor tasks. In this chapter, we will review and discuss the available information related to four pertinent questions: (1) Is the ability to be engaged in and practice motor tasks via imagery impaired in subjects with PD? (2) Is the brain activity during engagement in motor imagery different in persons with PD as compared with healthy subjects? (3) What is the effect of medical and surgical (deep brain stimulation) treatment on the motor imagery capacity in individuals with PD? (4) Is it beneficial to apply motor imagery training in the motor rehabilitation of individuals with PD?

Are individuals with Parkinson's Disease impaired in their ability to engage in and practice motor tasks via imagery?

It has been established that the mental rotation of objects requires visuospatial functions mediated by the parietal lobes, whereas the mental rotation of hands also engages frontal motor-system processes (Amick *et al.* 2006). Experimental paradigms aimed at testing the imagery capacity of hand rotation tasks in subjects with PD have been applied in several studies. Amick and colleagues showed that patients with PD were capable of normally performing the mental rotation of objects in space, from which the researchers concluded that the operation of visuospatial cognition in these patients was intact. Yet, individuals with right-sided onset made more errors in imagery rotation of the hands than did healthy control subjects or patients with left-sided PD onset (Amick *et al.* 2006).

Similarly, in a study of patients with PD (right dominant with right body side involvement) during the 'on' state, Dominey and colleagues measured reaction times for the accurate determination of (1) letters displayed in either normal or mirror face (non-motor imagery task), and (2) side of the hand (left or right) displayed on a screen in various orientations (motor imagery task). They noted slowness (bradykinesia) among the PD patients in comparison to the healthy controls for real as well as for mental letter and hand rotation. However, marked slowness of the right as compared with the left side was mainly observed for hand rotation, while performance was more symmetrical for letter rotation. In a second paradigm, the performance time of sequential finger movements was tested in the same patients. The findings pointed to slower execution times in the patients than in the controls, with marked asymmetry favouring the relative intact left hand in both real and imagery performances. The overall conclusion was that motor execution and motor imagery are similarly affected in PD. These results were attributed to the dysfunction of internal state transition mechanisms that underlie both imagery and real motor execution and are normally operated by basal ganglia-thalamic-frontal circuits. Based on the two tested paradigms, the researchers concluded that the basal ganglia participate not only in response selection to internal states, but also in maintaining the internal state and in controlling the orderly succession of transitions from one internal state to the next (Dominey *et al.* 1995).

In another study, PD patients with markedly right-lateralized symptoms employed motor imagery in order to determine the laterality of hand images rotated in either a lateral or medial orientation to their sagittal body axis. As determined by reaction times, the patients affected primarily on their right body side were markedly slower when judging images of the affected hand in lateral orientations than when judging images of the contralateral hand. It was observed that the lateralized PD patients, unlike the control group, had particular difficulty with simulating movements away from the body and involving the affected hand, a deficit that was also noted in real execution. Furthermore, based on fMRI during imagery of the affected hand while attempting to judge images in lateral orientations, the neurons in extra-striate visual areas were activated in addition to parieto-premotor activity. The researchers noted the correspondence between these observations and the known tendency of patients with PD to rely on visual cues (Helmich *et al.* 2007).

Specific deficits in kinaesthetic imagery in patients with PD during the on state were noted by Frak and colleagues during imagery of opposition in precision grasping among patients at Stage III of the Hoehn and Yahr scale (Hoehn and Yahr 1967). Thus, individuals with PD were able to perform grasping movements without difficulty in the preferred orientations, but displayed impairment in simulating grasping, either in preferred or non-preferred orientations. The authors attributed the difference between real and imagery performance in the patients to impairment in the kinaesthetic (rather than visual) imagery required for the simulation of grasping (Frak *et al.* 2004).

In order to determine whether imagining a motor task can facilitate the acquisition of movement features in real task execution, Yaguez and associates tested patients with PD and patients with Huntington's disease. They looked at actual performance of a graphomotor task following 10 minutes of imagery practice of that same task. The imagery training task employed visual and kinaesthetic rehearsal of drawing two ideograms in five different sizes. Testing of real drawing before and after imagery practice was done with a computerized digitizing tablet, which enabled the analysis of movement parameters and the comparison of pre- and post-training performance. The results showed that neither imagery nor real practice enhanced the performance of the patients with PD; yet patients with Huntington disease showed considerable improvement. It was therefore concluded that dopaminergic input via the nigrostriatal pathway is crucial for translating motor representations into motor performance. In other words, the authors surmised that the patients with PD are able to create representations of motor acts, though their dopaminergic deficiency prevents translation into actual performance. In addition, they suggested that deficits found in patients with PD might be related to limited attentional resources and difficulties in employing predictive motor strategies (Yaguez *et al.* 1999).

In the abovementioned studies, bradykinesia was observed both in real and in imagery motor performances. These observations were supported by additional studies in which slowness was measured during both real and imagery movement, with comparable and highly positively correlated durations (Sabate *et al.* 2007). Deficits in the timekeeping mechanism, including motor timing deficits, have been attributed to dopamine depletion. Pouthas and Perbal suggested deficits in working memory as the underlying cause of the inaccurate and variable duration judgements found among patients with PD, whereas long-term memory was not found to be different from that of age-matched controls (Pouthas and Perbal 2004). In contrast, Schnider and colleagues reported intact timing estimation and trajectory predictions, though execution in response to practice was found to be slower than in healthy controls (Schnider *et al.* 1995).

Conclusion

The prominent common denominator of the findings for the cited studies is the prevalence of bradykinesia and inaccuracies in the generation of motor imagery of self-body movements. The disorder in imagery was found to parallel the actual deficit in movement generation of the tested body side and part. The effect of motor imagery practice (training) on motor output was tested in only one study, which was limited to one session of 10 minutes. Based on current evidence, and similar to the practice of real movements, the presence of disorder(s) in imagery capacity does not justify reluctance to practice motor tasks by imagery.

How is the brain activity during engagement in motor imagery different in persons with PD as compared with healthy subjects?

Activation of the basal ganglia has been demonstrated during the preparation and execution of movement. Movement disorders in subjects with PD are thought to derive mainly from deprivation in the pre-SMA, the SMA, and the prefrontal cortex of normal input provided by the striato-frontal pathways. As a result, the functions (i.e., producing internally generated movements, generating and practicing motor imagery, making motor decisions) controlled by neurons at these sites are impaired (Bakker *et al.* 2007; Malouin *et al.* 2003). Such impairment should be reflected in the brain activity of individuals with PD who try to generate motor imagery and engage in its practice.

Tremblay and colleagues and Filippi and associates used transcranial magnetic stimulation (TMS) to study corticomotor excitability in patients with PD while engaged in motor imagery. Tremblay *et al.* found that imagery of a task involving hand movements had no effect on the EMG response of hand muscles in patients on medication, whereas imagery was associated with response facilitation in healthy subjects (Tremblay *et al.* 2008). Filippi *et al.* who studied patients with hemi-Parkinson, observed hemispheric asymmetry in the area of cortical representation of the contralateral abductor digiti minimi muscle (ADM), which was elicited by motor imagery. The area was reduced in the clinically affected hemisphere, but not in the unaffected hemisphere or in healthy control subjects. The authors concluded that the impairment in motor imagery processes for engaging sensorimotor brain areas is lateralized, thus partially accounting for the abnormalities in brain function of patients with PD (Filippi *et al.* 2001).

Thobois and colleagues used PET and $H_2^{(15)}O$ to determine whether motor imagery activation patterns depend on the hand used to complete the task. Measurements in controls and patients with predominantly right-sided Parkinson's were taken while subjects imagined a pre-determined unimanual externally cued sequential movement, using a joystick with either the left or the right hand and during a rest condition. In comparison to controls, motor imagery with the right affected (akinetic) hand in the patients with PD was characterized by lack of activation of the contralateral primary sensorimotor cortex and the cerebellum. However, activity was noted in the SMA and bilaterally in the superior parietal cortex. Brain activity during imagery with the left, less affected ('non-akinetic') hand was globally reduced, with reduced activation of the SMA as compared with that of controls. Thus, the observations related to the left, less affect-ed hand, showed that the activation pattern of the SMA in the patients with PD was impaired bilaterally even in cases of unilateral overt signs. Based on the unexpected observation of SMA activation during motor imagery with the right affected hand, the authors argued that motor imagery abnormalities in patients with PD seem to be dependent on the hand with which they imagine the task and that the a-priori hypoactivation of the SMA is not consistently found (Thobois *et al.* 2000).

In another PET study, preserved function of the SMA, in both the on and off states, was found during the performance of an auditory guided imagery opposition task. However, dysfunction of the pre-SMA as well as of the anterior cingulate and the dorsolateral prefrontal cortex (DLPFC) was observed. Notably, activity in these latter areas was more enhanced in the on than in the off-state. In addition, activity suggested as compensatory was reported in the ipsilateral premotor and inferior parietal cortex (Cunnington *et al.* 2001).

Findings of a third PET study showed that in patients with PD, imagery was associated with a relative reduction in the bilateral, dorsolateral, and mesial frontal cortex activation. These obser-vations support previously reported notions of the under-functioning of the mesial (SMA and pre-SMA) frontal and the DLPFC and allude to dysfunction of the frontal association areas as the underlying cause of impaired motor preparation in this patient group (Samuel *et al.* 2001).

Based on an fMRI study, the triggering of cortical compensatory mechanisms in patients with PD off medication was observed in patients who had to perform mental lateral rotation with the more affected right hand. It has been suggested that these patients have involvement of the right extrastriate body area (EBA) and occipito-parietal cortex, as well as their connectivity towards the left dorsal premotor cortex for the right (affected) hand in a lateral orientation (Helmich *et al.* 2007).

Taking the findings of the cited PET and fMRI study together, the emergent hypo-active brain sites in patients with PD appear to be the SMA and pre-SMA, the anterior cingulate area, and the dorsolateral prefrontal cortex. For the SMA, the findings are not unequivocal; yet, signs of disorder might be bilateral even if the overt motor symptoms are confined to one body side. The triggering of compensatory mechanisms was mainly inferred from observation of activity in the occipito-parietal areas that are involved in the processing of visual information.

It has been established that motor preparation state can be evaluated by integrated values of the late components of the contingent negative variation (late CNV), obtained by averaging electroencephalograms during the last 100ms of the preparatory period (Maeda and Fujiwara 2007).

In one study, the CNV was recorded in patients with PD and control subjects, both before and after the separate employment of 10 minutes of kinaesthetic and of visual imagery. In patients on medication, significant enhancement over the dorsolateral prefrontal regions was noted after the kinaesthetic imagery as compared to before, while no comparable change was observed in the controls. Visual imagery had no effect on the CNV in either group. The researchers suggested that the results point to kinaesthetic imagery as a promising tool for investigations into motor changes, with potential therapeutic use for patients with PD (Lim *et al.* 2006). These findings provide support for previous claims that impairment in kinaesthetic imagery dominates imagery deficits in patients with PD (Frak *et al.* 2004; Amick *et al.* 2006). According to Lim and associates, the enhancement of kinaesthetic imagery via practice could facilitate activation of the motor network, which includes the inferoparietal cortex, the SMA, the anterior cingulate cortex, the premotor cortex, the dorsolateral prefrontal cortex, and the cerebellum (Lim *et al.* 2006).

Kuhn and associates investigated the role of the subthalamic nucleus (STN) during bilateral deep brain stimulation by recording local field potential activity. The patients were tested when off dopaminergic medication while employing kinaesthetic imagery of a wrist extension (no peripheral feedback), as well as during the actual performance of a wrist extension. Several patients were also tested during visual imagery of a non-motor task (i.e., imagining the face of a relative). The findings pointed to comparable changes in the STN during kinaesthetic imagery and during real execution of the wrist extension (as manifested in event-related desynchronization (ERD) of oscillatory beta activity in the region of the STN). The ERD during motor imagery and real motor performance were both significantly larger than the ERD in the non-motor visual imagery. In contrast, event-related synchronization (ERS) was significantly smaller in trials of motor imagery than in real task execution, and visual imagery was associated with a small insignificant ERS. The authors concluded that neurons in the STN are active both during feedforward, that is, during engagement in kinaesthetic imagery (indexed by the ERD, not related to peripheral feedback) and during real movement execution (indexed by the ERS, which is dependent on sensorimotor feedback) (Kuhn *et al.* 2006).

Conclusion

Studies focusing on brain function in individuals with PD during motor imagery generation or practice are scarce and their protocols diverse. Overall, the deficits in patients with unilateral motor syndromes were consistently more conspicuous on the contralateral brain side. Hypo-activation of the pre-SMA, the dorsolateral prefrontal cortex, and the anterior cingulate area was repeatedly documented. The majority of the results also indicated reduced activity in the SMA and hypo-excitability of the primary sensoriomotor cortex. Also noted in some studies was an indication of compensatory activity in non-affected brain areas, such as the extrastriate and the occipitoparietal cortex.

What is the effect of medical and surgical (deep brain stimulation) treatment on the motor imagery capacity in individuals with PD?

The potential for employing motor imagery in patients with PD is closely linked to the ability for real motor execution. Specific tests to numerically grade motor imagery capacity, such as the Motor Imagery Questionnaire (MIQ; Hall and Martin 1997), or the Kinesthetic Visual Motor Imagery Questionnaire (KVMIQ; Malouin *et al.* 2007) have not yet been applied to subjects with PD. While it is generally agreed that their capacity to employ motor imagery is impaired, the effect of medical treatment on motor imagery is often inferred from its impact on brain activation.

Core information related to motor imagery and brain activity in patients with PD has been provided in the preceding section. In this section, the effects of being on and off medication, as well as the effects of deep brain stimulation on the ability to use imagery will be briefly addressed.

Dominey and colleagues noted that motor imagery was substantially enhanced in patients on dopaminergic treatment as compared to those in the off state, with the latter condition almost hindering motor imagery as well as motor execution (Dominey *et al.* 1995). These observations were corroborated by other reports showing, during the on-state, enhancement of activity in the brain areas that are crucial for the employment of motor imagery (i.e., the pre-SMA, the SMA, the anterior cingulate cortex, and the dorsolateral prefrontal cortex) (Yaguez *et al.* 1999; Cunnington *et al.* 2001; Lim *et al.* 2006).

The relationship between the effect of deep brain stimulation of the STN and the employment of motor imagery has been described in two studies. In one study, STN activity due to deep brain stimulation was enhanced during motor imagery in patients off dopaminergic medication (Kuhn *et al.* 2006). In the second, a PET study demonstrated that left STN stimulation during imagery enhanced the activity in the prefrontal cortex, including in the DLPFC bilaterally, as well as the activity in the left thalamus and putamen. In contrast, the activity in the left SMA and primary motor cortex decreased. It was concluded that STN stimulation during motor imagery (as well as during motor execution) tends to improve the functioning of the frontal-striatal-thalamic pathway and to reduce the recruitment of compensatory motor circuits in the motor, premotor, and parietal cortical areas (Thobois *et al.* 2002).

Conclusion

In correspondence with motor execution, the ability to engage in motor imagery is positively affected by dopaminergic medication. In addition, engagement in motor imagery enhances the therapeutic effects of STN stimulation. Thus, the practice of motor imagery during dopaminergic treatment or while receiving STN stimulation appears to contribute to the effects of either treatment mode.

Is it beneficial to apply motor imagery training in the motor rehabilitation of individuals with PD?

Two viewpoints about the application of motor imagery in individuals with PD can be differentiated. One viewpoint discourages motor imagery practice because the deficient capacity of these patients to employ imagery is perceived as rendering such treatment useless. For example, Tremblay and colleagues argued that patients with PD may experience major difficulties in engaging in motor imagery (Tremblay *et al.* 2008). Likewise, Yaguez and colleagues demonstrated that motor imagery practice in patients with PD is not beneficial for motor execution (Yaguez *et al.* 1999).

The other viewpoint supports the application of motor imagery practice despite deficient imagery capacity. This opinion is mainly based on the evidence that imagery in patients with PD is associated with the enhancement of activity in several brain areas. For example, prior practice of kinaesthetic imagery was found to be associated with enhancement in activity in the DLPFC (Lim *et al.* 2006). Similarly, motor imagery was found to enhance the positive effects of STN stimulation on activity in that area (Thobois *et al.* 2002).

Surprisingly, in contrast to other neurological dysfunctions (mainly stroke), the employment of motor imagery practice in the motor rehabilitation of patients with PD is rare. In an exclusive study, Tamir and colleagues (Tamir *et al.* 2007) applied combined (real and imagery) exercises to a group of patients with PD at Stages 2–3 of the Hoehn and Yahr scale (Hoehn and Yahr 1967). Their performance was compared to a control patient group that was treated with real exercises only. The programme was largely guided by the recommendation of Morris (Morris 2000), and was based on external cues to assist in motor imagery practice and on the integration of physical and imagery practice in each training session. Motor imagery exercises were comprised of kinaesthetic, auditory, and visual imagery scenes that either preceded or succeeded and then again preceded the real performance of comparable tasks. Imagery contents similar to the contents of real exercises were targeted to address body impairments and functional limitations. For example, for the purpose of increasing movement amplitudes, imagery exercises of single or several joint movements were practiced in isolation as well as in functional activities, such as rolling and walking. The performance of sequential movements was specifically addressed in imagery and in real exercises. External cues provided during real practice were also used in the imagery exercises. For example, listening to the pace of a metronome or a melody of a march was exercised in imagery practice as well as during real practice. Patients complied well with the request to employ imagery practice of functional tasks during group exercise and at home. The results of the 12-week intervention programme indicated that the patients in the experimental combined exercise group exhibited greater enhancement of the duration of sequential movement tasks as compared to the control group. These observations point, primarily, to the positive effect of imagery training on ameliorating bradykinesia. Also noteworthy is the superior improvement of the experimental patients in the performance of ADL activities.

Conclusions and recommendations

The positive contribution of motor imagery practice to real movement execution is well substantiated. As with real movements, movements that can be practiced via imagery vary in many different aspects and are associated with activity in specific relevant neuronal networks. In addition, motor imagery is associated with enhanced activity in some areas that are not shared with motor execution, namely the dorsal premotor cortex, the pre-SMA, and frontal eye fields – areas that are important to visuospatial information processing for subsequent actions (Hanakawa *et al.* 2008).

Given that the motor rehabilitation of patients with central neurological disorders is geared toward improving brain control of movements and that engagement in motor imagery involves neuronal activation in large brain areas, the paucity of its employment in patients with central neurological deficits is unfortunate.

Referring specifically to patients with PD, the benefits of real practice are well accepted. Many recent studies have suggested specific training procedures to enhance the functional motor performance of patients with PD (e.g., Schenkman *et al.* 1998; Farley and Koshland 2005a; Morris 2006; Ellis *et al.* 2008; Falvo *et al.* 2008; Fisher *et al.* 2008). These treatment and exercise repertoires could be enriched by adding imagery practice of the same recommended exercise routines. All imagery modes are relevant in this context. Kinaesthetic imagery in subjects with PD seems to be more impaired than visual imagery (Amick *et al.* 2006; Frak *et al.* 2004); however, its regular employment could enhance motor improvement (Lim *et al.* 2006). Auditory pacing (Mcintosh *et al.* 1997; Thaut *et al.* 1996) and music (De Bruin *et al.* 2008; Shankar *et al.* 2008; Tomaino 2006) are known to enhance gait in subjects with PD. Their employment via auditory imagery during non-ambulatory periods and immediately before real performance can potentially enhance execution, especially in the early stages of the disease.

The recently proposed method of 'training big' (Farley and Koshland 2002, 2005a,b), seems especially relevant for employment of imagery because it directly relates to the problem of movement amplitude perception and execution in this patient group. Also noteworthy is the distinction between imagery generation and, the control of imagery vividness over time (maintenance). That distinction, recently highlighted by Holmes, is especially relevant to patients with PD who are hampered in movement initiation (Holmes 2007). However, the translation of that distinction into imagery practice procedures during physical treatment awaits further research.

The negligible risk, cost, and ease of application make the integration of motor imagery practice into the physical therapy treatment of individuals with PD extremely appealing.

Experience from studies of other patient populations with central neurological deficits (Page *et al.* 2001; Jackson *et al.* 2004; Malouin *et al.* 2004b), indicates that the combined application of imagery and real exercises produces the largest gains. Therefore, unless otherwise indicated, this practice mode should be recommended for patients with PD.

References

Amick, M.M., Schendan, H.E., Ganis, G., and Cronin-Golomb, A. (2006). Frontostriatal circuits are necessary for visuomotor transformation: mental rotation in Parkinson's disease. *Neuropsychologia,* **44**, 339–49.

Annett, J. (1995). Motor imagery: perception or action? *Neuropsychologia,* **33**, 1395–417.

Bakker, M., Verstappen, C.C., Bloem, B.R., and Toni, I. (2007). Recent advances in functional neuroimaging of gait. *Journal of Neural Transmission,* **114**, 1323–31.

Braak, H. and Del Tredici, K. (2008). Cortico-basal ganglia-cortical circuitry in Parkinson's disease reconsidered. *Experimental Neurology,* **212**, 226–9.

Cunnington, R., Egan, G.F., O'sullivan, J.D., Hughes, A.J., Bradshaw, J.L., and Colebatch, J.G. (2001). Motor imagery in Parkinson's disease: a PET study. *Movement Disorders,* **16**, 849-57.

De Bruin, N., Bonfield, S., Hu, B., Suchowersky, O., Doan, J., and Brown, L. (2008). Walking while listening to music improves gait performance in Parkinson's disease. *Movement Disorders,* **23**, S220–S220.

Dominey, P., Decety, J., Broussolle, E., Chazot,G., and. Jeannerod, M. (1995). Motor imagery of a lateralized sequential task is asymmetrically slowed in hemi-Parkinson's patients. *Neuropsychologia,* **33**, 727–41.

Ellis, T., Katz, D.I., White, D.K., Depiero, T.J., Hohler, A.D., and Saint-Hilaire, M. (2008). Effectiveness of an inpatient multidisciplinary rehabilitation program for people with Parkinson disease. *Physical Therapy,* **88**, 812–9.

Falvo, M.J., Schilling, B.K., and Earhart, G.M. (2008). Parkinson's disease and resistive exercise: rationale, review, and recommendations. *Movement Disorders,* **23**, 1–11.

Farley, B.G. and Koshland, G.F. (2002). Think big: a new physical therapy intervention for bradykinesia. *Movement Disorders,* **17,** S72–S72.

Farley, B.G. and Koshland, G.F. (2005a). Learning big (TM): efficacy of a large-amplitude exercise approach for patients with Parkinson's disease-bradykinesia to balance. *Movement Disorders,* **20,** S137–S137.

Farley, B.G. and Koshland, G.F. (2005b). Training big to move faster: the application of the speed-amplitude relation as a rehabilitation strategy for people with Parkinson's disease. *Experimental Brain Research,* **167,** 462–7.

Filippi, M.M., Oliveri, M., Pasqualetti, P., *et al.* (2001). Effects of motor imagery on motor cortical output topography in Parkinson's disease. *Neurology,* **57,** 55–61.

Fisher, B.E., Wu, A.D., Salem, G.J., *et al.* (2008). The effect of exercise training in improving motor performance and corticomotor excitability in people with early Parkinson's disease. *Archives of Physical Medicine and Rehabilitation,* **89,** 1221–9.

Frak, V., Cohen, H., and Pourcher, E. (2004). A dissociation between real and simulated movements in Parkinson's disease. *Neuroreport,* **15,** 1489–92.

Gerardin, E., Sirigu, A., Lehericy, S., *et al.* (2000). Partially overlapping neural networks for real and imagined hand movements. *Cerebral Cortex,* **10,** 1093–104

Guillot, A., Collet, C., Nguyen, V.A., Malouin, F., Richards, C., and Doyon, J. (2008). Functional neuroanatomical networks associated with expertise in motor imagery. *Neuroimage,* **41,** 1471–83.

Hall, C. and Martin, K. (1997). Measuring movement imagery abilities: a revision of the movement imagery questionnaire. *Journal of Mental Imagery,* **21,** 143–54.

Hanakawa, T., Dimyan, M.A., and Hallett, M. (2008). Motor planning, imagery, and execution in the distributed motor network: a time-course study with functional MRI. *Cerebral Cortex,* **12,** 2775–88.

Hanakawa, T., Immisch, I., Toma, K., Dimyan, M.A., Van Gelderen, P., and Hallett, M. (2003). Functional properties of brain areas associated with motor execution and imagery. *Journal of Neurophysiology,* **89,** 989–1002.

Helmich, R.C., De Lange, F.P., Bloem, B.R., and Toni, I. (2007). Cerebral compensation during motor imagery in Parkinson's disease. *Neuropsychologia,* **45,** 2201–15.

Hoehn, M.M. and Yahr, M.D. (1967). Parkinsonism: onset, progression, and mortality. *Neurology,* **17,** 427–42.

Holmes, S. (2007). Theoretical and practical problems for imagery in stroke rehabilitation: an observation solution. *Rehabilitation Psychology,* **52,** 1–10.

Jackson, P.L., Doyon, J., Richards, C.L., and Malouin, F. (2004). The efficacy of combined physical and mental practice in the learning of a foot-sequence task after stroke: a case report. *Neurorehabilitation and Neural Repair,* **18,** 106–11.

Kosslyn, S.M., Ganis, G., and Thompson, W.L. (2001). Neural foundations of imagery. *Nature Reviews Neuroscience,* **2,** 635–42.

Kuhn, A.A., Doyle, L., Pogosyan, A., *et al.* (2006). Modulation of beta oscillations in the subthalamic area during motor imagery in Parkinson's disease. *Brain,* **129,** 695–706.

Lim, V.K., Polych, M.A., Hollander, A., Byblow, W.D., Kirk, I.J., and Hamm, J.P. (2006). Kinesthetic but not visual imagery assists in normalizing the CNV in Parkinson's disease. *Clinical Neurophysiology,* **117,** 2308–14.

Maeda, K. and Fujiwara, K. (2007). Effects of preparatory period on anticipatory postural control and contingent negative variation associated with rapid arm movement in standing posture. *Gait and Posture,* **25,** 78–85.

Malouin, F., Belleville, S., Richards, C.L., Desrosiers, J., and Doyon, J. (2004a). Working memory and mental practice outcomes after stroke. *Archives of Physical Medicine and Rehabilitation,* **85,** 177–83.

Malouin, F., Richards, C., Jackson, P., Lafleur, M., Durand, A., and Doyon, J. (2007). The Kinesthetic and Visual Imagery Questionnaire (KVIQ) for assessing motor imagery in persons with physical disabilities: a reliability and construct validity study. *Journal of Neurology and Physical Therapy, 31*, 20–9.

Malouin, F., Richards, C.L., Doyon, J., Desrosiers, J., and Belleville, S. (2004b). Training mobility tasks after stroke with combined mental and physical practice: a feasibility study. *Neurorehabilitation and Neural Repair, 18*, 66–75.

Malouin, F., Richards, C.L., Jackson, P.L., Dumas, F., and Doyon, J. (2003). Brain activations during motor imagery of locomotor-related tasks: a PET study. *Human Brain Mapping, 19*, 47–62.

Mcintosh, G.C., Brown, S.H., Rice, R.R., and Thaut, M.H. (1997). Rhythmic auditory-motor facilitation of gait patterns in patients with Parkinson's disease. *Journal of Neurology Neurosurgery and Psychiatry, 62*, 22–6.

Michelon, P., Vettel, J.M., and Zacks, J.M. (2006). Lateral somatotopic organization during imagined and prepared movements. *Journal of Neurophysiology, 95*, 811–22.

Morris, M.E. (2000). Movement disorders in people with Parkinson disease: a model for physical therapy. *Physical Therapy, 80*, 578–97.

Morris, M.E. (2006). Locomotor training in people with Parkinson disease. *Physical Therapy, 86*, 1426–35.

Munzert, J., Zentgraf, K., Stark, R., and Vaitl, D. (2008). Neural activation in cognitive motor processes: comparing motor imagery and observation of gymnastic movements. *Experimental Brain Research, 188*, 437–44.

Oullier, O., Jantzen, K.J., Steinberg, F.L., and Kelso, J.A.S. (2005). Neural substrates of real and imagined sensorimotor coordination. *Cerebral Cortex, 15*, 975–85.

Page, S.J., Levine, P., Sisto, S.A., and Johnston, M.V. (2001). Mental practice combined with physical practice for upper-limb motor deficit in subacute stroke. *Physical Therapy, 81*, 1455–62.

Pouthas, V. and Perbal, S. (2004). Time perception depends on accurate clock mechanisms as well as unimpaired attention and memory processes. *Acta Neurobiological Experimentalis (Wars), 64*, 367–85.

Rowe, J., Hughes, L., Ghosh, B., *et al.* (2008). Parkinson's disease and dopaminergic therapy differential effects on movement, reward and cognition keywords: Parkinson's disease; reward. *Brain,* advanced publication.

Sabate, M., Gonzalez, B. and Rodriguez, M. (2007). Adapting movement planning to motor impairments: the motor-scanning system. *Neuropsychologia, 45*, 378–86.

Samuel, M., Ceballos-Baumann, A.O., Boecker, H., and Brooks, D.J. (2001). Motor imagery in normal subjects and Parkinson's disease patients: an H2150 PET study. *Neuroreport, 12*, 821–8.

Schenkman, M., Cutson, T.M., Kuchibhatla, M., *et al.* .(1998). Exercise to improve spinal flexibility and function for people with Parkinson's Disease: a randomized, controlled trial. *Journal of the American Geriatrics Society, 46*, 1207–16.

Schnider, A., Gutbrod, K., and Hess, C.W. (1995). Motion imagery in Parkinson's disease. *Brain,* **118(Pt 2)**, 485–93.

Shankar, A., De Brain, N., Bonfield, S., *et al.* (2008). Benefit of music therapy in patients with Parkinson's disease: a randomized controlled trial. *Movement Disorders, 23*, S201–S201.

Stephens, B., Mueller, A.J., Shering, A.F., *et al.* (2005). Evidence of a breakdown of corticostriatal connections in Parkinson's disease. *Neuroscience, 132*, 741–54.

Szameitat, A.J., Shen, S., and Sterr, A. (2007). Motor imagery of complex everyday movements. An fMRI study. *Neuroimage, 34*, 702–13.

Tamir, R., Dickstein, R., and Huberman, M. (2007). Integration of motor imagery and physical practice in group treatment applied to subjects with Parkinson's disease. *Neurorehabilitation and Neural Repair, 21*, 68–75.

Tanner, C. and Goldman, S. (1996). Epidemiology of Parkinson's disease. *Neurologic Clinics, 14*, 317–35.

Thaut, M.H., Mcintosh, G.C., Rice, R.R., Miller, R.A., Rathbun, J., and Brault, J.M. (1996). Rhythmic auditory stimulation in gait training for Parkinson's disease patients. *Movement Disorders, 11*, 193–200.

Thobois, S., Dominey, P., Fraix, V., *et al.* (2002). Effects of subthalamic nucleus stimulation on actual and imagined movement in Parkinson's disease: a PET study. *Journal of Neurology,* **249**, 1689–98.

Thobois, S., Dominey, P.F., Decety, J., *et al.* (2000). Motor imagery in normal subjects and in asymmetrical Parkinson's disease: a PET study. *Neurology,* **55**, 996–1002.

Tomaino, C.M. (2006) Music therapy to benefit individuals with Parkinson's disease. *Movement Disorders,* **21**, S29–S29.

Tremblay, F., Leonard, G., and Tremblay, L. (2008). Corticomotor facilitation associated with observation and imagery of hand actions is impaired in Parkinson's disease. *Experimental Brain Research,* **185**, 249–57.

Yaguez, L., Canavan, A.G., Lange, H.W., and. Homberg, V. (1999). Motor learning by imagery is differentially affected in Parkinson's and Huntington's diseases. *Behavioural Brain Research,* **102**, 115–27.

Zimmer, H.D. (2008). Visual and spatial working memory: from boxes to networks. *Neuroscience and Biobehavioral Reviews,* **32**, 1373–95.

Chapter 13

Blindness and motor imagery

Luís Aureliano Imbiriba, Sylvia B. Joffily,
Erika Carvalho Rodrigues, and Claudia D. Vargas

The day was gorgeous! I was riding a horse along a beach right
beside the sea. As he moved I could feel the wind in my face and
the smell of the sea...
*Portuguese transcript of the oniric report made by a young
congenitally blind girl.*

Vision is the most highly developed sense in primates, and represents the doorway through which most of our knowledge of the external world arises. Many daily life activities are affected by visual loss, causing social, economical, and health problems. In 2002, more than 161 million people worldwide were estimated as being visually impaired, of whom about 37 million were completely blind (Resnikoff *et al.* 2004). On the past years most studies have focused on how blindness affects visual representations in the brain and much less is known about how action representations are influenced by complete visual loss. In this chapter we will start with an overview of how blindness affects sensory and motor representations, aiming then to contribute to the knowledge of its effects upon motor behaviour through the use of paradigms employing mental simulation of actions. We will summarize herein the findings of studies related to totally blind persons and with visual deficits of peripheral origin.

It has been suggested that a simulation (or 'S') state corresponds to any mental state involving an action content where brain activity seems to mimic or simulate all aspects of movement execution, except for the absence of any overt motor behaviour (Jeannerod 1994, 2001). Accordingly, S states were associated to a broad range of situations including intended actions, imagined actions, prospective action judgements, perceptually based decisions, observation of graspable objects, actions performed by others, and action in dreams – all of them recruiting sensory and motor representations but with departing levels of awareness. Having barely been exposed to visual information, congenitally blind subjects are an inspiring and invaluable source of information allowing establishing the relations among imagery, perception, and action. As will be extensively discussed below, visual and/or motor imagery in blind subjects might most probably require the retrieval of non-visual based (perhaps tactile, auditory, or multisensory) images, stored as more abstract representations (for recent reviews about visual imagery in blindness see Cattaneo *et al.* 2008 and Dulin *et al.* 2008). Investigating S states in blind subjects might help to understand the physiological and behavioural consequences of visual loss and to define strategies to cope with this disability.

Blindness-induced modifications in the brain
Blindness and brain plasticity
Individuals who become blind, during the course of their lifetime, have to adjust to the striking demands of no longer being able to rely on vision to interact with their environment.

Growing experimental evidence suggests that these adjustments not only implicate the remaining sensory modalities, such as touch and hearing, but also involve those parts of the brain once dedicated to vision itself (Théoret *et al.* 2004). Therefore, in blind subjects, brain areas commonly associated with the processing of visual information appear not to have been rendered 'silent' by visual deprivation but rather are recruited in a compensatory cross-modal manner, being now taken on by the remaining sensory modalities (Bavelier and Neville 2002; Théoret *et al.* 2004; Merabet *et al.* 2005). Many of these studies have also shown that visual-loss etiology (Kaski 2002) and time-ensuing loss occurrence (Hollins 1985) are critical to the investigation of brain reorganization that follows blindness.

Wanet-Defalque *et al.* (1988) were among the first to report brain functional changes in early blind subjects. Using the cerebral metabolic rate for glucose as a marker of neuronal function, the authors showed that long-standing visual deprivation led to higher regional glucose utilization in striate and prestriate cortical areas as compared to blindfolded sighted controls while carrying out object manipulative or auditory tasks. Veraart *et al.* (1990) compared glucose metabolism in early and late-blind individuals (i.e., in those with visual-loss occurrence after complete development of the visual system). They found that glucose utilization within the visual cortex of early blind subjects was elevated and comparable to normal-sighted controls (with the eyes open). Veraart *et al.* (1990) interpreted this surprising elevated metabolism to the persistence of a high synaptic density, hypothetically due to a lack of synaptic pruning in the early deafferented areas during brain development.

Functional imaging studies have confirmed that plastic reorganization occurs in response to blindness in unequivocal ways. Most notably, the deafferented visual cortex is activated by tactile and auditory stimulation in blind subjects (Kujala *et al.* 1995; Sadato *et al.* 1996; Cohen *et al.* 1997; Kujala *et al.* 2000; Burton *et al.* 2002; Sadato *et al.* 2002). In a PET study, Sadato *et al.* (1996) showed activation of primary and secondary visual cortical areas in blind subjects during tactile tasks, whereas normal controls showed deactivation. Later on, however, Büchel *et al.* (1998) demonstrated that congenitally blind subjects show task specific activation of extrastriate visual and parietal association areas during Braille reading, as compared to auditory word processing, whereas by employing the same tasks blind subjects who lost their sight after puberty showed additional activation in the primary visual cortex.

Employing fMRI, Amedi *et al.* (2003) found a robust activation in primary visual cortex (V1) of congenitally blind participants during a verbal-memory task as well as during verb generation and Braille reading. Transcranial magnetic stimulation (TMS) over V1 during the performance of these tasks precluded their completion in blind but not in normal subjects (Amedi *et al.* 2004), suggesting that the loss of vision during early infancy can even lead to top-down reorganizations. One interesting question arises: Are congenitally blind subjects able to perform the mental rehearsal of visual contents?

Blindness and visual imagery

Visual imagery can be defined as the representation of perceptual information in the absence of visual input (Kaski 2002). Whilst the sighted are able to use visual imagery to represent tangible objects mentally, including their own bodies (Parsons 1994), the existence of any similitude between blind and sighted subjects in mental imagery mechanisms was at first controversial. Early studies indicated a larger delay for image formation in blind subjects as compared to sighted ones (Marmor 1977; Kerr 1983). It has also been proposed that blind subjects might rely on other imagery modalities or use semantic representations to perform these imagery tasks (Zimler and Keenan 1983).

Current research confirms that, while intuitively unacceptable, congenitally blind subjects seem able to perform visual-spatial imagery tasks, with some aspects of mental imagery being evoked by multiple modalities (for example, auditory, tactile and haptic) and stored as abstract representations (Kerr 1983; Arditi *et al.* 1988; Vanlierde and Wanet-Defalque, 2004; Lambert *et al.* 2004; Monegato *et al.* 2007; Cattaneo *et al.* 2007, 2008). For instance, Vanlierde and Wanet-Defalque (2004) have employed a paradigm where subjects were instructed to generate a mental representation of verbally presented 2-D patterns that were placed in a grid and to indicate how many pattern elements were in corresponding positions in the two halves of the grid according to a specific grid axis (vertical or horizontal). The authors found that early and late-blind subjects were able to perform this visuo-spatial imagery task as well as sighted subjects although using different strategies: whilst both sighted and late-blind subjects took advantage of a visuo-spatial strategy by generating a mental image of the matrix and simplifying this image to maintain only the relevant information in their memory, early blind subjects encoded each element of the pattern by its location in an (X;Y) coordinate system without any visual representation.

In another line of evidence, Lambert *et al.* (2004) measured the fMRI activation in sighted and blind volunteers while they listened to a list of animal names from which they were instructed to generate a mental image. In the subjects blind from birth who were able to generate a mental image of an animal, most activation foci were found, as for blindfolded subjects, in the parieto-occipital area encompassing the precuneus (BA 19) and superior and inferior parietal areas (BA 7 and BA 40, respectively). For the authors, the fact that the dorsal pathway was activated also in blind people suggests that tactile experience strongly contributes to the formation of mental images in early blind subjects.

Blindness and dreaming with visual content

Dreams with visual content are considered to be expressions of visual imagery (Lopes Da Silva 2003). Whether the congenitally blind have dreams with visual content or not has been a controversial subject for a long time, and is still open to question. In a rigorous study of home dream reports, Hurovitz *et al.* (1999) have convincingly shown that congenitally blind dreamers and those who became blind at infancy do not have visual imagery in their dreams, whereas those blinded in adolescence or young adulthood often retain visual imagery both in their waking life and in their dreams. Hurovitz *et al.* (1999) also showed that about half of all dreams have auditory sensations and reported a high percentage of locomotion and transportation references in congenitally blind subjects. The findings on multimodal sensory reference frames and dreamer-involved misfortunes in locomotion/transportation dreams were interpreted by Hurovitz *et al.* (1999) as evidence of the continuity between dream content and waking cognition.

Against this idea, Bértolo *et al.* (2003) recorded EEG during sleep to assess whether dreams with visual contents occur in the congenitally blind. As for control subjects, the pattern of cortical activation during dreams with visual content was reported to be similar to that observed during visual imagery, and were reflected in a decrease of scalp EEG alpha-activity (8–12 Hz). However, as mentioned before, interactions between non-visual cortical areas and those predetermined to mediate visual perception seem to be established by cross-modal expansion of non-visual inputs in congenitally blind subjects (Büchel *et al.* 1998; Merabet *et al.* 2005). Therefore, the many similarities found in EEG states recorded during sleep in congenitally blind and sighted subjects preclude a definitive conclusion about whether alpha rhythms in the occipital pole are attributable to visual dream content in congenitally blind subjects (Lopes Da Silva 2003).

In conclusion, congenitally blind adults seem to preserve and process mental representations of spatial information both during imagery and dreaming, as occurs in sighted subjects.

Undoubtedly, knowledge about space can be obtained from numerous sources, including tactile, auditory, and kinaesthetic modalities (Kaski 2002). A cautionary note was raised by Théoret *et al.* (2004), who claimed that activity within occipital areas in congenitally blind people does not necessarily mean that the visual cortex is directly involved in the completion of tactile, auditory, or even cognitive behaviours, and that more experiments on the functional relevance of this 'occipital recruitment' should be addressed to attach behavioural significance to these activations.

Action representations and blindness

Actions occur in space. To act efficiently in space, our brain must not only localize any objects of interest in extrapersonal (out of reach) space but also hold a constantly updated status of the body shape and posture to act in peripersonal space (immediately surrounding the body). Most actions performed within peripersonal space involve both visual and somatosensory processing related to objects being manipulated within that space, although other sensory systems such as auditory and gustatory are also often involved. In contrast, when considering processing of objects some distance from the body (e.g., outside of reaching distance), it seems to be the visual system that does most of the perceiving (e.g., perceiving which object to act on next) – although, of course, audition is used to hear distant objects, and other systems might come into play to a lesser extent. Thus, with respect to peripersonal space, the visual and somatosensory systems are both primary (Franz 2007). As such, one might suppose that the lack of vision at early stages of development should affect the building and maintenance of both peripersonal and extrapersonal space representations.

In the process of moving our body in space, a series of sensorimotor transformations that translates visual and other sensory information about the location of the target and the body parts in space into a set of motor commands will bring us to the desired position (Wolpert and Miall 1996). It is now well established that these high level cognitive plans for movement are created in the brain by combining visual and kinaesthetic information and integrating it to the proper motor commands in order to create a common reference frame (Andersen and Buneo 2002) with these signals providing an estimate of impending movement. According to this view, different subregions within posterior parietal areas contain maps of intention related to the planning of different movements, such as those of the eye, and reaching and grasping movements (Andersen and Buneo 2002), revealing a contribution of these areas to the early stages of motor preparation before movement itself begins (reviewed in Blackemore and Sirigu 2003). These motor plans are built throughout motor development, when the central nervous system learns and maintains internal models of sensorimotor transformations to predict the consequences of motor commands and to determine the motor commands required to perform specific tasks (Wolpert *et al.* 2001).

Motor development without vision

Motor development investigation in blind children represents a straightforward way to have access to the consequences of blindness upon motor representations. Accordingly, blind infants should provide experimental evidence concerning the essential role of visual information in early motor development and how and when the absence of vision may be compensated for. Unfortunately, most data about motor development of blind infants is fragmentary and contradictory. This can be attributed to methodological problems including small and heterogeneous samples, in recent years, the increasing number of children with multiple handicaps besides blindness on account of improvements in survival rates in high-risk newborns, and inadequate diagnostic instruments to accurately define the onset and severity of blindness in the first years of life (Elisa *et al.* 2002).

Adelson and Fraiberg (1974) suggested that there are two stages in the motor development of a blind child. In the first stage, which corresponds to the first six months of life, gross-motor development is essentially the same as that of the sighted child. From six months of life onwards, normal motor development begins to be enhanced by a growing number of voluntary patterns, and motion assumes its full global character, giving support to the relational aspects of life (exploration, inquiry, etc.). At this stage, the motor performance of blind children starts to lag behind that of sighted children (Adelson and Fraiberg 1974).

Fraiberg (1971) concluded that postural items such as head and trunk control and postural functions that require neuromuscular maturation appeared in the blind within the expected range of sighted children. Although different studies have agreed that there is a delay in the initiation of mobility in a blind child (Jan and Scott 1974; Levtzion-Korach et al. 2000), Fraiberg (1971) hypothesized that the peculiar delay in motor development found in a blind child is to be attributed to the absence of 'incentive' that sight represents for all voluntary skills, and to the fact that, when sight is lacking, it is difficult to build up a picture of the world with which to interact. In conclusion, practice and exercise do not hasten the appearance of early motor skills that are determined by maturation, although lack of opportunity can cause retardation of development (Jan and Scott 1974). Does early blindness affect higher level motor representations?

Contribution of mental simulation of movements to the understanding of motor representations in blind subjects

The recent advance of new neuroimaging and non-invasive brain stimulation technologies have allowed researchers to propose a physiologic parallelism between motor imagery and execution (Roland et al. 1980; Decety and Michel 1989; Decety et al. 1994; Jeannerod 1994; Sirigu et al. 1996; Gerardin et al. 2000; Stippich et al. 2002). Furthermore, many studies employing TMS have demonstrated that motor imagery modulates the excitability of the primary motor cortex (M1) in an effector-specific manner (Yahagi et al.1996; Kasai et al. 1997; Kiers et al. 1997; Yahagi and Kasai 1998; Fadiga et al. 1999; Hashimoto and Rothwell 1999; Rossini et al. 1999; Stinear and Byblow 2003; Vargas et al. 2004).

As for motor planning, the mental simulation of an action also retrieves sensory representations and most importantly involves the prediction of the sensory consequences of a given action (Wolpert et al. 2001). Accordingly, lesions in the inferior parietal cortex impair the ability to mentally simulate a movement (Sirigu et al. 1996). Thus, when a subject is asked to perform the mental simulation of an action, he/she will naturally retrieve these stored sensory representations and build an estimate of the sensory consequences of the imagined action. In this process the subject can most commonly call for kinaesthetic, visual or a blend of the two representations (Hall et al. 1985). Kinaesthetic motor imagery involves imagining the 'feeling' or the body sensation that the actual task performance produces and visual motor imagery involves imagining 'visualizing oneself' performing the task. Therefore, as motor images are frequently built based on multisensory reference frames, people can perform imagery of movements using a visual/kinaesthetic perspective of themselves (internal or egocentric) or a predominantly visual perspective of themselves or someone else (external or allocentric) (Decety 1996).

Mentally simulating our own movements

Although neuroimaging studies indicate that the neural underpinning of motor imagery and motor execution are similar, differences across studies in reported instructional details and subjective experience make it difficult to discern what imagery modality is being measured.

For instance, it was shown that the strategy adopted to perform motor imagery in the first person (1P) seems to determine which cortical areas will be recruited. Employing fMRI, Dechent *et al.* (2004) showed that M1 activation in response to the imagination of a hand movement condition (without explicitly instructing subjects about which imagery mode should be employed) occurred only in one out of six subjects. The authors proposed that these discrepancies should be attributed to differences in the simulation strategy, as the movement imagery process often involves a blend of both kinaesthetic and visual form of imagination. Accordingly, in a PET study, subjects were asked to visualize (instead of feeling) the movement of their own fingers and this type of imagery did not recruit M1 (Deiber *et al.* 1998). Employing fMRI, Solodkin *et al.* (2004) asked a group of subjects to perform the kinaesthetic simulation of a hand movement and compared the activation pattern with a second group of subjects that simulated the same movement in a visual mode. Data modelling revealed activations in the primary sensorimotor cortex for the former but not for the latter group. More recently, Guillot *et al.* (2009) confirmed that movement-related cortical areas were more activated during kinaesthetic imagery than during visual imagery in good imagers. Stinear *et al.* (2006) have shown, in a TMS study, that corticospinal excitability is consistently higher when the mental simulation of one's own movement is performed in the kinaesthetic but not the visual mode.

While searching for a physiological modulation of motor imagery modes in normal volunteers, we investigated the effect of somato-motor and visual strategies during the mental simulation of a task that involved postural adjustments. Subjects were asked to stand up on a force platform and were instructed either to rest for 20 s or count mentally from 1 to 15, or imagine themselves executing a bilateral plantar flexion 15 times and execute the same movement 15 times. Subjects were told to report which imagery mode was employed to perform the task, and were further divided into visual and somato-motor groups. Analysis of the stabilometric parameters showed higher amplitude of displacement values in the antero-posterior (y) axis for the somato-motor as compared to the visual group (Rodrigues *et al.* 2003), suggesting that, when performed in 1P, each imagery mode activated a distinct subset of brain networks. Accordingly, mental simulation of a hand movement in the somato-motor mode was shown to recruit distinct brain regions as compared to the visual mode (Solodkin *et al.* 2004; Olsson *et al.* 2008; Guillot *et al.* 2009).

We then supposed that motor imagery should be dramatically affected by the existence and duration of previous visual experience: in the absolute lack of vision, motor imagery would be performed mainly in a kinaesthetic mode. In late-blind individuals, on the other hand, the adding of a visual component in movement planning and execution in early life could have led to a visuo-kinaesthetic motor imagery mode. To test this hypothesis, we employed the previously reported (Rodrigues *et al.* 2003) mental simulation of a postural task. Stabilometric (body sway), electro-myographic (EMG, lateral gastrocnemius) and eletrocardiographic (ECG) signals were acquired simultaneously during task performance in subjects with early- and late-blindness onset (Imbiriba *et al.* 2006). Using discriminant analysis, we found an overall correct classification of 100 and 90.9% between groups for stabilometric parameters and heart beats, respectively. This result was found only for the mental simulation task (Figure 13.1), being absent for resting, counting and executing tasks, thus confirming previous studies showing that motor simulation in a kinaesthetic mode strongly associates with somatic and autonomic changes (Decety *et al.* 1993; Decety 1996; Guillot and Collet 2005).

Röder *et al.* (2004) had shown that late but not congenitally blind people are impaired in tactile discrimination tasks by crossing their hands, suggesting the critical role played by childhood vision in modulating the perception of touch that may arise from the emergence of specific cross-modal links during development, and indicating that behavioural outcome critically depends on early childhood vision. It has been argued that because of the dominant role of vision in motor

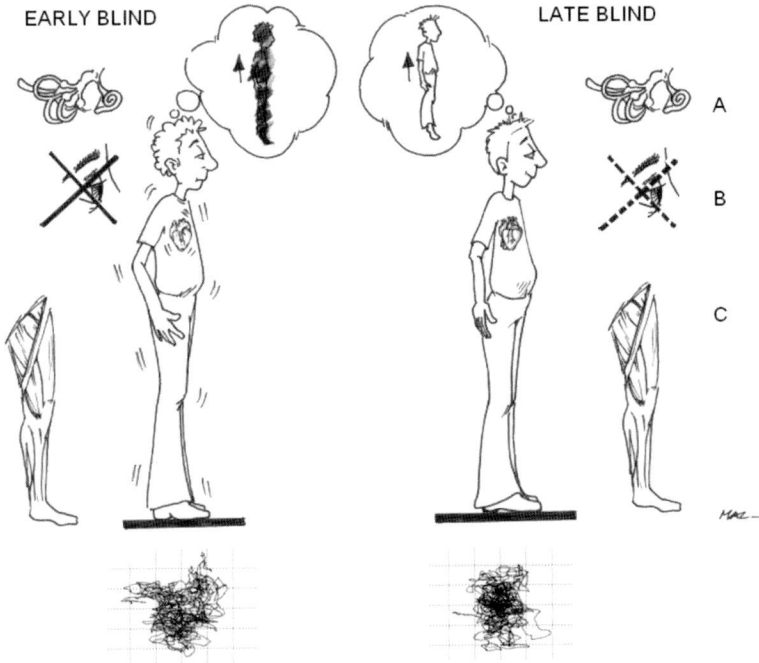

Fig. 13.1 Pictorial representation of the results gathered by Imbiriba *et al* (2006): analysis of stabilometric and heart rate parameters indicated that movement simulation tend to unfold with the use of body representations that are distinctly affected by the age of blindness onset. The cartoon illustrates the sensory modalities contributing to postural control in sighted subjects: (A) vestibular, (B) visual, and (C) proprioceptive information.

planning and execution, tactile stimuli are mapped into externally defined coordinates (predominantly determined by visual inputs) that take longer to achieve when external and body-centred codes (determined primarily by somatosensory/proprioceptive inputs) are in conflict. In a very interesting series of experiments employing a classical spatial compatibility ('Simon effect') paradigm, Röder *et al.* (2007) tested whether the default use of the external reference frame is innately determined or acquired instead during development primed by the increasing dominance of vision over manual control. Congenitally blind, late-blind and sighted adults had to press a left or right response key depending on the bandwidth of pink noise bursts presented from loudspeakers placed either on the left or on the right side. All participants responded more efficiently with uncrossed hands when the sound was presented from the same side as the responding hand. However, the congenitally blind responded faster than other participants when the hand was located contralateral to the sound source, suggesting that the default mapping of sensory inputs into external coordinates that reflects the dominance of vision in manual control was absent in congenitally blind participants. When, however, explicit matching of the sound location with the spatial position of the responding hand was required, congenitally blind participants showed a higher crossing deficit than sighted and late-blind adults, suggesting the existence of a stimulus-location/response-*hand mapping* in congenitally blind and a stimulation/response-*location mapping* in sighted and late-blind participants (Röder *et al.* 2007). In line with Röder *et al.* (2004, 2007), our results indicated that movement simulation in the 1P mode tended to unfold with the use of body representations that were distinctly affected by the age of the onset of blindness.

First versus third motor imagery mode and blindness

Subjects can be asked to perform an action in 1P or third-person (3P) mode. In a PET study, Ruby and Decety (2001) have employed mental simulation of action to explore patterns of brain activation while subjects simulated actions from either an 1P or a 3P perspective. Both conditions were associated with common activation in the supplementary motor area (SMA), the precentral gyrus, the precuneus and the MT/V5 complex. When compared to the 1P perspective, the 3P perspective recruited the right inferior parietal, precuneus, posterior cingulate, and frontopolar cortex. The opposite contrast revealed activation in the left inferior parietal and somatosensory cortex. Sirigu and Duhamel (2001) have also addressed this question by comparing the effect of a simple change in the phrasing of imagery instructions (1P or 3P imagery). The authors proposed that under instructions to seek the solution using imagery in 1P, subjects use primarily motor resources, and under instructions to seek the solution using imagery in 3P, they use primarily visual resources (Sirigu and Duhamel 2001).

Jackson *et al.* (2006) suggested that motor representation based on 1P perspective might involve more kinaesthetic components than that based on 3P perspective. On the other hand, Anquetil and Jeannerod (2007) have shown that response times were similar when subjects had to mentally simulate an action either in 1P or 3P mode, and Fourkas *et al.* (2006a) did not find any difference in corticospinal excitability whenever the mental simulation of a hand movement was performed either in 1P or 3P mode, indicating that the effect of both imagery modalities is comparable, at least for simple motor tasks and in spite of explicit instructions prior to each condition to concentrate on specific visual or kinaesthetic information. Fourkas *et al.* (2006b) also confirmed that there was no evidence that 1P visual and kinaesthetic imagery leads to different levels of corticospinal excitability per se. Hence, one might expect 1P imagery, which incorporates kinaesthetic components in addition to visual components, to be more closely associated with motor control as it creates a more 'real' representation, and therefore the combination of modalities would produce a better action representation (Fourkas *et al.* 2006b).

In a preliminary study (Imbiriba *et al.* 2008), in order to investigate the contribution of vision on perspective taken during movement planning, we recorded the brain activity that precedes mental simulation of a given action (readiness potentials – RP) in normal and early-blind subjects. The RP, which starts about 1s before movements, is associated with the preparation to act in the near future (Shibasaki and Hallett 2006). In the simulation trials, blind and sighted subjects had either to imagine themselves performing the middle-finger extension from their own perspective (1P) or in the perspective of another person sitting in front of them performing the same action (3P).

Our analysis for Cz channel (corresponding most likely to supplementary motor area) has shown that, in blind subjects, RPs associated with imagining movements in the 1P perspective were similar to those of execution, and clearly departed from those of execution in the 3P perspective. In the sighted group there was no difference between 1P and 3P, and execution. Moreover, there was no main effect difference between the blind and sighted groups.

The lack of difference between 1P and 3P conditions found for sighted subjects suggest that they might have used a visuo-kinaesthetic strategy to perform both tasks, confirming that the representation used to simulate the action of another person (3P) must be close to the representation built for performing that same action (1P) (Anquetil and Jeannerod 2007). Congenitally blind people, however, seem to use a completely different strategy to simulate an action in 1P or 3P perspectives. In 1P, RPs were similar to those of execution, suggesting that they were representing movements using mostly kinaesthetic information. As suggested by Vanlierde and Wanet-Defalque (2004) for visuo-spatial tasks, congenitally blind subjects might have used an abstract strategy to mentally simulate an action in 3P perspective. Interestingly, both for sighted and blind subjects the 1P perspective was considered to be easier to perform than the 3P and the anticipatory heart rate did not differ between groups either (Imbiriba *et al.* 2008).

The identification of oneself as the origin of an action may seem a relatively simple task when movements are overtly executed. In this condition, sensory signals arise from the moving limbs and from the effects of the movement on the external world: these signals can be compared to those resulting from the action generation mechanism, and the outcome of this comparison can be used to label the action as self-generated. What makes self-identification and the role of the sense of agency less easy to understand is the existence of a number of situations where the action generation mechanism is activated, but where the action remains covert. One of these situations is that of imagined actions (motor images) (Jeannerod 2006). In normal volunteers, motor imagery performed in the 3P mode is assumed to draw itself at least partially from one's 1P motor resources, being however also strongly dependent on the visual content of the imagined action (Ruby and Decety 2001). In congenitally blind subjects, our results suggest that motor planning and execution occur likewise in the 1P but not in the 3P mode, suggesting the existence of an alternative (non-visual and non-somesthesic), and probably higher level strategy to perform this task.

One strongly impairing effect of early blindness was recently pointed out by Théoret and Fecteau (2005). Congenitally blind individuals seem to display autism-like characteristics (Hobson and Bishop 2003), performing at lower levels than normal subjects on theory-of-mind tasks (Minter *et al.* 1998). These results raise interesting questions regarding the development of the parieto-frontal circuits related to action observation and understanding (Rizzolatti and Craighero 2004). In blind individuals, the lack of visual input would derail the normal mechanism matching action-perception and execution within the visual system. A motor resonance mechanism could still operate through the auditory modality (Kohler *et al.* 2002), but in an obviously limited manner due to lack of visual input. Therefore, our results (Imbiriba *et al.* 2008) and those of others (Minter *et al.* 1998; Hobson and Bishop 2003) suggest that early blindness can lead to changes in motor cognition.

Conclusions and perspectives

In conclusion, the perceptual and behavioural consequences of blindness are still being debated and many questions remain as to the underlying neural reorganization that occurs within the brain. Thus, especially in the case of blind children, it seems crucial to promote the development of body awareness while enabling them to handle and understand the existence and nature of the world.

Acknowledgement

We acknowledge the financial support by CNPq, FAPERJ, PRONEX, IBN-NET/FINEP.

References

Adelson, E. and Fraiberg, S. (1974). Gross motor development in infants blind from birth. *Child Development*, **45**, 114–26.

Amedi, A., Raz, N., Pianka, P., Malach, R., and Zohary, E. (2003). Early 'visual' cortex activation correlates with superior verbal memory performance in the blind. *Nature Neuroscience*, **6**, 758–66.

Amedi, A., Floel, A., Knescht, S., Zohary, E., and Cohen, L.G. (2004). Transcranial magnetic stimulation of the occipital pole interferes with verbal processing in blind subjects. *Nature Neuroscience*, **7**, 1266–70.

Andersen, R.A. and Buneo, C.A. (2002). Intentional maps in posterior parietal cortex. *Annual Review of Neuroscience*, **25**, 189–220.

Anquetil, T. and Jeannerod, M. (2007). Simulated actions in the first and third person perspectives share common representations. *Brain Research*, **1130**, 125–9.

Arditi, A., Holtzman, J.D., and Kosslyn, S.M. (1988). Mental imagery and sensory experience in congenital blindness. *Neuropsychologia*, **26**, 1–12.

Bavelier, D. and Neville, H.J. (2002). Cross-modal plasticity: where and how? *Nature Reviews Neuroscience*, **3**, 442–52.

Bértolo, H., Paiva, T., Pessoa, L., Mestre, T., Marques, R., and Santos, R. (2003). Visual dream content, graphical representation and EEG alpha activity in congenitally blind subjects. *Cognitive Brain Research*, **15**, 277–84.

Blakemore, S.J. and Sirigu, A. (2003). Action prediction in the cerebellum and in the parietal lobe. *Experimental Brain Research*, **153**, 239–45.

Büchel, C., Price, C., Frackowiak, R.S.J., and Friston, K. (1998). Different activation patterns in the visual cortex of late and congenitally blind subjects. *Brain*, **121**, 409–19.

Burton, H., Snyder, A.Z., Conturo, T.E., Akbudak, E., Ollinger, J.M., and Raichle, M.E. (2002). Adaptive changes in early and late blind: a fMRI study of Braille reading. *Journal of Neurophysiology*, **87**, 589–607.

Cattaneo, Z., Vecchi, T., Cornoldi, C., *et al.* (2008). Imagery and spatial process in blindness and visual impairment. *Neuroscience and Biobehavioral Reviews*, **32**, 1346–60.

Cattaneo, Z., Vecchi, T., Monegato, M., Pece, A., and Cornoldi, C. (2007). Effects of late visual impairment on mental representations activated by visual and tactile stimuli. *Brain Research*, **1148**, 170–6.

Cohen, L.G., Celnik, P., Pascual-Leone, A., *et al.* (1997). Functional relevance of cross-modal plasticity in blind humans. *Nature*, **389**, 180–3.

Decety, J. and Michel, F. (1989). Comparative analysis of actual and mental movement times in two graphic tasks. *Brain Cognition*, **11**, 87–97.

Decety, J. (1996). The neurophysiological basis of motor imagery. *Behavioural Brain Research*, **77**, 45–52.

Decety, J., Jeannerod, M., Durozard, D., and Baverel, G. (1993). Central activation of autonomic effectors during mental simulation of motor actions in man. *Journal of Physiology*, **461**, 549–63.

Decety, J., Perani, D., Jeannerod, M., *et al.*(1994). Mapping motor representations with positron emission tomography. *Nature*, **371**, 600–2.

Dechent, P., Merboldt, K.D., and Frahm, J. (2004). Is the human primary motor cortex involved in motor imagery? *Cognitive Brain Research*, **19**, 138–44.

Deiber, M.P., Ibañez, V., Honda, M., Sadato, N., Raman, R., and Hallett, M. (1998). Cerebral process related to visuomotor imagery and generation of simple finger movements studied with positron emission tomography. *Neuroimage*, **7**, 73–85.

Dulin, D., Hatwell, Y., Pylyshyn, Z., and Chokron, S. (2008). Effects of peripheral and central visual impairment on mental imagery capacity. *Neuroscience and Biobehavioral Reviews*, **32**, 1396–1408.

Elisa, F., Josée, L., Oreste, F.G., *et al.* (2002). Gross motor development and reach on sound as critical tools for the development of the blind child. *Brain and Development*, **24**, 269–75.

Fadiga, L., Buccino, G., Craighero, L., Fogassi, L., Gallese, V., and Pavesi, G. (1999). Corticospinal excitability is specifically modulated by motor imagery: a magnetic stimulation study. *Neuropsychologia*, **37**, 147–58.

Fourkas, A.D., Avenanti, A., Urgesi, C., and Aglioti, S.M. (2006a). Corticospinal facilitation during first and third person imagery. *Experimental Brain Research*, **168**, 143–51.

Fourkas, A.D., Ionta, S., and Aglioti, S.M. (2006b). Influence of imagined posture and imagery modality on corticospinal excitability. *Behavioural Brain Research*, **168**, 190–6.

Fraiberg, S. (1971). Intervention in infancy. *Journal of the American Academy of Child Psychiatry*, **10**, 390–4.

Franz, E.A. (2007). Considering general organizational principles for dorsal-ventral systems within an action framework. *Behavioral and Brain Sciences*, **30**, 207–8.

Gerardin, E., Sirigu, A., Lehericy, S., *et al.* (2000). Partially overlapping neural networks for real and imagined hand movements. *Cerebral Cortex*, **10**, 1093–104.

Guillot, A. and Collet, C. (2005). Contribution from neurophysiological and psychological methods to the study of motor imagery. *Brain Research Reviews*, **50**, 387–97.

Guillot, A., Collet, C., Nguyen, V. A., Malouin, F., Richards, C., and Doyon, J. (2009). Brain activity during visual versus kinesthethic imagery: an fMRI study. *Human Brain Mapping*, **30**, 2157–72.

Hall, C., Pongrac, J., and Buckholz, E. (1985). The measurement of imagery ability. *Human Movement Science*, **4**, 107–18.

Hashimoto, R. and Rothwell, J.C. (1999). Dynamic changes in corticospinal excitability during motor imagery. *Experimental Brain Research*, **125**, 75–81.

Hobson, R.P. and Bishop, M. (2003). The pathogenesis of autism: insights from congenital blindness. *Philosophical Transactions of the Royal Society of London B*, **358**, 335–44.

Hollins, M. (1985). Styles of mental imagery in blind adults. *Neuropsychologia*, **23**, 561–6.

Hurovitz, C.S., Dunn, S., Domhoff, G.W., and Fiss, H. (1999). The dreams of blind men and women: a replication and extension of previous findings. *Dreaming*, **9**, 183–93.

Imbiriba, L.A., Rodrigues, E.C., Magalhães, J., and Vargas, C.D. (2006). Motor imagery in blind subjects: the influence of the previous visual experience. *Neuroscience Letters*, **400**, 181–5.

Imbiriba, L.A., Oliveira, L.A., Russo, M.M., *et al.* (2008). Movement-related brain potentials in blind subjects. *Clinical Neurophysiology*, **40**, 181.

Jackson, P.L., Meltzoff, A.N., and Decety, J. (2006). Neural circuits involved in imitation and perspective-taking. *Neuroimage*, **31**, 429–39.

Jan, J.E. and Scott, E.S. (1974). Hypotonia and delayed early motor development in congenitally blind children. *The Journal of Pediatrics*, **84**, 929–30.

Jeannerod, M. (1994). The representing brain – neural correlates of motor intention and imagery. *Behavioral and Brain Sciences*, **17**, 187–202.

Jeannerod, M. (2001). Neural simulation of action: a unifying mechanism for motor cognition. *Neuroimage*, **14**, 103–9.

Jeannerod, M. (2006). *Motor Cognition: What Actions Tell the Self*. Oxford: Oxford University Press.

Kasai, T., Kawai, S., Kawanishi, M., and Yahagi, S. (1997). Evidence of facilitation of motor evoked potentials (MEPs) induced by motor imagery. *Brain Research*, **744**:147–50.

Kaski, D. (2002). Revision: is visual perception a requisite for visual imagery? *Perception*, **31**, 717–31.

Kerr, N.H. (1983). The role of vision in visual imagery experiments: evidence from the congenitally blind. *Journal of Experimental Psychology*, **112**, 265–77.

Kiers, L., Fernando, B., and Tomkins, D. (1997). Facilitatory effect of thinking about a movement on magnetic motor evoked potentials. *Electroencephalography Clinical Neurophysiology*, **105**, 262–8.

Kohler, E., Keysers, C, Umiltá, M.A., Fogassi, L, Gallese, V., and Rizzolatti, G. (2002). Hearing sounds, understanding actions: action representation in mirror neurons. *Science*, **297**, 846–8.

Kujala, T., Huotilainen, M., Sinkkonen, J., *et al.* (1995). Visual cortex activation in blind humans during sound discrimination. *Neuroscience Letters*, **183**, 143–6.

Kujala, T., Alho, K., and Näätänen, R. (2000). Cross-modal reorganization of human cortical functions. *Trends in Neuroscience*, **23**, 115–20.

Lambert, S., Sampaio, E., Mauss, Y., and Scheiber, C. (2004). Blindness and brain plasticity: contribution of mental imagery? An fMRI study. *Cognitive Brain Research*, **20**, 1–11.

Levtzion-Korach, O., Tennenbaum, A., Schnitzer, R., and Ornoy, A. (2000). Early motor development of blind children. *Journal of Paediatrics*, **36**, 226–9.

Lopes Da Silva, F.H. (2003). Visual dreams in the congenitally blind? *Trends in Cognitive Sciences*, **7**, 328–30.

Marmor, G.S. (1977). Age at onset of blindness and the development of visual imagery. *Perceptual and Motor Skills*, **45**, 1031–4.

Merabet, L.B., Rizzo, J.F., Amedi, A., Somers, D.C., andPascual-Leone, A. (2005). What blindness can tell us about seeing again: merging neuroplasticity and neuroprostheses. *Nature Reviews Neuroscience*, **6**, 71–7.

Minter, M., Hobson, R.P., and Bishop, M. (1998). Congenital visual impairment and theory of mind. *British Journal of Developmental Psychology*, **16**, 183–96.

Monegato, M., Cattaneo, Z., Pece, A., and Vecchi, T. (2007). Comparing the effects of congenital and late visual impairments on visuospatial mental abilities. *Journal of Visual Impairment and Blindness*, **101**, 278– 95.

Olsson, C.J., Jonsson, B., Larsson, A., and Nyberg, L. (2008). Motor representations and practice affect brain systems underlying imagery: an fMRI study of internal imagery in novices and active high jumpers. *The Open Neuroimaging Journal*, **2**, 5–13.

Parsons, L.M. (1994). Temporal and kinematic properties of motor behavior reflected in mentally simulated action. *Journal of Experimental Psychology: Human Perception and Performance*, **20**, 709–30.

Resnikoff, S., Pascolini, D., Etya'ale, D., *et al.* (2004). Global data on visual impairment in the year 2002. *Bulletin of the World Health Organization*, **82**, 844–51.

Rizzolatti, G. and Craighero, L. (2004). The mirror neuron system. *Annual Review of Neuroscience*, **27**, 169–92.

Röder, B., Kusmierek, A., Spence, C., and Schicke, T. (2007). Developmental vision determines the reference frame for the multisensory control of action. *Proceedings of the National Academy of Sciences*, **104**, 4753–8.

Röder, B., Rösler, F., and Spence, C. (2004). Early vision impairs tactile perception in the blind. *Current Biology*, **14**, 121–4.

Rodrigues, E.C., Imbiriba, L.A., Leite, G.R., Magalhães, J., Volchan, E., and Vargas, C.D. (2003). Efeito da estratégia de simulação mental sobre o controle postural. *Revista Brasileira de Psiquiatria*, **25**, 33–5 (in Portuguese).

Roland, P.E., Skinhoj, E., Lassen, N.A., and Larsen, B. (1980). Different cortical areas in man in organization of voluntary movements in extrapersonal space. *Journal of Neurophysiology*, **43**, 137–50.

Rossini, P.M., Rossi, S., Pasqualetti, P., and Tecchio, F. (1999). Corticospinal excitability modulation to hand muscles during movement imagery. *Cerebral Cortex*, **9**, 1047–3211.

Ruby, P and Decety, J. (2001). Effect of subjective perspective taking during simulation of action: a PET investigation of agency. *Nature Neuroscience*, **4**, 546–50.

Sadato, N., Pascual-Leone, A., Grafman, J., *et al.* (1996). Activation of the primary visual cortex by braille reading in blind subjects. *Nature*, **380**, 526–8.

Sadato, N., Okada, T., Honda, M., and Yonekura, Y. (2002). Critical period for cross-modal plasticity in blind humans: a functional MRI study. *Neuroimage*, **16**, 389–400.

Shibasaki, H. and Hallett, M. (2006). What is the bereitschaftspotential? *Clinical Neurophysiology*, **117**, 2341–56.

Sirigu, A. and Duhamel, J.R. (2001). Motor and visual imagery as two complementary but neutrally dissociable mental processes. *Journal of Cognitive Neuroscience*, **13**, 910–9.

Sirigu, A., Duhamel, J.R., Cohen, L., Pillon, B., Dubois, B., and Agid, Y. (1996). The mental representation of hand movements after parietal cortex damage. *Science*, **273**, 1564–8.

Solodkin, A., Hlustik, P., Chen, E.E., and Small, S.L. (2004). Fine modulation in network activation during motor execution and motor imagery. *Cerebral Cortex*, **14**, 1246–55.

Stinear, C.M. and Byblow, W.D. (2003). Motor imagery of phasic thumb abduction temporally and spatially modulates corticospinal excitability. *Clinical Neurophysiology*, **114**, 909–14.

Stinear, C.M., Byblow, W.D., Steyvers, M., Levin, O., and Swinnen, S.P. (2006). Kinesthetic, but not visual, motor imagery modulates corticomotor excitability. *Experimental Brain Research*, **168**, 157–64.

Stippich, C., Ochmann, H., and Sartor, K. (2002). Somatotopic mapping of the human primary ensorimotor cortex during motor imagery and motor execution by functional magnetic resonance imaging. *Neuroscience Letters*, **331**, 50–54.

Théoret, H., Merabet, L, and Pascual-Leone, A. (2004). Behavioral and neuroplastic changes in the blind: evidence for functionally relevant cross-modal interactions. *Journal of Physiology*, **98**, 221–33.

Théoret, H. and Fecteau, S. (2005). Making a case for mirror-neuron system involvement in language development: what about autism and blindness? *Behavioral and Brain Sciences*, **28**, 145–6.

Vanlierde, A. and Wanet-Defalque, M.C. (2004). Abilities and strategies of blind and sighted subjects in visuo-spatial imagery. *Acta Psychologica*, **16**, 205–22.

Vargas, C.D., Olivier, E., Craighero, L., Fadiga, L., Duhamel, J.R., and Sirigu, A. (2004). The influence of hand posture on corticospinal excitability during motor imagery: a transcranial magnetic stimulation study. *Cerebral Cortex*, **14**, 1200–6.

Veraart, C., De Volder, A., Wanet-Defalque, M.C., Bol, A., Michel, C., and Goffinet, A.M. (1990). Glucose utilization in human visual cortex is abnormally elevated in blindness of early onset but decreased in blindness of late onset. *Brain Research*, **510**, 115–21.

Wanet-Defalque, M.C.; Veraart, C.; De Volder, A., *et al.* (1988). High metabolic activity in the visual cortex of early blind human subjects. *Brain Research*, **446**, 369–73.

Wolpert, D.M., Ghahramani, Z., and Flanagan, J.R. (2001). Perspectives and problems in motor learning. *Trends in Cognitive Sciences*, **5**, 487–94.

Wolpert, D.M. and Miall, R.C. (1996). Forward models for physiological motor control. *Neural Network*, **9**, 1265–79.

Yahagi, S. and Kasai T. (1998). Facilitation of motor evoked potentials (MEPs) in first dorsal interosseous (FDI) muscle is dependent on different motor images. *Electroencephalography and Clinical Neurophysiology*, **109**, 409–17.

Yahagi, S., Shimura, K., and Kasai, T. (1996). An increase in cortical excitability with no change in spinal excitability during motor imagery. *Perceptual and Motor Skills*, **83**, 288–90.

Zimler, J. and Keenan, J.M. (1983). Imagery in the congenitally blind: how visual are visual images? *Journal of Experimental Psychology: Learning, Memory and Cognition*, **8**, 269–82.

Chapter 14

EEG-based brain–computer communication

Gert Pfurtscheller and Christa Neuper

What is a brain–computer interface and who needs it?

A brain–computer interface (BCI) is a novel communication system that translates human thoughts or intentions into a control signal without using any muscle activity. In this way, a BCI provides a new non-muscular communication or control channel which can be used either to assist people with severe motor disabilities (Birbaumer *et al.* 1999; Wolpaw *et al.* 2002; Pfurtscheller *et al.* 2006a), or to support biofeedback training in people suffering from epilepsy or stroke (Birbaumer and Cohen 2007). Today the world of BCI application is expanding and new fields are opening. One benefit is to use the BCI to control multimedia applications (Scherer 2008), another is to use the BCI for user authentication (Pfurtscheller and Neuper 2006; Marcel and Millan 2007).

Each mental activity, for example decision making, intention to move, simulation of movement, mental arithmetic and others, is accompanied by excitation of distributed neural structures or networks. As a consequence of this, electrical potentials, magnetic fields, and (with a delay of some seconds) also the metabolic supply changes can be recorded with adequate sensors, when the population of activated neurons exceeds some critical mass. Consequently, a BCI can be based on a variety of signals at its input, as, for example, electrical potentials, magnetic fields, or metabolic/hemodynamic changes.

When we talk about a BCI, several components have to be considered. The signal recordings can either be invasive or non-invasive, appropriate signal features must be analyzed and classified, a suitable mental strategy used for control has to be chosen as well as the type of operation and the type of feedback.

Till date, many BCI systems have employed motor imagery tasks to generate modulation of sensorimotor EEG activity, which are then used to operate an external device. Because motor imagery results in somatotopically organized activation patterns, mental imagination of different movements (e.g., hand, foot, tongue) represents an efficient strategy to operate a BCI (Pfurtscheller *et al.* 1997; Neuper *et al.* 1999; Pfurtscheller and Neuper 2001; Cincotti *et al.* 2003; Neuper *et al.* 2005, 2006; Blankertz *et al.* 2007; Mellinger *et al.* 2007). A further advantage of using motor imagery (instead of other cognitive tasks) in BCI is that it produces changes in sensorimotor brain oscillations that occur naturally in movement planning and execution (Pfurtscheller and Neuper 1997). Because these rhythms are generated in cortical areas, most directly connected to the brain's normal motor output channels, they are particularly suitable for assistive device control.

Suitable brain signals

Recording electrical potentials with electrodes placed directly on the cortex (subdural or epidural) and the subsequent analysis of the electrocorticogram (ECoG) is an example of an invasive method (Leuthard *et al.* 2006). Alternatively, the neural firing of a small population of neurons can be recorded with a multi-unit electrode array placed directly in the cortex (Hochberg *et al.* 2006). Both types of signals have a superior signal-to-noise ratio, need less user training and are suitable for replacing or restoring lost motor functions in patients with damaged neuronal system parts.

On the other hand, non-invasive BCIs can use a variety of brain signals as input such as the electroencephalogram (EEG), the magnetoencephalogram (MEG), the blood oxygen level dependent (BOLD) signal, as well as the concentration of (de)oxyhemoglobin. With MEG weak magnetic fields are detected, which are caused by current flows in the cortex. These small magnetic fields, in the range of some pT to fT are measured with multichannel superconducting quantum interference device (SQUID) gradiometers in a shielded environment. This technique combines excellent time resolution with a moderate spatial resolution and was used to realize a MEG-based BCI (Kauhanen *et al.* 2006). Both, the BOLD signal obtained with functional magnetic resonance imaging (fMRI) and (de)oxyhemoglobin changes, measured with near infrared spectroscopy (NIRS), are hemodynamic responses with a poor time resolution. NIRS is an optical technique which uses light in the near infrared spectrum (typically between wavelengths of 630–1350 nm) to determine the oxygenation of the tissue and has recently been applied to the field of BCI research (Coyle *et al.* 2004). Weiskopf *et al.* (2004) reported on an fMRI-based BCI.

EEG-based BCI systems

The EEG is the most widely used brain signal for operating a BCI system. Two types of changes can be extracted from the ongoing EEG signals: one change is time and phase-locked (evoked) to an externally or internally paced event, the other is non-phase-locked (induced). To the former belong the event-related potentials or ERPs including the P300, the slow cortical potential (SCP) shifts and the steady state visual evoked potentials (SSVEP). To the latter belong the event-related desynchronization (ERD) and synchronization (ERS). This means we can differentiate between two types of systems one, is based on a predefined mental task and classifying induced brain activities (Figure 14.1A) the other is based on sensory stimulation (e.g., visual) and classifying evoked changes (Figure 14.1B).

The P300-BCI

The P300 is the positive component of the evoked potential at a latency of 300 ms evoked by randomly presented target stimuli. Donchin and his colleagues made use of the P300 to develop a communication system. This BCI is based on the presentation of a 6*6 letter matrix in which, in short intervals (125 ms), one of the rows or one of the columns flashes. The user's focusation to a

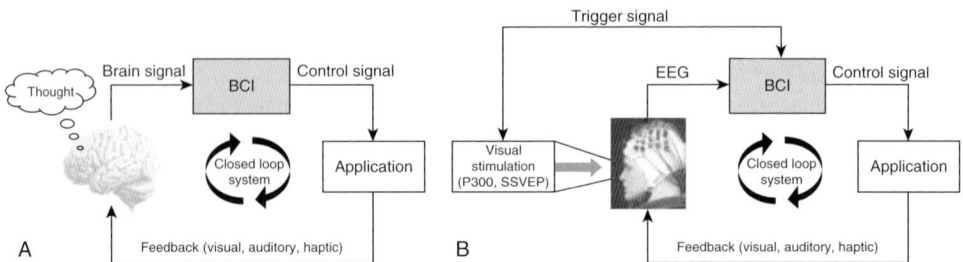

Fig. 14.1 A. Principal schemes of BCIs operated with motor imagery. B. visual- or gaze-directed attention to visual stimulation. See colour plate section.

certain item produces larger P300 amplitude for the desired letter compared to the other possible choices. With this system, a communication rate of approximately seven items per minute can be obtained (Donchin *et al.* 2000). An advantage is that the training time is relatively short allowing much faster selection of letters than any other BCI system. Another interesting application of the P300-BCI is the control of a robot (Bell *et al.* 2008).

The SCP-BCI

Beginning in 1979, Birbaumer and coworkers published a series of experiments demonstrating operant control of SCPs (see Birbaumer *et al.* 1990 for review). Operant conditioning is a learning process with the goal of the self-regulation of brain potentials (e.g., SCP shifts) or brain waves (e.g., sensorimotor rhythms) with the help of suitable feedback. This process does not require continuous feedback, but a reward for achieving the desired brain potential (wave) change is necessary. Operant conditioning was used to realize a communication system for completely paralysed (locked-in) patients (Birbaumer *et al.* 1999).

The SSVEP-BCI

Steady-state evoked potentials (SSEP) occur when sensory stimuli are repetitively delivered at high enough rates so that the relevant neuronal structures are prevented to return to their resting states. Ideally, the discrete frequency components remain constant in amplitude and phase within an infinitely long time period. They have the same fundamental frequency as the frequency of the stimulus, but often they also include higher and/or sub-harmonic frequencies.

In a BCI application, the user gazes at one of several lights whereby each flickers at a different rate. The gaze-directed flickering light evokes SSVEP over the visual cortex that can be detected and used for control. Multiple flickering lights are necessary to enable higher dimensional discrimination. Cheng *et al.* (2002) described a BCI with 13 flickering lights and a high information transfer rate of 27 bits per minutes. Recently, Müller-Putz and Pfurtscheller (2008) reported on the control of an electrical prosthesis with an SSVEP-BCI.

The ERD-BCI

Sensorimotor rhythms can either display an event-related amplitude decrease or ERD or an event-related amplitude increase or ERS (Pfurtscheller and Lopes da Silva 1999). A localized ERD can be viewed as an electrophysiological correlate of an activated cortical network. On the opposite, a localized ERS in the alpha band can be seen, at least under certain circumstances, as a correlate of a deactivated or even inhibited cortical network and would correspond to a disengaged or de-activated state.

The term ERD-BCI describes all different types of BCIs, analysing and classifying the dynamics (ERD, ERS) of either one single frequency component (e.g., mu-rhythm-based BCI, Wolpaw *et al.* 2002; beta-rhythm-based BCI, Bai *et al.* 2008) or 2 or more components of sensorimotor rhythms (Pfurtscheller *et al.* 2006b; Blankertz *et al.* 2007; Scherer 2008). Also, the sensorimotor rhythm BCI of Birbaumer (Birbaumer and Cohen 2007) uses the mentally induced increase (ERS) and/or decrease (ERD) of sensorimotor rhythms to control a hand orthosis.

One of the first papers reporting on on-line classification of different motor imagery induced ERD/ERS patterns was published by Pfurtscheller *et al.* (1993). At this time, beside others, the Wadsworth BCI (Wolpaw *et al.* 2002), the Berlin BCI (Blankertz *et al.* 2007), the Graz BCI (Pfurtscheller *et al.* 2006a), and variants of the Tübingen BCI (Birbaumer and Cohen 2007) used the ERD/S as features for single trial EEG classification. The bit-rates reported are between around 3 and up to 35 bits per minutes (Krausz *et al.* 2003; Blankertz *et al.* 2007). It has to be noted that the ERD-BCI can operate in two different modes: either cue-based in a synchronous mode or self-paced (at free will) in an asynchronous mode with continuous data processing.

Motor imagery as mental strategy

Motor imagery is a conscious mental process defined as mental simulation of a specific movement. According to the present view, motor imagery is based on similar activation/deactivation processes to those that are involved in programming and preparing actual actions (Jeannerod 2001). The main difference between action execution and imagination of the same action is that in the latter case, the motor output would be blocked at some cortico-spinal level. For further elaboration and discussion of the inhibition of the motor command during imagined actions see Chapters 4 and 6.

Summarizing, motor imagery can induce the following different EEG changes that can be utilized for BCI control (see also Chapter 5):

1 Desynchronization (ERD) of sensorimotor rhythms (mu and central beta oscillations) during motor imagery (Pfurtscheller *et al.* 1997)

2 Synchronization (ERS) of mu and beta oscillations in non-attended cortical body-part areas during motor imagery (Pfurtscheller *et al.* 2006b)

3 Synchronization of beta oscillations in attended body-part areas during motor imagery (Pfurtscheller *et al.* 2000)

4 Short-lasting beta oscillations after termination of motor imagery (Pfurtscheller *et al.* 2005)

For the control of an external device based on single-trial classification of brain signals, it is essential that motor imagery related brain activity can be detected in ongoing EEG and classified in real-time. Even though it has been documented that the imagination of simple body-part movements elicits predictable temporally stable changes in the sensorimotor rhythms with a small intra-subject variability (Pfurtscheller *et al.* 2006b), there are also participants who do not show the expected imagination-related EEG changes. Moreover, a diversity of time-frequency patterns (i.e., high inter-subject variability), especially with respect to the reactive frequency components, is found when studying the dynamics of oscillatory activity during movement imagination (see, e.g., Neuper *et al.* 2005). Therefore, motor imagery based SMR-BCIs have to cope with a high inter-subject variability as well as with changes in the individual's brain processes between successive experimental sessions (e.g., due to feedback, fatigue, change of task involvement; cf. Pfurtscheller and Neuper 2001; Wang *et al.* 2004; Shenoy *et al.* 2006; Blankertz *et al.* 2007). Though little is known about the neurophysiological or psychological causes of this variability, there is some evidence that the observed individual differences in imagination-related EEG changes may be explained by varieties of the cognitive processes involved in motor imagery. For example, different ERD/ERS patterns can be expected with different types of motor imagery, involving either a visual-motor or kinaesthetic experience (Neuper *et al.* 2005). In general, an amplitude increase in the EEG activity in form of an ERS can be easier and more accurately detected in single trials than an amplitude decrease (ERD).

Self-paced and cue-based BCI systems

The mode of operation determines the type of data processing, either in a predefined time window of some seconds following a cue stimulus (synchronous or cue-based BCI) or continuously sample-by-sample (asynchronous or self-paced BCI). The cue contains either information for the users (e.g., indication for left- or right-hand motor imagery during training) or is neutral. In the latter case, the users are free to choose one of the predefined mental tasks after the cue. However, using a synchronous BCI system, control commands come only into operation within the cue-based processing window. In the asynchronous mode no cue is necessary, hence the system is continuously available to the users for control so they can decide at free will when they wish to generate a control signal. Such a system is more complex and demanding. The great challenge is to maximize the intentional control (true positives), while simultaneously minimizing the non-intentional control (false positives) at the output. Such an asynchronous BCI was used successfully to operate a spelling device and to navigate in a virtual environment (Millán and Mouriño 2003; Scherer *et al.* 2004; Müller and Blankhertz 2006).

How training and feedback is organized

Before a BCI can be used successfully, the user has to perform a number of training sessions with the goal of obtaining control over his/her brain waves and maximizing the classification accuracy of different brain states, respectively. In general, the training starts with one or two predefined mental tasks repeated periodically in a cue-based mode. In predefined time windows after the cue, the brain signals are recorded and used for off-line analyses. In this way, the computer 'learns' to recognize the mental task-related brain patterns of the users. This process of learning is highly subject-specific and requires that each user must undergo a training process. This learning phase produces a classifier which may be used to classify the brain patterns on-line and suitable feedback can be provided to the users.

Feedback about performance is typically provided by both (i) a continuous feedback signal (e.g., cursor movement) and (ii) the outcome of the trial (i.e., discrete feedback about success or failure). It is important to note, that the operation of an ERD-BCI in trained subjects is not dependent on the sensory input provided by the feedback signal. For example, McFarland *et al.* (1998) reported that well-trained subjects still displayed EEG control when feedback (cursor movement) was removed for some periods of time. In general, when a naïve user starts to practice hand motor imagery, a contralaterally dominant desynchronization pattern is found. In the course of a number of training sessions, in which he or she receives feedback about the performed mental task, changes of the relevant EEG patterns can be expected (Neuper *et al.* 1999, 2008).

Evidence has accumulated that visual feedback has an especially high impact on the dynamics of brain oscillations and can not only facilitate, but – under certain circumstances – also deteriorate the learning process. A recent study demonstrates that visual BCI feedback clearly modulates sensorimotor EEG rhythms. In contrast to a sole motor imagery task, motor imagery and simultaneous processing of visual feedback increased ERD over sensorimotor areas, i.e., significant larger and more widespread ERD was found during on-line BCI operation (with visual feedback) compared to motor imagery without feedback (Neuper *et al.* 2008). The training phase is relatively short with SSVEP-BCIs or P300-BCIs, but can last weeks or even months with ERD-BCIs.

Frequency band and electrode selection

Developing SMR-BCIs for home application and for use in every-day life, the system must be robust, light-weighted, wireless, and simple to use. The latter means the system should consist of preferably only one or two EEG channels. To achieve this it is of interest to compare the classification results of multichannel (full-head) EEG studies where either all channels are considered compared to the use of only one or two EEG channels. The standard method for processing multichannel data and discrimination between two brain states is the common spatial pattern (CSP) algorithm (Müller-Gerking *et al.* 1999). Using the CSP algorithm applied to 30-channel

EEG of 10 naïve subjects, Scherer (2008) reported a classification accuracy of 88.8% ±5.5 for discrimination between hand and foot MI. In the case of only 1 subject-specific Laplacian EEG derivation, the corresponding accuracy was 81.4%±8.7. This is surprising, that with one channel only such superior classification accuracy can be achieved. The prerequisite is that features such as electrode locations and frequency bands have to be carefully selected and optimized (Pregenzer *et al.* 1996). Similarly, Blankertz *et al.* (2008) reported a classification accuracy of about 80% for the discrimination between right hand and foot MI with a 55-electrode EEG montage. With two individually-selected bipolar EEG channels the classification accuracy was about 10% lower.

Some BCI application

An EEG-based BCI can be used to control spelling systems or neuroprosthesis in severely para-lysed patients but also to optimize the feedback therapy with the goal to reduce epileptic seizures to treat attentional deficit disorders or to restore movement in chronic stroke (see e.g., Birbaumer and Cohen 2007). Able-bodied subjects can control computer games, multimedia applications, and others (Nijholt and Tan 2007). Another application is the use of the EEG activity pattern as biometric measure and the EEG-based BCI for person identification and user authentication ('pass thought'; Pfurtscheller and Neuper 2006; Marcel and Milan 2007). Three applications are explained in more detail:

1. Control of spelling systems in severely paralyzed patients

Completely paralyzed patients without any conscious control of muscle activity can communi-cate with their environment when, through the use of a BCI, an electronic spelling device is con-trolled. Spelling systems are communication aids which allow users to express themselves by selecting letters or items of an alphabet and thus form words and sentences. The simplest case is to use a binary control signal requiring two distinctive mental activities. Patients suffering from amyotrophic lateral sclerosis (ALS) can learn to control their own SPCs (SCP-BCI) and so to operate the Thought Translation Device, a spelling device (Birbaumer *et al.* 1999; Kübler *et al.* 1999). By using the same dichotomous selection strategy, an ALS patient and a patient suffering from severe cerebral palsy (Neuper *et al.* 2003) learned to operate the virtual keyboard spelling application (Obermaier *et al.* 2003). This spelling device is based on the detection and classifica-tion of motor imagery related EEG patterns. This means that the patient uses the imagination of specific movements (e.g., left-hand versus right-hand movement) to indicate the position of the desired letter on a computer monitor (e.g., left versus right half of the screen). The spelling rates in these studies varied from 0.15 to approximately 1.0 letter per minute. An example for such a spelling system with an ERD-BCI is displayed in Figure 14.2B. The Wadsworth speller, based on mu and beta activity (ERD-BCI), for example, divides the alphabet into four parts (Wolpaw *et al.* 2003). In Millán and Mouriño (2003), an average spelling rate of about 3.0 letters per minute was reported by using a 3-class BCI. A novel spelling concept, possible due to the asynchronous pro-tocol, was introduced in Scherer *et al.* (2004). Another efficient selection strategy was introduced recently in Müller and Blankertz (2006). The Hex-O-Spell application combines asynchronous 2-class ERD-BCI control and divides the alphabet into six parts. This raised the average spelling rate up to about 6.0 letters per minute.

2. Control of neuroprosthesis to restore grasp function

The development of BCI systems grounded on the idea to bypass interrupted motor pathways and, therewith, allow restoration of movement in paralysed patients. Systems for functional electrical stimulation (FES) – so-called neuroprostheses – are able to restore lost control/motor

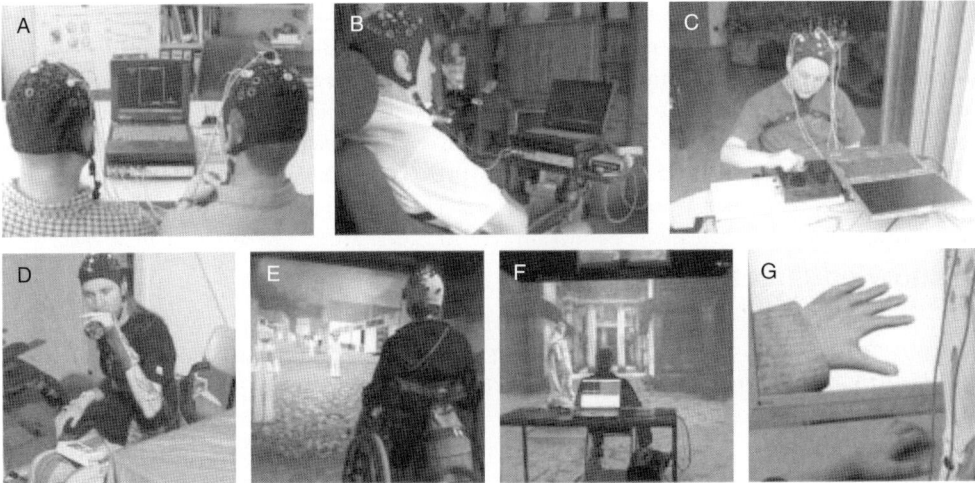

Fig. 14.2 A Two students playing table tennis; B. ALS patient operating a spelling system at home; C. thought-based control of a neuroprosthesis through implanted functional electrical stimulation (FES) of hand muscles; D. thought-based control of a neuroprosthesis through FES of hand muscles using surface electrodes; E. 'wheel chair movement' in a virtual environment; F. navigation through thought in a virtual library; G. and opening/closing of a virtual hand through hand motor imagery. See colour plate section.

functions of body parts after spinal cord injury (SCI) with the use of electrical impulses. By combining such a neuroprosthesis with a BCI system the operation of the prosthetic device can be triggered by the detection of the user's motor intents or movement imaginations. The control signal generated by the BCI switches the FES on/off. Pfurtscheller *et al.* (2000) reported a first attempt on EEG-based control systems to restore the hand grasping function in a tetraplegic patient by using an electrically driven hand orthosis. Later on, in the same patient, the control of hand grasp was realized by FES controlled through foot motor imagery (Figure 14.2D; Müller-Putz *et al.* 2005). An implantable neuroprostheses, known as the Freehand™ system (Keith *et al.* 1989), was coupled with an ERD-BCI and used in a tetraplegic male patient to perform a grasp sequence (Müller-Putz *et al.* 2005).

3. Control of virtual reality

Virtual reality (VR) provides an excellent training and testing environment for rehearsal of scenarios or events that are otherwise too dangerous or costly – or even currently impossible in physical reality. Such an event is, for example, the control of wheel chair movement through brain waves. In this case the output signal of the ERD-BCI is used to control not the wheel chair movement itself but the movement of the immersive virtual environment (Figure 14.2E), and simulates therewith the real wheel chair movement as realistically as possible (Leeb *et al.* 2007; Pfurtscheller *et al.* 2008). By this way, the thought-based wheel chair control can be optimized and validated.

Future prospects

The BCI technology is a relative new, fast growing field of research and applications with the potential to improve the quality of life in severely disabled people. Before a BCI can be used for communication and control at home several problems have to be solved. So, for example, it is of importance to automatically select electrode locations and frequency components in a motor imagery task, use the fewest number of recording electrodes and channels, respectively (the optimum is one EEG channel), minimize the training time through game-like feedback, to automatically detect artefacts, to perform output response verification, and to establish protocols for the easy BCI set-up and use. Of importance could be also the simultaneous analyses of other physiological signals as the heart rate (hybrid BCI) and the monitoring of the brain state to avoid fatigue.

Acknowledgements

The authors of BCI research has been supported by EU projects PRESENCIA (IST-2001-37927) and PRESENCCIA (IST-2006-27731), the Lorenz-Böhler Foundation, the 'Allgemeine Unfallversicherungsanstalt (AUVA)', and the WINGS for Life Spinal Cord Research Foundation.

References

Bai, O., Lin, P., Vorbach, S., Floeter, M.K., Hattori, N., and Hallett, M. (2008). A high performance sensorimotor beta rhythm-based brain–computer interface associated with human natural motor behavior. *Journal of Neural Engineering*, **5**, 24–35.

Bell, C. J., Shenoy, P., Chalodhorn, R., and Rao, R.P.N. (2008). Control of a humanoid robot by a non-invasive brain–computer interface in humans. *Journal of Neural Engineering*, **5**, 214–20.

Birbaumer, N., Elbert, T., Canavan, A.G., and Rockstroh, B. (1990). Slow potentials of the cerebral cortex and behavior. *Physiological Reviews*, **70**, 1–41.

Birbaumer, N., Ghanayim, N., Hinterberger, T., *et al.* (1999). A spelling device for the paralysed. *Nature*, **398**, 297–98.

Birbaumer, N., and Cohen, L.G. (2007). Brain–computer interfaces: communication and restoration of movement in paralysis. *The Journal of Physiology*, **579**, 621–36.

Blankertz, B., Dornhege, G., Krauledat, M., Müller, K.R., and Curio, G. (2007). The non-invasive Berlin Brain–Computer Interface: fast acquisition of effective performance in untrained subjects. *NeuroImage*, **37**, 539–50.

Blankertz, B., Losch, F., Krauledat, M., Dornhege, G., Curio, G., and Müller, K. R. (2008). The Berlin-Brain–Computer Interface: accurate performance from first-sessions in BCI-naive subjects. *IEEE Transactions on Biomedical Engineering*, **55**, 2452–62.

Cheng, M., Gao, X., Gao, S., and Xu, D. (2002). Design and implementation of a brain–computer interface with high transfer rates. *IEEE Transactions on Neural Systems and Rehabilitation Engineering*, **49**, 1181–6.

Cincotti, F., Mattia, D., Babiloni, C., et al. (2003). The use of EEG modifications due to motor imagery for brain–computer interfaces. *IEEE Transactions on Rehabilitation Engineering*, **11**, 131–3.

Coyle, S., Ward, T., Markham, C., and McDarby, G. (2004). On the suitability of near-infrared (NIR) systems for next-generation brain–computer interfaces. *Physiological Measurement*, **25**, 815–22.

Donchin, E., Spencer, K.M., and Wijesinghe, R. (2000). The mental prosthesis: assessing the speed of a P300-based brain–computer interface. *IEEE Transactions on Rehabilitation Engineering*, **8**, 174–9.

Hochberg, L.R., Serruya M.D., Friehs, G.M., *et al.* (2006). Neural ensemble control of prosthetic devices by a human with tetraplegia. *Nature*, **442**, 164–71.

Jeannerod, M. (2001). Neural simulation of action: a unifying mechanism for motor cognition. *NeuroImage*, **13**, 103–9.

Kauhanen, L., Nykopp, T., Lehtonen, J., *et al.* (2006). EEG and MEG brain–computer interface for tetraplegic patients. *IEEE Transactions on Neural Systems and Rehabilitation Engineering*, **14**, 190–3.

Keith, M.W., Peckham, P.H., Thrope, G.B., *et al.* (1989). Implantable functional neuromuscular stimulation in the tetraplegic hand. *The Journal of Hand Surgery*, **14**, 524–30.

Krausz, G., Scherer, R., Korisek, G., and Pfurtscheller, G. (2003). Critical decision-speed and information transfer in the 'Graz Brain–Computer Interface'. *Applied Psychophysiology and Biofeedback*, **28**, 233–40.

Kübler, A., Kotchoubey, B., Hinterberger, T., *et al.* (1999). The thought translation device: a neurophysiological approach to communication in total motor paralysis. *Experimental Brain Research*, **124**, 223–32.

Leeb, R., Friedman, D., Müller-Putz, G.R., Scherer, R., Slater, M., and Pfurtscheller, G. (2007). Self-paced (asynchronous) BCI control of a wheelchair in virtual environments: a case study with a tetraplegics. *Computational Intelligence and Neuroscience*, **2007**, Article ID 79642.

Leuthard, E.C., Miller, K. J., Schalk, G., Rao, R.P., and Ojemann, J.G. (2006). Electrocorticography-based brain interface – the Seattle experience *IEEE Transactions on Neural Systems and Rehabilitation Engineering*, **14**, 194–8.

Marcel, S. and Millan, J. (2007), Person authentication using brainwaves (EEG) and maximum a posteriori model adaption. *IEEE Transactions on Pattern Analysis and Machine Intelligence*, **29**, 743–8.

McFarland, D.J., McCane, L.M., and Wolpaw, J.R. (1998). EEG-based communication and control: short-term role of feedback. *IEEE Transactions on Rehabilitation Engineering*, **6**, 7–11.

Mellinger, J., Schalk, G., Braun, C., *et al.* (2007). An MEG-based brain–computer interface (BCI). *NeuroImage*, **36**, 581–93.

Millán, J. and Mouriño, J. (2003). Asynchronous BCI and local neural classifiers: an overview of the Adaptive Brain Interface project. *IEEE Transactions on Neural Systems and Rehabilitation Engineering*, **11**, 159–61.

Müller, K.R. and Blankertz, B. (2006). Toward noninvasive brain computer interfaces. *Signal Processing Magazine*, **23**, 125–8.

Müller-Gerking, J., Pfurtscheller, G., and Flyvbjerg, H. (1999). Designing optimal spatial filters for single-trial EEG classification in a movement task. *Clinical Neurophysiology*, **110**, 787–98.

Müller-Putz, G.R., Scherer, R., Pfurtscheller, G., and Rupp, R. (2005). EEG-based neuroprosthesis control: a step into clinical practice. *Neuroscience Letters*, **382**, 169–74.

Müller-Putz, G. and Pfurtscheller, G. (2008). Control of an electrical prosthesis with an SSVEP-based BCI. *IEEE Transactions on Biomedical Engineering*, **55**, 361–4.

Neuper, C., Schlögl, A., and Pfurtscheller, G. (1999). Enhancement of left–right sensorimotor EEG differences during feedback-regulated motor imagery. *Journal of Clinical Neurophysiology*, **16**, 373–82.

Neuper, C., Müller, G.R., Kübler, A., Birbaumer, N., and Pfurtscheller, G. (2003). Clinical application of an EEG-based brain–computer interface: a case study in a patient with severe motor impairment. *Clinical Neurophysiology*, **114**, 399–409

Neuper, C., Scherer, R., Reiner, M., and Pfurtscheller, G. (2005). Imagery of motor actions: differential effects of kinesthetic and visual-motor mode of imagery in single-trial EEG. *Brain Research. Cognitive Brain Research*, **25**, 668–77.

Neuper, C., Mueller-Putz, G.R., Scherer, R., and Pfurtscheller G. (2006). Motor imagery and EEG-based control of spelling devices and neuroprostheses. *Progress in Brain Research*, **159**, 393–409.

Neuper, C., Scherer, R., Wriessnegger, S.C., and Pfurtscheller, G. (2009). Motor imagery and action observation: modulation of sensorimotor brain rhythms during mental control of a brain–computer interface. *Clinical Neurophysiology*, **120**, 239–47.

Nijholt, A. and Tan, D. (2007). Playing with your brain: Brain–Computer Interfaces and Games. Workshop at ACE 2007, June 13–15, Salzburg, Austria.

Obermaier, B., Müller, G.R., and Pfurtscheller, G. (2003). 'Virtual keyboard' controlled by spontaneous EEG activity. *IEEE Transactions on Neural Systems and Rehabilitation Engineering*, **11**, 422–6.

Pfurtscheller, G., Kalcher, J., and Flotzinger, D. (1993) A new communication device for handicapped persons. The brain–computer interface, in E. Ballabion, I. Placencia-Porrero, and R. Puig de la Bellacasa (eds) *Rehabilitation Technology*. Vol. **9**. pp. 123–27. Amsterdam: IOS Press.

Pfurtscheller, G. and Neuper, C. (1997). Motor imagery activates primary sensorimotor area in humans. *Neuroscience Letters*, **239**, 65–8.

Pfurtscheller, G. and Neuper C. (2001). Motor imagery and direct brain–computer communication, *Proceedings of the IEEE (Special Issue); Neural Engineering: Merging Engineering and Neuroscience*, **89**, 1123–34.

Pfurtscheller, G., Neuper, C., Flotzinger, D., and Pregenzer, M. (1997). EEG-based discrimination between imagination of right and left hand movement. *Electroencephalography and Clinical Neurophysiology*, **103**, 642–51.

Pfurtscheller, G. and Lopes da Silva, F.H. (1999). Event-related EEG/MEG synchronization and desynchronization: basic principles. *Clinical Neurophysiology*, **110**, 1842–57.

Pfurtscheller, G., Guger, C., Müller, G., Krausz, G., and Neuper, C. (2000). Brain oscillations control hand orthosis in a tetraplegic. *Neuroscience Letters*, **292**, 211–4.

Pfurtscheller, G., Leeb, R., Friedman, D., and Slater, M. (2008). Centrally controlled heart rate changes during mental practice in immersive virtual environment: a case study with a tetraplegic. *International Journal of Psychophysiology*, **68**, 1–5.

Pfurtscheller, G., Neuper, C., Brunner, C., and Lopes da Silva, F.H. (2005). Beta rebound after different types of motor imagery in man. *Neuroscience Letters*, **378**, 156–9.

Pfurtscheller, G., Brunner, C., Schlögl, A., and Lopes da Silva, F. H. (2006b). Mu rhythm (de) synchronization and EEG single-trial classification of different motor imagery tasks. *NeuroImage*, **31**, 153–9.

Pfurtscheller, G., Müller-Putz, G.R., and Schlögl, A., *et al.* (2006a). 15 years of BCI research at Graz University of Technology: current projects. *IEEE Transactions on Neural Systems and Rehabilitation Engineering*, **14**, 205–10.

Pfurtscheller, G. and Neuper, C. (2006) Future prospects of ERD/ERS in the context of brain–computer interface (BCI) developements, in C. Neuper and W. Klimesch (eds), *Event-Related Dynamics of Brain Oscillations*. Progress in Brain Research. Vol. **159**. pp. 19–27. Amsterdam: Elsevier.

Pregenzer, M., Pfurtscheller, G., and Flotzinger, D. (1996). Automated feature selection with a distinction sensitive learning vector quantizer. *Neurocomputing*, **11**, 19–29.

Scherer, R., Müller, G.R., Neuper, C., Graimann, B., and Pfurtscheller, G. (2004). An asynchronously controlled EEG-based virtual keyboard: improvement of the spelling rate. *IEEE Transactions on Biomedical Engineering*, **51**, 979–84.

Scherer, R. (2008). Towards practical Brain–Computer Interfaces: Self-paced operation and reduction of the number of EEG sensors. PhD Thesis. Graz: Graz University of Technology.

Shenoy, P., Krauledat, M., Blankertz, B., Rao, R. P. N., and Müller, K. R. (2006). Towards adaptive classification for BCI. *Journal of Neural Engineering*, **3**, R13–R23.

Wang, T., Deng, H., and He, B. (2004). Classifying EEG-based motor imagery tasks by means of time-frequency synthesized spatial patterns. *Clinical Neurophysiology*, **115(12)**, 2744–53.

Weiskopf, N., Mathiak, K., Bock, S.W., *et al.* (2004). Principles of a brain–computer interface (BCI) based on real-time functional magnetic resonance imaging (fMRI). *IEEE Transactions on Biomedical Engineering*, **51**, 966–70.

Wolpaw, J.R., Birbaumer, N., McFarland, D.J., Pfurtscheller, G., and Vaughan, T. M. (2002). Brain–computer interfaces for communication and control. *Clinical Neurophysiology*, **113**, 767–91.

Wolpaw, J.R., McFarland, D.J., Vaughan, T.M., and Schalk, G. (2003). The Wadsworth Center brain–computer interface (BCI) research and development program. *IEEE Transactions on Neural Systems and Rehabilitation Engineering*, **11**, 204–07.

Motor imagery in learning processes

Chapter 15

Motor imagery and motor performance: Evidence from the sport science literature

Aymeric Guillot, Ursula Debarnot, Magali Louis, Nady Hoyek, and Christian Collet

Mental imagery is the general ability of representing different types of images, even when the original stimulus is out of sight. In other words, mental imagery is like perceiving, but in the absence of the appropriate external stimulus, and can occur in any sense mode (Kosslyn *et al.* 1990). The process of imagining motor execution forms is known as motor imagery, requiring the mental representation of an overt action without any concomitant movement (Jeannerod 1994). A wide range of idiomatic ways of referring to these specific cognitive processes exists, albeit they do not provide substantial additional details regarding the intrinsic nature of the mental representation (for extensive reviews, see Morris *et al.* 2005; Cumming and Ramsey 2008). There has been a great deal of research on imagery processes for well over a century (Kosslyn *et al.* 2006), and there is now compelling evidence that motor imagery substantially contributes to improve motor learning and motor performance (Feltz and Landers 1983; Driskell *et al.* 1994; Cumming and Ramsey 2008; Guillot and Collet 2008), and can further be used as a therapeutic tool to improve motor recovery during rehabilitation (e.g. Butler and Page 2006; Zimmerman *et al.* 2008; see also Section 3 of this book).

The aim of the present chapter is to examine the use of imagery in sport, to provide an overview the specific imagery effects that may be achieved by the athletes, as well as to contribute to better understanding the potential additional benefits brought by motor imagery as compared to actual motor performance, more especially by considering the degree of similarity between these two processes. From such viewpoint, we should underline how to make additional theoretical progress within the scope of using motor imagery.

Imagery modalities and perspectives

This is now well-established that imagery is a multi-sensory construct based on different sensory modalities. In light of this assumption, and despite the organization of the central nervous system, integrating primary information from each sensorial system into parallel pathways combining cues from different sources, it is possible to focus on a specific imagery modality or perspective, in regards to the situation in which imagery is performed. This latter ability has been supported by recent neuroimaging experiments (Ruby and Decety 2001; Solodkin *et al.* 2004; Jackson *et al.* 2006; Guillot *et al.* 2009; Lorey *et al.* 2009). It also remains possible for imagers to combine the different forms of imagery. Hence, imagers can selectively perform visual, kinaesthetic, auditory, tactile, olfactory, and gustatory imagery, as well as some other declinations including healing and pain imagery, body-related, metaphorical and anatomical imagery, or even spatial imagery and mental rotation. Diary imagery studies showed that about two-thirds of our mental images are visual in nature, which may explain the lack of research on the other imagery modalities (Kosslyn *et al.* 1990; Moran 2002). When considering the sport imagery literature *per se*, the vast majority of the experimental investigations dealing with the motor imagery experience have primarily focused on visual and kinaesthetic imagery. The former can still be divided into two different sub-modalities. In the first-person perspective, performers visualize the action as how they would experience it happen in the real-life situation, while in the third-person perspective, they imagine, as spectators, the action that somebody (themselves or another person) is performing. As well, kinaesthetic imagery involves the sensations of how it feels to perform an action, including the force and effort perceived during movement and balance (Callow and Waters 2005), hence suggesting to consider the body as a generator of forces (Jeannerod 1994).

Early, researchers have been interested in evaluating the selective effectiveness of the imagery modalities and perspectives. The respective efficiency of each modality and perspective may depend on the nature of the task being imagined (Driskell *et al.* 1994; Morris *et al.* 2005). Feltz and Landers (1983) reported earlier that the increase in performance would be greater for tasks with strong cognitive components, requiring fine visuo-motor adjustments than for motor tasks. The imagery research also suggests that imagery is frequently used and very effective in 'bio-informational' motor skills. For example, shooters and archers often use motor imagery during training, as well as just before pulling the trigger during the concentration phase, the quality of the mental images being highly detrimental to their subsequent performance (Deschaumes-Molinaro *et al.* 1991, 1992; Guillot *et al.* 2004a). On the other hand, imagery would be less common in 'energetic' sporting activities, but might rather depend on individual characteristics. For instance, Bolliet *et al.* (2003) reported that shot putters do not practice visualization right before a throw when competing, while weightlifters often mentally rehearse a technical difficulty during the concentration phase (Collet *et al.* 2000). Furthermore, and even though some researchers disagreed with this assumption (Isaac and Marks 1994), another way of comparison can be drawn with regard to the effectiveness of different types and perspectives of motor imagery in closed versus open skills. Historically, Poulton (1957) suggested a classification system for motor skills which was based on environment uncertainty in which the skill was performed. When the environment is stable, i.e. predictable, the skill is classified as closed. If, on the other hand, the skill involves an ever-changing, unpredictable environment, the skill is open. While in closed skills it is critical that the performer reliably produces the standardized pattern, the outcome of the movement is what must be effectively produced and a standardized motor pattern is rarely of assistance in open skills. Some researchers did not find any significant effect on performance based on imagery perspective both in closed and open skills, even if some individual preferences were reported in the use of visual perspectives (e.g. Epstein 1980; Spittle and Morris 2000; Boron 2002). Highlen and Bennett (1979), however, argued that it might be easier using imagery in closed skills as performers can imagine in their own time without the distraction of an opponent and without taking into account the probability of unexpected events. White and Hardy (1995) further reported that external visual imagery is more effective on motor skills that depend heavily on form for their successful execution. Accordingly, the athlete can easily visualize the global positions and movements that are required for successful performance. Hardy and Callow (1999) later suggested that internal imagery is more effective in closed skills, while external imagery improves performance of open skills. Hardy (1997) further argued that kinaesthetic imagery is more effective that either external or internal visual imagery, as it enables the athlete to match the feel of movements and its timing. Even if some researchers agree with this hypothesis, this latter argument related to timing has been challenged by some mental chronometry data (see Guillot and Collet 2005a). Hardy and Callow (1999) also confirmed that external visual imagery is more effective than internal visual imagery on form-based tasks. Their results finally offered some support to the hypothesis stating that, regardless of the visual imagery perspective, kinaesthetic imagery contributes an additional beneficial effect to performance once athletes have acquired a certain degree of physical expertise. More recently, Cohelo *et al.* (2007) suggested that imaging a positive outcome may be more powerful in improving performance of closed skill movements than of open skill movements.

In another study dealing with this research area, Guillot *et al.* (2004b) investigated whether gymnasts, who often control movements through somesthetic cues, and tennis players, who are mainly dependent on the visual information from the environment, might benefit to a great extent from kinaesthetic and visual imagery, respectively. Their results, however, were not quite so clear, as individual characteristics were found to be combined with the characteristics of the motor tasks. Consequently, explaining how each type of imagery was more or less effective remained unclear. The lack of superiority of a given type of imagery has also been reported in the recent study by Taktek *et al.* (2008) in a closed motor skill, whereas Farahat *et al.* (2004) found that each type of imagery had differential effects for learning to produce a graphic task using a stylus, visual imagery being superior during the retention phase, but not at the end of learning. Taken together, and although many directions have to be considered with regard to the results mentioned above, it seems premature to draw final conclusions regarding the comparative effects of the different types and perspectives of imagery. In particular, one additional factor which should be considered is the intrinsic characteristics of each individual – some people being more sensitive to visual information, while others are more likely to process somaesthetic information. This may be summarized with reference to the field dependence/independence (Witkin, 1950). In other words, more research is needed to better understand the influence of both imagery types and imagery perspectives on sport skills performance (Morris *et al.* 2005).

The degree of similarity between motor imagery and motor performance

The analytic framework for imagery effects by Paivio (1985) early suggested that motor imagery might serve both cognitive and motivational functions operating on general and specific levels. In this theory, the motivational components refer to the use of goal-oriented responses and the management of arousal level, while the cognitive components tap into skill improvement and refer to the imagery of game strategies. Especially, the cognitive functions involve the rehearsal of skills (cognitive-specific imagery) and strategies of play (cognitive general imagery). The motivational-specific imagery involves imagining outcomes and how to achieve these goals, while the motivational-general imagery relates to physiological arousal. Hall *et al.* (1998) further subdivided the motivational-general imagery into two sub-components (motivational-general arousal and motivational-general mastery). Research examining this issue often revealed that athletes primarily used imagery for motivational purposes. Even though such classification shows several obvious strengths, however, it has been criticized for its imprecision (Abma *et al.* 2002). In a recent meta-analysis, MacIntyre and Moran (2007) also provided evidence that the motivational functions of imagery were usually overstated, and that cognitive imagery emerged consistently in athletes' self-reports. Basically, other authors argued that a given mental image could serve either one or several distinct functions (e.g. Short *et al.* 2002; Murphy *et al.* 2008 for review).

Based on these data, an important number of imagery models and guidelines have been developed over the past decade with the aim to depict in greater details why, when, where, and how athletes should use imagery, as well as what is the imagery content. In a first model, Munroe *et al.* (2000) examined the four Ws of imagery: *what, where, why* and *when*. This qualitative approach

...a six-stage model describes how athletes may integrate imagery in sport in an effective ...ere distinguishes training from competition, whereas *when* separates the use of imagery ...g sporting activity from outside practice, as well as before, during, and after competing. ...refers to the use of cognitive and/or motivational functions, and *what* athletes should imag-...ne (length and frequency, effectiveness, nature, surrounding, and controllability of imagery) is the next stage. Finally, the last two levels include some other key-components such as the imagery type (e.g. visual, kinaesthetic, auditory), the imagery perspective (external or internal visual imagery), or the use of positive/facilitative and negative/debilitative mental images. As far as the sporting situation is concerned, this complete and robust model frequently serves as a guide for the development of applied imagery interventions during training sessions and contest. The major strength is that an important number of key-components of imagery use emerged from the questionnaires collected by the authors in elaborating their framework, even if they do not consider the specificity of each key-component with regards to the athletes' outcomes, as well as the therapeutic use of imagery in recovering motor functions during the rehabilitation process.

Later, the well-known PETTLEP model was proposed by Holmes and Collins (2001). The model includes seven elements (physical, environment, task, timing, learning, emotion, and perspective) derived from neuroscientific and behavioural equivalences between motor imagery and motor performance (see also Chapter 18). Although the model is not intended to be exclusive, its conceptual validity is strong and well documented (e.g. Callow *et al.* 2006; Smith *et al.* 2007). *Physical* relates to the physical nature of imagery (i.e. increased arousal or being relaxed), while *Environment* refers to the use of stimulus materials that mimic motor performance. *Timing* relates to the importance of imagining in real-time, i.e. similar imagined and actual times. *Task* includes the nature of imagery to be performed, the expertise level, and the imagery perspective. *Learning* relates to the use of imagery in the acquisition of new motor skills and for the correction of the technical aspects of the movement. *Emotion* refers to the individual integration of emotional components in mental images. Finally, *Perspective* provides guidance for the use of a given visual imagery perspective depending on the situation. The authors also highlight the major interactions among these components. The PETTLEP model covers a large and important aspect of imagery use, but the therapeutic effects of MI in the rehabilitation process are once again not directly considered.

More recently, Guillot and Collet (2008) proposed the motor imagery integrative model in sport (MIIMS), which should be considered a global guiding framework for motor imagery studies and experimentation, to develop more effective imagery interventions. By examining the impressive number of studies designed to investigate motor imagery, as well as the empirical applications implemented by the coaches, the authors finally considered four distinct imagery outcomes: (i) motor learning and performance, (ii) motivation, self-confidence, and anxiety, (iii) strategies and problem-solving, and (iv) injury rehabilitation. Interestingly, the model also takes into account the main key-components that need to be carefully controlled to ensure the effectiveness of motor imagery to achieve each individual goal within these imagery outcomes. Hence, the strength of the model is that it gives a detailed description of the rules and conditions of MI training in different kinds of scenarios where imagery can be used.

Overall, the imagery models mentioned above are based on the assumption that motor imagery and motor performance share some parallel characteristics. Interestingly, in the emerging field of motor cognition (Jeannerod 2006), the imagery experience is no more artificially decoupled from the action itself. Rather, motor imagery is placed along a continuum extending from the overt movement to its mental representation. Such approach has led researchers to consider that motor imagery could be performed not only before, or after the actual movement, but also *during* its physical execution, serving both the concentration phase and the anticipation of the forthcoming events (Vergeer and Roberts 2006; see also Chapter 16). Therefore, motor imagery is close to action simulation, which includes the representation of the future and some prospective judgments. In other words, motor imagery includes the goal of the action, how it could be reached, and how it will affect the individual and the external world (Olsson 2008). In a well-known review, Willingham (1998) argued that motor learning might occur only if a movement is executed, as learning is based on the actual execution of the motor act, so movement must be performed for learning to occur. He further claimed that learning by motor imagery should be strategic learning because proprioceptive feedback is not available under this condition, and proprioception cues are essential for sequencing or learning perceptual-motor compatibility. As mentioned previously, however, there is now compelling evidence that learning can take place using motor imagery, i.e. without concomitant body movement, nor actually intending to perform the action, although this latter point should be discussed, particularly when novice imagers are involved in mental rehearsal sessions. To improve the effectiveness of motor imagery in learning a new motor skill in novices, we propose using go/no-go paradigms to reinforce the ability of building the representation of the action. This proposal is mainly based on the fact that motor imagery implies that mental practice must be, to some extent, similar to motor execution, hence referring to the principle of functional equivalence (Holmes and Collins 2001; Murphy et al. 2008). Accordingly, there is a certain degree of overlap between the neuronal processes mediating both actual and imagined motor performance. More generally, it is assumed that motor images should ideally preserve many properties of the actual performance of the same movement. More generally, indirect evidence in support of this theory are derived from various neuroimaging and behavioural experimental designs, as well as interference paradigms, investigating the degree of similarity between motor performance and motor imagery for speed, biomechanical constraints, as well as patterns of cerebral activations.

These parallel characteristics have been a centrepiece of many chapters in the present book, and will thus be reviewed only briefly here. First, the time course of mentally simulated actions is highly correlated with the time taken to execute the same movement (e.g. Decety et al. 1989). This temporal equivalence, however, is not systematic as several factors (e.g. task duration and difficulty, instructions given to subjects, or the way in which attention is focused on a specific aspect of the mental image) may lead to an over- or underestimation of the imagined movement duration (Guillot and Collet 2005a,b; Grealy and Shearer 2007; Slifkin 2008). Second, peripheral activity of the autonomic nervous system has been found to show similar responses during both motor imagery and the motor execution of actions. For example, heart rate and pulmonary frequencies are known to co-vary with the degree of imagined effort (Decety et al. 1991, 1993; Fusi et al. 2005). Furthermore, increases in ventilation and systolic blood pressure have been reported during motor imagery of dumbbells lifting (Wang and Morgan 1992; Wuyam et al. 1995), while similar electrodermal and thermovascular responses are elicited during imagined and actual movements (Guillot et al. 2004b, 2005).

Generally speaking, brain imaging and brain-damaged patient data have provided evidence that similar cerebral structures are involved during motor imagery and motor performance. These neural networks notably include the motor systems, as well as the inferior and superior parietal lobules (e.g. Decety et al. 1994; Mellet et al. 1998; Lotze et al. 1999; Gerardin et al. 2000; Guillot et al. 2008; Munzert et al. 2009). Interestingly, the data also contributed to distinguish between the neural substrates mediating different types of imagery (Martinez 2000; Ruby and Decety 2001; Solodkin et al. 2004; Neuper et al. 2005; Jackson et al. 2006; Guillot et al. 2009; Lorey et al. 2009), as well as those involved during motor imagery in participants with high and poor imagery abilities (Lotze et al. 2003; Guillot et al. 2008). Interference paradigm experiments are also of particular interest to demonstrate cases for overlap/differences between the active cognitive processes (Smyth and Waller 1998; Stevens 2005).

Motor imagery has further been shown to be influenced by the biomechanical and the motor constraints (Parsons 1987, 1994; Petit et al. 2003; Petit and Harris 2005; Munzert et al. 2009). Accordingly, the time course of decision of body part orientation is increased for anatomical uncorrected positions, and the motor imagery experience reflects the biomechanics of the imagined limb. In fact, motor imagery timing is finally affected by the same influencing factors than actual actions, such as biomechanical constraints and awkwardness of action. Finally, in a recent novel line of research, Debarnot et al. (2009a,b) have confirmed the degree of similarity between motor imagery and motor performance by providing evidence that the participants engaged in motor imagery practice did improve their motor performance after a night of sleep. Based on sleep data and motor skill learning literature, these findings suggest that the consolidation processes remain effective following mental practice as well, thus assuming that a night of sleep after motor imagery practice results in similar motor memory consolidation than following physical practice. Interestingly, the authors also demonstrated that offline delayed gains were not related to the imagery content *per se*, as imagery practice voluntarily performed at a faster pace did not provide additional benefits in actual movement time after a night of sleep, as compared to real-time imagery training.

Individual differences

The ability to form accurate mental images (i.e. which are very close to the actual experience) is not universal (Isaac and Marks 1994). Many individual differences have thus been suggested to govern the best way to perform imagery and the best perspective to use (Murphy et al. 2008). For example, research has found that imagery use varies among sporting activities (Hall 2001). Among the other factors, expertise level and imagery ability have been subjected to many researches. While imagery has been shown to be effective in all learning stages, the best imagers usually tend to perform better (Goss et al. 1986; Vadocz et al. 1997; Murphy and Martin 2002; Robin et al. 2007), and kinaesthetic imagery appeared to be beneficial only with an adequate degree of expertise (Hardy and Callow 1999; Guillot et al. 2004b). Many experimental studies agree with this latter result, hence providing compelling evidence that elite athletes use more frequently imagery than novices (Hall et al. 1998; Nordin and Cumming 2007), and most especially kinaesthetic imagery (Barr and Hall 1992). Overall, more experienced athletes have usually imagery sessions of better quality (Vealey and Walter 1993). Novice athletes still benefit from imagery sessions but may be constrained due to lack of experience either in using imagery or with the motor skill itself (Hall 2001). For example, Salmon et al. (1994) found that even though both novice and elite football players benefited from imagery use, elite football players reported using more imagery, regardless of function, than novice football players. Therefore, there seems to be a positive linear relationship between the experience level of the athlete and the frequency of imagery use. It has even been suggested that a cyclical relationship may exist between imagery use and ability (Vadocz et al. 1997), i.e. participants with high imagery abilities are more likely to use motor imagery, while performing imagery subsequently bolsters imagery ability. Similarly, many studies have investigated the frequency of internal versus external visual imagery use. While being criticized, the early study by Mahoney and Avener (1977) suggested that successful gymnasts used internal imagery more often than external imagery, whereas less successful novice skiers were found to use external imagery more frequently (Rotella et al. 1980). Conversely, other researchers reported that athletes performed either visual imagery perspectives equally (Highlen and Benett 1979; Meyers et al. 1979; Hall et al. 1990; Barr and Hall 1992). Finally, numerous

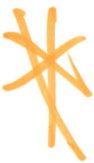

studies demonstrated that athletes with high level of expertise might easily switch between perspectives (Gordon *et al.* 1994; Collins *et al.* 1998; Holmes and Collins 2001).

From a neurophysiological viewpoint, the neuroimaging data support the differences within the level of expertise of the participants. For example, expertise-related differences were reported in mental scanning paradigms requesting participants to learn a map of an island, and then to reconstruct the mental image of this map to mentally explore the distances separating the landmarks (Charlot *et al.* 1992; Cocude *et al.* 1999). Accordingly, high visuo-spatial imagers yielded increased patterns of activation in the left temporo-occipital region during imagery, whereas the low visuo-spatial imagers showed much less clearly differentiated peaks of activation. Neuroimaging studies dealing with mental and motor imagery also showed that the neural networks activated by the execution of the task differed as a function of the individual expertise level. For example, Lotze *et al.* (2003) compared the patterns of brain activation during auditory imagery in experienced and novice musicians, with the professionals reporting high vividness and frequent use of imagery. Interestingly, the authors showed that the experienced musicians recruited very few cerebral areas, while amateurs exhibited a more widely distributed activation map. In the professional group, however, more activation was observed in the supplementary motor area, the superior premotor cortex, the superior parietal lobule, and the cerebellum. Even though there are very few studies looking at this issue in motor imagery, similar observations were reported in the neural network activations between novice and expert athletes (Milton *et al.* 2008). As suggested, both the consistency and reproducibility for the preparation period before the movement play a crucial role in many sporting activities. This specific phase, which is also called 'pre-shot routine', often contributes to differentiate experts from novices. A brain-mapping study by Ross *et al.* (2003) compared brain activations of six golfers of various handicaps during motor imagery of a golf swing using the first-person perspective. They found an inverse relationship between brain activity and skill level, i.e. decreased activations occurring with increased golf skill level, especially for the supplementary motor area and the cerebellum. Also, golf swing motor imagery produced little activation of basal ganglia and cingulate gyri across all skill levels. Milton *et al.* (2007) later reported that brain regions were activated in novices but not in elite golfers, hence suggesting that the neural networks involved in motor planning and motor imagery are dependent upon the individual skill level, i.e. the degree to which the motor skill have been automated.

Guillot *et al.* (2008) also compared the pattern of cerebral activations in 13 skilled and 15 unskilled imagers, during both physical execution and imagery of a finger movement sequence. While both groups manifested similar peaks of activation in many cerebral regions, good imagers activated more the parietal and ventrolateral premotor regions, known at playing a crucial role in the formation of the mental images. In contrast, poor imagers recruited the cerebellum, the orbito-frontal, and posterior cingulate cortices. With reference to the motor sequence learning literature (Doyon and Ungerleider, 2002; Doyon and Benali, 2005; Doyon, 2008), these findings support that the neural networks mediating expertise in motor imagery are not identical in high- and low-skilled individuals. In line with such hypothesis, Lafleur *et al.* (2002) and Jackson *et al.* (2003) demonstrated that the cerebral plasticity occurring during the incremental acquisition of a motor sequence was also reflected during motor imagery. The patterns of dynamic changes in cerebral activity were different when comparing both early and more-advanced learning phases of imagined sequential foot movements. In particular, Lafleur *et al.* (2002) observed significant differences medially in the rostral portion of the anterior cingulate and orbito-frontal cortices, as well as in the striatum, bilaterally. Jackson *et al.* (2003) confirmed the robustness of these findings by a regression analysis, which showed a positive correlation between the increase in cerebral blood flow within the right medial orbito-frontal cortex and the individual performance enhancement.

Taken overall, these data strongly support the existence of distinct neural mechanisms of expertise in motor imagery, as a function of the individual skill level and independently of the imagery type. Interestingly, the brain plasticity which occurs during learning of a motor skill is similar to that observed during learning through mental practice. Hence, even if this is too early to draw final conclusions regarding the neural substrates mediating the expertise in imagery, the hypothesis that dynamic changes elicited by the mental repetition of a given task will contribute to reduce the general cortical activation should be verified. Dynamic changes should become more refined and circumscribed with practice, just as during the learning process of motor tasks. Despite such general map of activity, however, some discrete differences in the patterns of activations should still be observed in expert and professionals as compared to amateurs, which will directly depend on the intrinsic nature of the task.

References

Abma, C.L., Fry, M. D., Li, Y., and Relyea, G. (2002). Difference in imagery content and imagery ability between high and low confident track and field athletes. *Journal of Applied Sport Psychology,* **14**, 67–75.

Barr K. and Hall C.R., (1992), The use of imagery by rowers. *International Journal of Sport Psychology,* **23**, 243–61.

Bolliet O., Collet C., and Dittmar A., (2003), Effect of preparation duration diminution on shot put performance through neurovegetative activity. *Biology of Sport,* **20**, 289–301.

Boron J.M., (2002), Imagery use in fencing. Unpublished doctoral dissertation, West Virginia University, USA.

Butler A.J. and Page S.J. (2006). Mental practice with motor imagery: evidence for motor recovery and cortical reorganization after stroke. *Archives in Physical and Medicine Rehabilitation,* **87**, 2–11.

Callow, N. and Waters, A. (2005). The effect of kinaesthetic imagery on the sport confidence of flat-race horse jockeys. *Psychology of Sport and Exercise,* **6**, 443–59.

Callow, N., Roberts, R., and Fawkes, J.Z. (2006). Effects of dynamic and static imagery on vividness of imagery skiing performance, and confidence. *Journal of Imagery Research in Sport and Physical Activity,* **1**, 1–15.

Charlot, V., Tzourio, N., Zilbovicius, M., Mazoyer, B., and Denis, M. (1992). Different mental imagery abilities result in different regional cerebral blood flow activation patterns during cognitive tasks. *Neuropsychologia,* **30**, 147–54.

Cocude, M., Mellet, E., and Denis, M. (1999). Visual and mental exploration of visuo-spatial configurations: behavioral and neuroimaging approaches. *Psychological Research,* **62**, 93–106.

Cohelo, R.W., De Campos, W., Da Silva, S.G., Okazaki, F.H.A., and Keller, B. (2007). Imagery intervention in open and closed tennis motor skill performance. *Perceptual and Motor Skills,* **105**, 458–68.

Collet, C., Roure, R., Dittmar, A., and Vernet-Maury, E. (2000). Autonomic nervous system activity as a witness mental imagery in sport and its role in motor performance and learning. *Science and Sports,* **15**, 261–3.

Collins, D.J., Smith, D., and Hale B.D. (1998). Imagery perspectives and karate performance. *Journal of Sports Sciences,* **16**, 103–04.

Cumming J. and Ramsey, R. (2008). Sport imagery interventions, in S. Mellalieu and S. Hanton (eds), *Advances in Applied Sport Psychology: A Review.* London: Routledge.

Debarnot U., Creveaux T., Collet C., *et al.* (2009a). Sleep-related improvements in motor learning following mental practice. *Brain and Cognition,* **69**, 398–405.

Debarnot U., Creveaux T., Collet C., Doyon J., and Guillot A. (2009b). Sleep contribution to motor memory consolidation: a motor imagery study. *Sleep,* 32.

Decety, J., Jeannerod, M., and Prablanc, C. (1989). The timing of mentally represented actions. *Behavioural Brain Research,* **34**, 35–42.

Decety, J., Jeannerod, M., Germain, M., and Pastene, J., (1991), Vegetative response during imagined movement is proportional to mental effort. *Behavioural Brain Research*, **42**, 1–5.

Decety, J., Jeannerod, M., Durozard, D., and Baverel, G., (1993), Central activation of autonomic effectors during mental simulation of motor actions in man. *Journal of Physiology*, **461**, 549–63.

Decety, J., Perani, D., Jeannerod, M. *et al.* (1994). Mapping motor representations with positron emission tomography. *Nature,* **371**, 600–2.

Deschaumes-Molinaro, C., Dittmar, A., and Vernet-Maury, E. (1991). Relationship between mental imagery and sporting performance. *Behavioural Brain Research*, **45**, 29–36.

Deschaumes-Molinaro C., Dittmar A., and Vernet-Maury E. (1992). Autonomic nervous system response patterns correlate with mental imagery. *Physiology and Behavior*, **51**, 1021–27.

Doyon, J. (2008). Motor sequence learning and movement disorders. *Current Opinion in Neurology,* **21**, 478–83.

Doyon, J. and Benali, H. (2005). Reorganization and plasticity in the adult brain during learning of motor skills. *Current Opinion in Neurobiology*, **25**, 161–7.

Doyon, J. and Ungerleider, L.G. (2002). Functional anatomy of motor skill learning, in L.R Squire and D.L. Schacter (eds), *Neuropsychology of Memory*. pp. 225–38. New York: Guilford Press.

Driskell, J. E., Copper, C., and Moran, A. (1994). Does mental practice enhance performance? *Journal of Applied Psychology*, **79**, 481–92.

Epstein, M.L. (1980). The relationship of mental imagery and mental rehearsal to performance of a motor task. *Journal of Sport Psychology*, **2**, 211–20.

Farahat, E., Ille, A., and Thon, B. (2004). Effect of visual and kinaesthetic imagery on the learning of a patterned movement. *International Journal of Sport Psychology*, **35**, 119–32.

Feltz, D.L. and Landers, D.M. (1983). The effects of mental practice on motor skill learning and performance: a meta-analysis. *Journal of Psychology,* **5**, 25–57.

Fusi, S., Cutuli, D., Valente, M.R., Bergonzi, P., Porro, C.A., and Di Prampero, P.E. (2005) Cardioventilatory responses during real or imagined walking at low speed. *Archives Italiennes de Biologie*, **143**, p. 223–8.

Gerardin, E., Sirigu, A., Lehericy, S. *et al.* (2000). Partially overlapping neural networks for real and imagined hand movements. *Cerebral Cortex*, **10**, 1093–104.

Gordon S., Weinberg R.S., and Jackson A., (1994). Effects of internal and external imagery on cricket performance. *Journal of Sport Behavior*, **17**, 60–76.

Goss, S., Hall, C.R., Buckolz, E., and Fishburne, G. (1986). Imagery ability and the acquisition and retention of movements. *Memory and Cognition*, **14**, 469–77.

Grealy, M. and Shearer G. (2007). Timing processes in motor imagery. *European Journal of Cognitive Psychology*, **20**, 867–92.

Guillot, A. and Collet, C. (2005a). Duration of mentally simulated movement: a review. *Journal of Motor Behavior*, **37**, 10–9.

Guillot, A. and Collet, C. (2005b). Contribution from neurophysiological and psychological methods to the study of motor imagery. *Brain Research Reviews*, **50**, 387–97.

Guillot, A. and Collet, C. (2008). Construction of the motor imagery integrative model in sport: a review and theoretical investigation of motor imagery use. *International Review of Sport and Exercise Psychology*, **1**, 31–44.

Guillot, A., Collet, C., Molinaro, C., and Dittmar, A. (2004a) Expertise and peripheral autonomic activity during the preparation phase in shooting events. *Perceptual and Motor Skills*, **98**, 371–81.

Guillot, A., Collet, C., and Dittmar, A. (2004b). Relationship between visual vs kinaesthetic imagery, field dependence-independence and complex motor skills. *Journal of Psychophysiology*, **18**, 190–8.

Guillot A., Haguenauer M., Dittmar A., and Collet C. (2005). Effect of a fatiguing protocol on motor imagery accuracy. *European Journal of Applied Physiology*, **95**, 186–90.

Guillot, A., Collet, C., Nguyen, V.A., Malouin, F., Richards, C., and Doyon, J. (2008). Functional neuroanatomical networks associated with expertise in motor imagery ability. *NeuroImage*, **41**, 1471–83.

Guillot, A., Collet, C., Nguyen, V.A., Malouin, F., Richards, C., and Doyon, J. (2009). Brain activity during visual vs. kinesthetic imagery: an fMRI study. *Human Brain Mapping*, **30**, 2157–72.

Hall, C. R. (2001). Imagery in sport and exercise, in R.N. Singer, H.N. Hausenblas, and C. Janelle (eds), *Handbook of Sport Psychology*. 2nd Edition. pp. 529–49. New York: Wiley.

Hall, C.R., Rodgers, W.M., and Barr, K., (1990). The use of imagery by athletes in selected sports. *The Sport Psychologist*, **4**, 1–10.

Hall, C.R., Mack, D.E., Paivio, A., and Hausenblas, H.A., (1998). Imagery use by athletes: development of the sport imagery questionnaire. *International Journal of Sport Psychology*, **29**, 73–89.

Hardy, L., (1997). Three myths about applied consultancy work. *Journal of Applied Sport Psychology*, **9**, 277–94.

Hardy, L. and Callow, N. (1999). Efficacy of external and internal visual imagery perspectives for the enhancement of performance on tasks in which form is important. *Journal of Sport and Exercise Psychology*, **21**, 95–112.

Highlen, P.S. and Bennett, B.B. (1979), Elite divers and wrestlers: a comparison between open and closed skill athletes. *Journal of Sport Psychology*, **1**, 123–37.

Holmes, P. S. and Collins, D.J. (2001). The PETTLEP approach to motor imagery: a functional equivalence model for sport psychologists. *Journal of Applied Sport Psychology*, **13**, 60–83.

Isaac, A.R. and Marks, D.F. (1994). Individual differences in mental imagery experience: developmental changes and specialization. *British Journal of Psychology*, **85**, 479–500.

Jackson, P.L., Lafleur, M.F., Malouin, F., Richards, C.L., and Doyon, J. (2003). Functional cerebral reorganization following motor sequence learning through mental practice with motor imagery. *NeuroImage*, **20**, 1171–80.

Jackson, P.L., Meltzoff, A.N., and Decety, J. (2006). Neural circuits involved in imitation and perspective-taking. *NeuroImage*, **31**, 429–39.

Jeannerod, M. (1994). The representing brain: neural correlates of motor intention and imagery. *Behavioural Brain Sciences*, **17**, 187–202.

Jeannerod, M. (2006). *Motor Cognition*. New York: Oxford University Press.

Kosslyn, S.M., Segar, C., Pani, J., and Hillger, L.A. (1990). When is imagery used in everyday life? A diary study. *Journal of Mental Imagery*, **14**, 131–52.

Kosslyn, S. M., Thompson, W. L., and Ganis, G. (2006). *The Case for Mental Imagery*. New York: Oxford University Press.

Lafleur, M.F., Jackson, P.L., Malouin, F., Richards, C.L., Evans, A.C., and Doyon, J. (2002). Motor learning produces parallel dynamic functional changes during the execution and imagination of sequential foot movements. *NeuroImage*, **2**, 142–57.

Lorey, B., Bischoff, M., Pilgramm, S., Stark, R., Munzert, J., and Zentgraf, K. (2009). The embodied nature of motor imagery: the influence of posture and perspective. *Experimental Brain Research*, **194**, 233–43.

Lotze, L., Montoya, P., Erb, M. *et al.* (1999). Activation of cortical and cerebellar motor areas during executed and imagined hand movements: an fMRI study. *Journal of Cognitive Neuroscience*, **11**, 491–501.

Lotze, M., Scheler, G., Tan, H.R.M., Braun, C., and Birbaumer, N. (2003). The musician's brain: functional imaging of amateurs and professionals during performance and imagery. *NeuroImage*, **20**, 1817–29.

MacIntyre, T., and Moran, A. (2007). A qualitative investigation of meta-imagery processes and imagery direction among in elite athletes. *Journal of Imagery Research in Sport and Physical Activity*, **2(1)**, article 4.

Mahoney, M.J. and Avener, M., (1977). Psychology of the elite athlete: an exploratory study. *Cognitive Therapy and Research*, **1**, 135–41.

Martinez, R.K. (2000). Changes in the frequency power spectrum of the human EEG during visual and kinesthetic imagery. *Dissertation Abstracts International*, **61**, 545.

Mellet, E., Petit, L., Mazoyer, B., Denis, M., and Tzourio, N. (1998). Reopening the mental imagery debate: lessons from functional anatomy. *NeuroImage, 8*, 129–39.

Meyers, A.W., Cooke, C.J., Cullen, J., and Liles, L., (1979). Psychological aspects of athletic competitors: a replication across sports. *Cognitive Therapy and Research, 3*, 331–6.

Milton, J., Small, S.L., and Solodkin, A. (2008). Imaging motor imagery: methodological issues related to expertise. *Methods, 45*, 336–41.

Milton, J., Solodkin, A., Hlustik, P., and Small, S.L. (2007). The mind of expert motor performance is cool and focused. *NeuroImage, 35*, 804–13.

Moran, A. (2002). In the mind's eye. *The Psychologist, 15*, 414–5.

Morris, T., Spittle, M., and Watt, A.P. (2005). *Imagery in Sport*. Champaign, IL: Human Kinetics.

Munroe, K.J., Giacobbi, P.R., Hall, C., and Weinberg, R. (2000). The four Ws of imagery use: where, when, why and what. *The Sport Psychologist, 14*, 119–37.

Munzert, J., Lorey, B., and Zentgraf, K. (2009). Cognitive motor processes: the role of motor imagery in the study of motor representations. *Brain Research Reviews, 60*, 306–326.

Murphy, S.M. and Martin, K.A. (2002). The use of imagery in sport, in T.S. Horn (ed.), *Advances in Sport Psychology*. 2nd Edition. Champaign, IL: Human Kinetics.

Murphy, S., Nordin, S.M., and Cumming, J. (2008). Imagery in sport, exercise and dance, in T.S. Horn (ed.), *Advances in Sport Psychology*. pp. 306–15. Champagne, IL: Human Kinetics.

Neuper, C., Scherer, R., Reiner, M., and Pfurtscheller, G. (2005). Imagery of motor actions: differential effects of kinaesthetic and visual-motor mode of imagery in single-trial EEG. *Cognitive Brain Research, 25*, 668–77.

Nordin, S.M. and Cumming, J. (2007). When, where and how: a quantitative account of dance imagery. *Research Quarterly for Exercise and Sport, 78*, 390–5.

Olsson, C.J., Jonsson, B., and Nyberg, L. (2008). Internal imagery training in active high jumpers. *Scandinavian Journal of Psychology, 49*, 133–40.

Paivio, A. (1985). Cognitive and motivational functions of imagery in human performance. *Canadian Journal of Applied Sport Science, 10*, 22S–28S.

Parsons, L.M. (1987). Imagined spatial transformation of one's body. *Journal of Experimental and Psychological Genetics, 116*, 172–91.

Parsons, L.M. (1994). Temporal and kinematic properties of motor behavior reflected in mentally simulated action. *Journal of Experimental Psychology: Human Perception and Performance, 20*, 709–30.

Petit, L.S., Pegna, A.J., Mayer, E., and Hauert, C.A. (2003). Representation of anatomical constraints in motor imagery: mental rotation of a body segment. *Brain and Cognition, 51*, 95–101.

Petit, L.S. and Harris, I.M. (2005). Anatomical limitations in mental transformations of body parts. *Visual Cognition, 12*, 737–58.

Poulton, E.C., (1957). On prediction in skilled movements. *Psychological Bulletin, 54*, 467–78.

Robin, N., Dominique, L., Toussaint, L., Blandin, Y., Guillot, A., and Le Her, M. (2007). Effects of motor imagery training on returning serve accuracy in tennis: the role of imagery ability. *International Journal of Sport and Exercise Psychology, 2*, 177–88.

Ross, J.S., Tkach, J., Ruggieri, P.M., Lieber, M., and Lapresto, E. (2003). The mind's eye: functional MR imaging of golf motor imagery. *American Journal of Neuroradiology, 24*, 103–1044.

Rotella, R.J., Gansneder, B., Ojala D., and Billing, J., (1980). Cognitions and coping strategies of elite skiers: an exploratory study of young developing athletes. *Journal of Sport Psychology, 2*, 350–4.

Ruby, P. and Decety, J., (2001), Effect of subjective perspective taking during simulation of action: a PET investigation of agency. *Nature Neuroscience, 4*, 546–50.

Salmon, J., Hall, C.R., and Haslam, I.R., (1994). The use of imagery by soccer players. *Journal of Applied Sport Psychology, 6*, 116–33.

Short, S.E., Bruggeman, J.M., Engel, S.G., *et al.* (2002). The effect of imagery function and imagery direction on self-efficacy and performance on a golf-putting task. *The Sport Psychologist, 16*, 48–67.

Slifkin, A.B. (2008). High loads induce differences between actual and imagined movement duration. *Experimental Brain Research*, **185**, 297–307.

Smith, D., Wright, C., Allsopp, A., and Westhead, H. (2007). It's all in the mind: PETTLEP-based imagery and sport performance. *Journal of Applied Sport Psychology*, **19**, 80–92.

Smyth, M.M. and Waller, A. (1998). Movement imagery in rock climbing: patterns of interference from visual, spatial and kinaesthetic secondary tasks. *Applied Cognitive Psychology*, **12**, 145–57.

Solodkin, A., Hlustik, P., Chen, E.E., and Small, S.L. (2004). Fine modulation in network activation during motor execution and motor imagery. *Cerebral Cortex*, **14**, 1246–55.

Spittle, M. and Moris, T. (2000). Imagery perspectives preferences and motor performance. *Australian Journal of Psychology*, **52S**, 112.

Stevens, J.A. (2005). Interference effects demonstrate distinct roles for visual and motor imagery during the mental representation of human action. *Cognition*, **95**, 329–50.

Taktek, K., Zinsser, N., and St-John, B. (2008). Visual versus kinesthetic mental imagery: efficacy for the retention and transfer of a closed motor skill in young children. *Canadian Journal of Experimental Psychology*, **62**, 174–87.

Vadocz, E.A., Hall, C.R., and Moritz, S.E., (1997). The relationship between competitive anxiety and imagery use. *Journal of Applied Sport Psychology*, **9**, 241–53.

Vealey, R. S. and Walter, S. M. (1993). Imagery training for performance enhancement and personal development, in J.M. Williams (ed.), *Applied Sport Psychology: Personal Growth to Peak Performance*. 2nd Edition. pp. 200–224. Mountain View, CA: Mayfield.

Vergeer, E. and Roberts, J. (2006). Movement and stretching imagery during flexibility training. *Journal of Sports Sciences*, **24**, 197–208.

Wang, Y. and Morgan, W.P. (1992). The effects of imagery perspectives on the physiological responses to imagined exercise. *Behavioural Brain Research*, **52**, 167–74.

White, A. and Hardy, L. (1995). Use of different imagery perspectives on the learning and performance of different motor skills. *British Journal of Psychology*, **86**, 191–216.

Willingham, D.B. (1998). A neuropsychological theory of motor skill learning. *Psychological Review*, **105**, 558–84.

Witkin, H.A. (1950). Individual differences in ease of perception of embedded figures. *Journal of Personality*, **19**, 1–15.

Wuyam, B., Moosavi, S.H., Decety, J., Adams, L., Lansing, R.W., and Guz, A. (1995). Imagination of dynamic exercise produced ventilatory responses which were more apparent in competitive sportsmen. *Journal of Physiology*, **482**, 713–24.

Zimmerman-Schlatter, A., Schuster, C., Puhan, M.A., *et al.* (2008). Efficacy of motor imagery in post-stroke rehabilitation: a systematic review. *Journal of Neuroengineering and Rehabilitation*, **5**, 8.

Chapter 16

Meta-imagery processes among elite sports performers

Tadhg MacIntyre and Aidan Moran

I picked out three numbers in the stand behind the posts. I can still picture them perfectly. That was my target. I visualized the ball going through and kept that image.
Ireland and Lions rugby player speaking out his last minute drop-goal to win the 2009 'grand slam' for Ireland, Ronan O'Gara cited in Walsh, 2009, p. 9.

You have to see the shots and feel them through your hands.
Golfer Tiger Woods, quoted in Pitt, 1998, p. 5.

This visualisation technique is a sort of clarified daydream with snippets of the atmosphere from past matches included to enhance the sense of reality…The game will throw up many different scenarios but I am as prepared in my own head for them as I can be. If you have realistically imagined situations, you feel better prepared and less fearful of the unexpected.
Former England and Lions rugby player, Jonny Wilkinson, 2006, p. 58.

Visualising things is massively important. If you don't visualise, then you allow other negative thoughts to enter your head. Not visualising is almost like having a satellite navigation system in your car, but not entering your destination into it. The machinery can only work if you put everything in there.
Golfer Darren Clarke, 2005, p. 3

Introduction

As the above quotations show, recent years have witnessed a plethora of anecdotal testimonials from elite athletes such as golfers (e.g., Tiger Woods, Darren Clarke) and rugby players (e.g., Ronan O'Gara, Jonny Wilkinson) about the value of 'seeing' and 'feeling' themselves, performing key skills in their mind's eye before actually executing them in competition. For such athletes, motor imagery, commonly defined as 'the mental rehearsal of voluntary movement without accompanying body movement' (e.g., Milton *et al.* 2008, p. 336), is important for success. Stronger evidence to support this claim comes from psychometric studies showing that imagery-based techniques are used extensively by athletes, coaches, and psychologists for a variety of different purposes such as skill learning and execution (Morris *et al.* 2005). Augmenting anecdotal and psychometric evidence, a wealth of experimental research evidence now exists on the nature and application of mental imagery in sport (e.g., see review by Weinberg 2008).

Unfortunately, despite its popularity, research on imagery in sport is hampered by at least three unresolved issues. First, few studies in this field have actually been conducted on 'elite' athletes – as defined by the criterion of having competed at international level in their specialist sport (Vanden Auweele *et al.* 1993). As a result, relatively little is known about how top-class sports performers use or experience imagery in training and/or competition. Inspection of the research literature on imagery in athletes shows that most studies are based on samples of novice athletes (e.g., Short *et al.* 2002), students (e.g., Cumming *et al.* 2006; Nordin and Cumming 2005a) or youth-level competitors (e.g., Munroe-Chandler *et al.* 2005). Nevertheless, some imagery studies (e.g., Driediger *et al.* 2006; Evans *et al.* 2006; Shearer *et al.* 2007) involving elite participants have been published. In general, however, Morris *et al.* (2005) bemoaned the fact that 'research on imagery … has focused largely on studies using novice of beginner performers' (p. 316). A second weakness in this field concerns the fact that due to the popularity of quantitative self-report imagery measures, there have been relatively few qualitative investigations of imagery processes in athletes (but see White and Hardy 1998; Munroe *et al.* 2000; MacIntyre and Moran 2007a,b). As a result, a great deal remains to be discovered about the complexity and flexibility of athletes' use of imagery. Finally, and most relevant to the present chapter, imagery researchers in sport have largely neglected 'meta-imagery' processes or athletes' knowledge of, and control over, their *own* mental imagery skills and experiences (Moran 2002). The neglect of what athletes know about and do with their own imagery processes is surprising in view of the abundance of anecdotal insights available from athletes on this topic.

Against this background, and in an effort to address the preceding unresolved issues, the purpose of the present chapter is to investigate meta-imagery processes in elite sports performers. We shall proceed as follows. To begin with, we shall explore the nature and types of meta-cognition that have been postulated by researchers. After that, we shall review research on meta-cognitive processes in athletes. Then, we shall articulate some of the possible reasons for the neglect of meta-imagery and subsequently describe some preliminary investigations of meta-imagery processes in athletes. Finally, we shall consider the neglected role of meta-imagery processes in current theoretical models of imagery processes in athletes.

Meta-cognition: nature and types

A unique feature of the human species is that people not only think – but also *reflect upon* their own thinking. This self-reflective activity – 'thinking about thinking' – lies at the heart of the construct of *meta-cognition* (see Dunlosky and Metcalfe 2008, for a recent overview of this topic). As the prefix of this term, 'meta', literally means 'above', it is clear that the cornerstone of meta-cognition is the proposition that some cognitive processes appear to operate at a higher level than other such processes. For example, most adults can not only *read* (a cognitive process) but are also able to evaluate the degree to which they *understand* the meaning of what they read ('meta-comprehension' – a meta-cognitive process). So, the term 'meta-cognition' refers to 'the scientific study of the mind's ability to monitor and control itself or, in other words, the study of our ability to know about our knowing' (Van Overschelde 2008, p. 47). But it goes further than that. Thus Halpern (2003) defines meta-cognition not only as 'our knowledge of what we know' (p. 19) but also as 'the use of this knowledge to direct further learning activities'. So, in summary, the construct of meta-cognition refers to people's knowledge and monitoring of, and ability to exert strategic control over, their own mental processes (Moran 2004).

Just as different cognitive processes exist, so also can different types of meta-cognitive phenomena be identified. For example, meta-cognitive researchers have investigated such topics as 'meta-memory' (knowledge about our own memory and learning processes), 'meta-attention' (knowledge about our own attentional processes), 'meta-comprehension' (knowledge about our comprehension), 'visual meta-cognition' (knowledge about our perceptual processes; Levin and Angelone 2009), and 'meta-imagery' (cognition about our own imagery experiences) – the focus of this chapter. To explain this latter term, meta-imagery processes refer to 'people's knowledge about, and control over, their own mental imagery processes' (Moran 2004, p. 285). Early discussions of meta-imagery may be found in Cornoldi *et al.* (1996), Denis and Carfantan (1985), and Moran (2002).

In general, researchers distinguish between three types of meta-cognitive processes (Dunlosky *et al.* 2007). To begin with, 'meta-cognitive knowledge' involves people's declarative knowledge ('knowing that') and beliefs about how their minds work. In sport, this may involve athletes' belief about their concentration system – such as that it resembles a shower which one can turn on or off as one requires (Moran 2004). Second, 'meta-cognitive monitoring' refers to people's ability to check or reflect on some aspect of their thinking. For example, athletes might check from time to time that their mind is relaxed during a competitive event. Finally, 'meta-cognitive control' denotes any strategy that a person uses in attempting to regulate and/or improve his or her skills or performance. For example, athletes might deliberately switch their focus of attention from external factors onto their breathing when they begin to feel tired during a marathon. Meta-cognitive control processes are especially valuable because they allow people to change their behaviour strategically in accordance with task demands. With these distinctions in mind, let us now consider some research findings on meta-cognitive activity in sport.

Research on meta-cognitive processes in athletes

Only a handful of studies have been conducted on meta-cognitive processes in athletes although the application of meta-cognitive theory to sport performance was anticipated over two decades ago by Flavell (1987) who referred to 'attempts to monitor one's own motor activity in a motor skill situation' (p. 21). These studies have addressed different types of meta-cognitive processes as follows.

Meta-cognitive knowledge in athletes

To begin with, McPherson and Thomas (1989) discovered that skilful young tennis players (aged 10–13) possessed more sophisticated tennis-specific knowledge with regard to patterns and options available to them on court than did less proficient players. Likewise, Huber (1997) investigated knowledge differences between elite and less-proficient springboard divers. He found that the elite athletes 'possessed a large body of knowledge that was specific, densely interrelated, well-organised, and readily activated' (p. 156). By contrast, the knowledge base of the non-elite performers was sparser, less organized and less accessible. In a similar vein, Williams and Davids (1995) compared the soccer-based knowledge of three groups of participants: A highly skilled group, a lower skilled group, and a group of physically disabled spectators (who had watched an average of 600 soccer matches but who had never played the game). Results showed that the highly skilled participants scored significantly higher than the other two groups on their ability to recall, recognize, and anticipate soccer movements – even though all three groups had equivalent amounts of soccer experience either as competitors or as spectators. The conclusion from this study is that playing soccer facilitates the acquisition of sport-specific knowledge in a way that is not possible through the accumulation of vicarious experience (e.g., by observation only).

Meta-cognitive monitoring in athletes

Strategic processes in sports performers have attracted interest from researchers over the past decade. For example, McPherson (2000) compared the use of planning strategies by highly skilled versus less-skilled tennis players. Having asked participants to describe their thoughts between points in a tennis match, she discovered that the highly skilled players reported using *three times* as many planning strategies as did their less skilled counterparts. These strategies included designated actions to be followed under certain circumstances as well as a variety of regulatory statements arising from the way in which the players monitored their performance. By contrast, less-experienced tennis players tended to report task-irrelevant thoughts between points.

Meta-cognitive control in athletes

Turning to the final component of the tri-partite construct of meta-cognition, some research has been published on athletes' use of cognitive behavioural strategies to regulate or control their ongoing mental skills or actions. Typically, such studies have been conducted within the 'expert-novice' paradigm (Hodges *et al.* 2007). To illustrate, Cleary and Zimmerman (2001) discovered significant differences between expert, non-expert, and novice basketball players in self-regulatory processes exhibited during practice sessions. Specifically, the expert players were found to plan their practice sessions better than did other groups by choosing specific, technique-oriented processes (e.g., 'to bend my knees').

Meta-imagery processes

Although a great deal of research has been conducted on mental imagery processes for well over a century (Kosslyn *et al.* 2006), surprisingly few studies have examined people's knowledge and beliefs about their *own* imagery experiences. However, a seminal paper on this topic was published by Denis and Carfatan (1985). Briefly, these researchers investigated what a sample of undergraduate students knew about imagery findings in psychology. More precisely, they presented participants with a 15-item questionnaire that required them to (a) use their tacit knowledge to predict the outcomes of various imagery experiments that were described but not formally named (e.g., Is memory for pictures better than memory for words?) and (b) interpret certain experimental results from imagery studies (e.g., 'Can the structure of mental images be said to reflect the spatial organisation of the objects they refer to?'). Results showed that the majority of participants predicted correctly that imagery would have significantly beneficial effects on learning of verbal material and also on spatial and deductive reasoning. However, very few people were able to predict accurately the results of mental rotation experiments (whereby more time is required to accomplish greater amounts of rotation of images) or mental scanning studies (whereby longer distances between points in an image take longer to scan than shorter distances). Perhaps the most intriguing finding of Denis and Carfantan's (1985) study for the present chapter, however, was the discovery that a majority of participants regarded as implausible the idea that mental imagery could enhance the performance of motor skills. This latter finding led these researchers to note 'how counterintuitive the idea is that motor skills may be affected by purely mental practice' (p. 56). Interestingly, the authors acknowledge an important potential flaw in their study. Specifically, they concede that the tacit knowledge required to govern behaviour in certain imagery experiments (e.g., mental rotation and mental scanning studies) is likely to emerge only when respondents are actually engaged in these tasks – not when they merely think about them in a self-report questionnaire. Despite this objection, Denis and Carfantan's (1985) research is relevant to sport psychology because it suggests that people have intuitive theories about imagery phenomena – some of which are accurate and while some are patently false. But since these respondents were students with little exposure to the theory and practice of imagery in action, What could a more expert athletic sample tell us about their experiences of imagery techniques? It is to this question that we now turn.

Meta-imagery processes in elite athletes

Over two decades since the paper by Denis and Carfantan (1985), only two published studies (MacIntyre and Moran, 2007a,b) can be located in which 'meta-imagery' processes were investigated explicitly in athletes. Why have sport psychologists neglected this higher order construct while at the same time exploring extensively its lower order equivalent (i.e., imagery processes) in athletes? Our answer to this question is that imagery research in sport has largely been atheoretical, until recently, and that the conceptual and methodological tools for investigating meta-imagery processes (e.g., an understanding of meta-cognitive theory) were unavailable to typical researchers in this field. Interestingly, the dominant question for early research on imagery in sport was simply 'Does imagery work?' This question was driven largely by 'mental practice' research involving the study of the circumstances in which 'seeing' and 'feeling' actions in one's mind's eye leads to significant improvements in skilled performance (see review by Driskell *et al.* 1994). Subsequently, surveying imagery use became *de rigueur* and was subject to over 20 published research papers by Hall and colleagues (see Short *et al.* 2006). While this latter literature has tangentially touched upon the concept of meta-imagery (see later in chapter), the *modus operandi* of employing pencil and paper instruments (e.g., Sport Imagery Questionnaire; Hall *et al.* 2005) by default largely overlooks subtleties in an individual's cognitions and/or meta-cognitions. Only qualitative approaches to imagery would appear to be capable of doing justice to the rich, detailed and personal accounts of athletes' imagery experiences (see MacIntyre and Moran 2007a,b; Munroe *et al.* 2000; White and Hardy 1998). Another possible reason for the apparent neglect of meta-imagery processes in athletes is that until recently, psychologists have largely overlooked the study of human movements – leaving it to the domain of motor control and bio-mechanics (Rosenbaum 2005). However, over the past decade, a new sub-field of psychology called 'motor cognition' has emerged (Jeannerod 2006; Moran and MacIntyre 2008). This field explores how the mind plans and produces skilled actions and movements. More precisely, it is concerned with the 'preparation and production of actions as well as the processes involved in recognizing, anticipating, predicting and interpreting the actions of others' (Jackson and Decety 2004, p. 259). A key tenet of this field is the idea that motor imagery is functionally equivalent to action because it has been shown to share common neurological mechanisms and substrates (see Section 2). An important implication of the motor cognition paradigm is that it returns the study of action to psychology. It also overcomes the problem whereby the study of imagery has been artificially decoupled from that of action – a problem which is apparent in the traditional assumption that imagery is usually practiced in the absence of movement among athletes. As a result, it places imagery on a continuum where intentional movement is at one end and representation is at the opposite end. In passing, it is notable that the motor cognitive approach challenges certain common assumptions of imagery theory in sport psychology – most notably, the traditional definition of imagery as a cognitive activity that occurs only in the *absence* of movement. Interestingly, at least one contemporary model of imagery in athletes postulates that movement *is* possible during imagined action (Holmes and Collins 2001). We will return to this issue of motor imagery coupled with motor execution based on evidence from recent findings.

But let us now turn back to meta-imagery processes in athletes. Here, a potentially relevant body of work has been conducted by Hall and his colleagues on imagery *use* by sport performers. This latter topic is important for the present chapter because it has an indirect bearing on two key components of the construct of meta-imagery – imagery *monitoring* and imagery *control* processes. Interestingly, Weinberg *et al.* (2003) were among the first researchers to explore athletes' beliefs about the relationship between imagery use and imagery effectiveness. They found that, as expected, athletes generally used those types of imagery that they perceived to most effective – thereby showing a rudimentary awareness of meta-cognitive control processes. Weinberg *et al.*'s study was extended recently by Nordin and Cumming (2008) who surveyed a large sample of athletes ($N = 155$) about the perceived effectiveness of a various types of imagery allegedly serving different functions. They found that athletes who used imagery more frequently reported that imagery was more effective and easier to engage in than counterparts who used imagery less frequently. At this stage, it is important to examine in more detail the way in which imagery use has been studied by sport psychologists. In general, such investigators have employed either descriptive or theoretical approaches to this topic. Briefly, whereas the descriptive approach is typically concerned with establishing the *incidence* of certain kinds of imagery use in athletes, the theoretical approach explores specific *categories* of imagery use in such performers. Using the 'descriptive' approach, special survey instruments were designed to assess the extent to which various athletic populations reported using imagery as part of their training. Thus Murphy (1994) reported that 90% of a sample of elite athletes at the US Olympic Training Centre claimed to use imagery regularly. Similarly, Orlick and Partington (1988) discovered that almost 99% of Canadian athletes at the 1984 Olympic Games reported using mental imagery regularly in their training. Clearly, imagery is ubiquitous among expert athletes. By contrast, Cumming and Hall (2002) found that recreational sport performers tended to use imagery less frequently, and rated it less favourably, than more proficient counterparts (e.g., provincial-level and international athletes). Similarly, successful athletes appear to use imagery more frequently than do less-successful competitors (Calmels *et al.* 2003; Durand-Bush *et al.* 2001). Although this type of descriptive research provided valuable 'baseline' data on imagery use in athletes, it did not elucidate the precise *functions* for which athletes employed imagery. To fill this gap, a more theoretical approach was required. And so, in the late 1990s, Hall *et al.* (1998) postulated a taxonomy of imagery use in athletes based on Paivio's (1985) theory that imagery affects both motivational and cognitive processes. This taxonomy proposes five categories of imagery use: (i) 'motivation general-mastery' (MG-M; e.g., imagining being mentally tough and focused in a forthcoming match), (ii) 'motivation general-arousal' (MG-A; e.g., imagining the feelings of excitement that accompany competitive performance), (iii) 'motivation-specific' (MS; e.g., imagining the achievement of a goal such as winning a race), (iv) cognitive general (CG; e.g., imagining a specific strategy or game-plan in a match) and (v) 'cognitive specific' (CS; e.g., mentally rehearsing a skill such as a golf putt or a penalty kick in football). Although this taxonomy is valuable in allowing researchers to explore the relationship between theoretically-derived imagery functions and subsequent athletic performance, it has been criticized for the apparent vagueness of its categorical boundaries.

For example, Abma *et al.* (2002) pointed out that athletes who use 'cognitive specific' imagery regularly (e.g., in rehearsing a particular skill) may be classified as using 'motivation general-mastery' if they believe that mental practice is the best way to boost their confidence. A similar criticism may be directed at Paivio's (1985) seminal paper. For example, in order to support his claim about different cognitive components of imagery, Paivio referred to two well-known examples of reported imagery by elite sports performers. The first example cited is that of Jean-Claude Killy, who, whilst apparently injured and physically unable to ski, reportedly engaged in imagery of an alpine ski run to assist with his competition preparation (Suinn 1980). This anecdotal evidence is contrasted with Jack Nicklaus' widely cited quote on his use of imagery: 'I never hit a shot, even in practice, without having a very sharp, in-focus picture of it in my head … First, I 'see' the ball where I want it to finish…and I 'see' the ball going there; its path, trajectory, and shape, even its behavior on landing' (Nicklaus and Boden 1974, p.79). Although Paivio (1985) classified this quote as an example of 'skill rehearsal' (p. 25S), we disagree. Thus if we examine the Killy and Nicklaus quotations more carefully, we can see that they may have more in common than is evident at first glance. Specifically, they both appear to represent the 'cognitive general' use of imagery. Perhaps the most serious limitation of Hall *et al.*'s model, however, is that it fails to address adequately the issue of negative (or 'debilitative') imagery in athletes. This omission is surprising because Paivio (1985) admitted that most people routinely 'experience positive and negative emotions along with the imagined successes or failures' (p. 23S). Nevertheless, Hall (2001) concluded that 'athletes seldom imagine themselves losing … therefore, practitioners probably should not be overly concerned with negative imagery' (p. 536). In our view, this latter conclusion is debatable as many athletes (especially performers in individual activities such as golf) complain of being plagued by negative imaginary scenarios (such as driving the ball out of bounds on tee-shots). More generally, evidence has emerged recently to suggest that debilitative images *do* occur in athletes (Cumming *et al.* 2006; Hanton *et al.* 2005) with adverse consequences for skilled performance (Nordin and Cumming 2005a; Woolfolk *et al.* 1985).

Turning finally to *explicit* investigations of meta-imagery in athletes, contemporary research has investigated meta-imagery processes among a small sample of elite performers in canoe-slalom, gymnastics, rugby, fencing, golf, and motor-racing (MacIntyre 2007; MacIntyre and Moran 2007a,b). Almost all of these athletes were truly 'elite' as they had represented their country in international competition. The key findings from these studies are elaborated upon in terms of the aforementioned three types of meta-cognitive processes: (i) meta-cognitive knowledge; (ii) meta-cognitive monitoring, and (iii) meta-cognitive control.

Firstly, the aspects of meta-imagery knowledge that appear to be most relevant to sport participants include ideas, for example, about the 'mental practice' effect (i.e., the discovery that under certain circumstances, the cognitive rehearsal of a skill or movement can improve its actual execution), the 'mental travel' effect (i.e., the fact that for expert athletes in certain sports, there is a high degree of concordance between imagined and actual time to execute key skills), and the multi-modality nature of imagery representations (the fact that one can use any sensory system to create an imagery experience). Probing athletes' knowledge about imagery more deeply, consider the frequently encountered advice that athletes should employ imagery both in practice and competition environments (see Hall 2001). In a series of experimental studies involving mental travel, MacIntyre (2007) utilized a modified version of the Denis and Carfantan (1985) questionnaire to examine athlete-specific meta-imagery processes. The findings indicated that the majority of athletes (elite athlete samples from canoe-slalom and gymnastics) were aware of the mental practice effect and also of the idea that imagery could engage numerous sensory modalities. Furthermore, they showed an understanding of the 'mental travel' principle – the idea that, in general, when one imagines a movement it should last the same duration as the actually executed action. Recall from earlier, in Denis and Carfantan's (1985) study, only a small proportion of the participants (students) was aware of the mental practice effect. Clearly, this contrast between these researchers' findings and those of MacIntyre (2007) highlights the importance of sample selection in exploring meta-imagery processes in people.

Turning to qualitative analyses of meta-imagery processes, MacIntyre (2007) investigated athletes' definitions of imagery, the role of perspective, and the multi-modality nature of their imagery. Briefly, results showed that athletes typically defined imagery as multi-modal in nature; they employed different perspectives for strategic reasons and even switched perspective at appropriate times. These findings add to the wealth of information that has accumulated on imagery use (e.g., Short *et al.* 2006) and are consistent with the idea that elite athletes possessed a great deal of meta-cognitive knowledge about how to apply imagery to enhance performance.

The second meta-imagery process on which some data exist is *monitoring* – or people's ability to reflect on and/or experience some aspect of their ongoing imagery processes. For example, when athletes experience a debilitative image (e.g., missing a putt) they can, by monitoring their imagery content, choose to stop the imagery, rewind it, and attempt to 'see' the desired action or outcome (i.e., a successful putt). Accounts from some elite athletes (see MacIntyre and Moran 2007a,b) support this specific example. For instance, one participant stated the following: 'I can see some mistake and I think, the thing is, you sort of have to be, like, holding a remote control and hit the re-wind and pep yourself up and play it again 'til you get it right'.

Augmenting this example, a content analysis of interview data from elite sports performers revealed a complex picture of athletes' experience of negative imagery content. To illustrate, athletes sometimes gave examples of how they could use an image of a poor performance in an effort to enhance future performance (i.e., negative imagery content being facilitative). Results also showed that elite athletes used their motor imagery to generate 'what-if' scenarios. For instance one golfer stated the following: 'I try and rehearse the ideal but then you'll always have the bad thoughts coming in as well. So you'll kind of say well, there's a bunker to the left so if I am going to miss the target I don't want to miss it left, so I will allow for a certain amount of error'. Curiously, imagining *errors* was also undertaken deliberately by some participants – suggesting that the intentional use of negative visualization may have an adaptive role for some performers. In sum, the imagining of 'worst case' scenarios may assist athletes to be ready for what is to be done if things go wrong in competitive situations strategy to regulate, and this represents an example of meta-cognitive control (any strategy that a person uses in attempting to regulate and/ or improve his or her skills or performance).

Another novel instance of meta-imagery control relates to applying imagery to facilitate physical performance. Specifically, one rugby player indicated that he created an imaginary target to help him in line-kicking: 'If I'm kicking for touch, I'm looking for someone in the crowd and I'm focusing on that guy and I'm kicking the ball to that guy on a Monday night at training . . . There's probably about 10,000 in the crowd and I'm not kicking to everyone, I'm just kicking to that guy with the red hat'.

The qualitative studies conducted by MacIntyre and Moran (2007a,b) focused on the role of kinaesthetic processes during imagery and the consequent findings are pertinent to our discussion of meta-imagery control. In particular, athletes reported employing several strategies to enhance the kinaesthetic sensations during imagery. These strategies included holding relevant sporting implements during imagery, and engaging in movement as they visualized. To explain, an elite golfer reported that during imagery 'you've got the club in your hand and you've got the weight there as well, the weight is a big thing really. I mean swinging a pen, you can still imagine it but if you've got a club in your hand it's a lot easier'. This insight from a top golfer corroborates anecdotal reports of elite canoe-slalom athletes holding their paddles during mental practice of course runs (Mantle 1996). Support for the value of this latter idea comes from Guillot *et al.* (2005) who found that imagery content was more accurate when athletes performed visualization in contexts that resembled training or competition environments compared with laboratory conditions.

Interestingly, canoe-slalom athletes' movements were of two different types. Firstly, *synchronous* movement included movements during imagery that are similar to the actual body and limb movements in the activity. As one competitor explained 'it can help … if you move your arms in a similar motion as you're going to move them in the boat, it can help with the timing a little bit more and you can sort of feel how you're anticipating'. One the other hand, asynchronous movement is when during imagery they use their body to represent the movement of an external object. The participants from canoe-slalom and motor-racing tilted their hands to convey changes in the orientation of the kayak or monocoque, respectively. In other words, the participants were using their hands to represent the orientation of an object, rather than moving their hand in synchrony with their expected limb position to perform a paddle stroke or drive a racing car. Thus for elite level athletes meta-imagery control, based on these initial findings, would appear to be vital.

Interestingly, the above findings call into question some of our underlying assumptions about imagery and pose challenge for researchers in terms of both practice and theory. While practitioners may see the benefit of movement during imagery (e.g., advocates of a PETTLEP approach), the application of either synchronous or asynchronous movement during imagery, while plausible, has not been tested adequately for it to be adopted on a widespread basis. Next, the theoretical ramifications are two-fold. Firstly, if motor imagery and action are occurring simultaneously, is the imagery primarily visual (or other senses) and the motor execution merely supplementing this input or alternatively, is motor imagery *per se* leading to the motor execution itself? Some evidence for the latter process is derived from research by Nikulin *et al.* who attempted to classify motor imagery into simulation without the intention to move or as volitional movements which are minimized by the subject to such an extent that finally they become undetectable by objective measures, termed *quasi-movements* (Nikulin *et al.* 2008). Furthermore, a fundamental premise of motor imagery is that it occurs in the absence of movement, for example, Zimmerman-Schlattler *et al.* describe it as active process during which a specific action is reproduced within working memory without any real movements (Zimmerman-Schlattler *et al.* 2008). However, given that athletes may be augmenting their motor imagery with quasi-movements or executed movements, it may be worth re-visiting our definitions of motor imagery to encompass the movements that occur during imagery. A motor cognition approach would facilitate the study of motor imagery, quasi-movements, and execution as it postulates that they are all on a representation-action continuum (Jeannerod 2006). Interestingly, contemporary researchers have advocated a re-examination of the approach that views imagery in different modalities as being distinct and separable in absolute terms (Munzert 2009). Similarly, at least in practice, evidence exists that distinguishing between overt movements and motor imagery may not always be possible.

So far, we have discussed some preliminary findings on aspects of meta-imagery processes in athletes. However, just as we pointed out above the limitations of a descriptive approach to imagery use research, we must also acknowledge that without an underlying theoretical foundation, we are limited in our ability to explain, test, and predict how meta-imagery interacts with other components of imagery to facilitate athletic performance. Therefore, in an effort to address this gap, we shall now consider some recent theoretical models of imagery processes in athletes.

Models of imagery processes in elite athletes: the role of meta-imagery

At least seven theoretical models of imagery processes in athletes have been postulated over the past decade (see Table 16.1). These models include the Applied Model of Imagery Use in Sport

Table 16.1 Recent theoretical accounts of mental imagery in sport

Authors	Model	Findings
Martin *et al.* (1999)	AMIUS	Focuses on content as key determinant in imagery effectiveness, in light of research indicating motivational use of imagery, so timely
Holmes and Collins (2001)	PETTLEP	Focus on motor imagery and provides guidelines for application. Some research indicates PETTLEP oriented interventions more effective than MP, but need for examination of interpretation of functional equivalence
Watt *et al.* (2004)	Sport Imagery Ability Model	Concentrates on role of different modalities in imagery, or the quality and nature of the image, rather than the content. Requires further research to test components of model
Fournier *et al.* (2008)	Tripartite Working Model	Emphasis on function, characteristics and situation of the image for the athlete. Qualitative studies guided development of model but relative importance of the three factors needs to be determined
Murphy *et al.* (2008)	Neurocognitive Model of Imagery in Sport, Exercise and Dance	Comprehensive, moves beyond application to explore cognitive processes, function, outcomes, and interaction with self-talk. Laudable in its aims and breadth, it even includes spontaneous imagery; but while it describes and accounts for findings in the field, it does not strictly provide testable hypotheses
Guillot and Collet (2008)	Motor Imagery Integrative Model in Sport	The authors include a role for imagery in rehabilitation and explore the role of environmental factors, individual differences including the level of expertise of the athlete

(AMIUS; Martin *et al.* 1999), the PETTLEP model (Holmes and Collins 2001), the Sport Imagery Ability Model (Watt *et al.* 2004), the Tripartite Working Model (Fournier *et al.* 2008), the Neurocognitive Model of Imagery in Sport, Exercise and Dance (Murphy *et al.* 2008), and the Motor Imagery Integrative Model in Sport (MIIMS; Guillot and Collet 2008). The key features of these models may be summarized in chronological order as follows.

First, influenced by Hall *et al*'s (1998) ideas, the AMIUS proposed that there are five different categories of imagery use in sport (recall the descriptions provided earlier in this chapter): motivational general-mastery (MG-M), motivational general-arousal (MG-A), motivational specific (MS), CG, and CS. These categories of imagery use are central to the model – along with imagery ability (e.g., visual, kinaesthetic), the outcome of imagery use (e.g., skill learning), and the sport situation in question (training or competition). Although this model has received some empirical support (see Watt *et al.* 2008), its neglect of individual differences has been noted (Nordin and Cumming 2008). Second, the PETTLEP model attempts to provide theory-based guidelines for the optimal implementation of imagery interventions for motor skills. The letters PETTLEP are an acronym representing specific dimensions of imagery, namely: Physical (P: e.g., the athlete's stance, clothing or equipment), Environmental (E: the place in which the imagery will be performed), Task (T: the task or skill to be imagined), Timing (T: the pace at which imagery is conducted by the performer), Learning (L: the adaptation of imagery content to the stage of expertise of the person involved), Emotion (E: the emotions associated with the image), and Perspective (P: whether the image is experienced from an 'internal' or first person or from an 'external' or third person perspective). While predictions from this model have not yet been tested adequately, there is preliminary evidence (Smith *et al.* 2007) that an imagery intervention based on the PETTLEP approach produced significantly improved performance in a gymnastics jumping skill relative to a traditional imagery intervention. Furthermore, while the authors of the PETTLEP model use the term *functional equivalence* in the title of their paper, contemporary researcher has called into question whether there is consensus on this term between sport psychologists (e.g., Ramsay *et al.* 2008) and proponents of functional equivalence theory (see Moran 2009*)*.

Next, the Sport Imagery Ability Model (Watt *et al.* 2004) again proposes a three-tier structure with a general imagery ability factor leading to image generation (e.g., vividness, control), image feeling (e.g., tactile, emotional), and imagery in a single sense (e.g., smell, taste). While the multi-faceted nature of this model is impressive, it has yet to be extensively tested and, for example, the grouping of both emotional content and kinaesthetic aspects of imagery under the 'image feeling' heading has to determined.

In 2008, Fournier *et al.* proposed a tri-partite working model, based on the primacy of the function of the imagery, but including the content, situation, and the characteristics of the imagery. Although this is a working model and has not been subject to rigorous theory testing, it is based on a series of qualitative studies and thus concentrates on the individual characteristics of the athlete. However, given that the underlying assumption is that imagery content and type are based on the intended function, it does not encompass *spontaneous* imagery which has been shown to be reported frequently both among athletes (see MacIntyre 2007), dancers (Nordin and Cumming 2005b) and non-athletes (Kosslyn *et al.* 1990). Furthermore, the authors have yet to provide detail on the role of different characteristics and their relative importance for athletes.

One researcher who has consistently argued for sport psychologists to engage in theory development in understanding imagery is Shane Murphy. Recently, Murphy *et al.* proposed a new model which is the most comprehensive account of imagery in sport to date (Murphy *et al.* 2008). It includes cognitive elements including working memory, attention, long-term memory and both the functions and outcomes of imagery. At this stage its only drawback is that it has not been adequately tested and perhaps that it does not account for meta-imagery differences among athletes.

Finally, the MIIMS (Guillot and Collet 2008) is a global conceptual framework that highlights four distinct 'imagery outcomes' or applications in sport: (i) motor learning and performance (ii) motivation, self-confidence, and anxiety (iii) strategies and problem-solving, and (iv) injury rehabilitation. Guillot and Collet (2008) divided each of these four outcomes into sub-categories (e.g., 'mental and physical practice' is examined under motor learning and performance. It is a notable advance on models, i.e., AMIUS) that were based on Paivio's orthogonal model of imagery use, as the authors outline a possible role for imagery in rehabilitation. They also explore the role of environmental factors, individual differences and the stage the learner is at in terms of skill acquisition in developing an appropriate imagery intervention.

Although each of these models is valuable both in making specific predictions and in integrating theory and practice, as a whole, they do appear to overlook the issue of meta-imagery. While the components of several models (e.g., Fournier *et al.* 2008; Holmes and Collins 2001; Murphy *et al.* 2008; Watt *et al.* 2004) are sufficiently detailed as to encompass multiple aspects of imagery as well as learner or athlete characteristics, only PETTLEP and MIMMS explicitly deal with factors that are relevant to meta-imagery both in terms of declarative knowledge (meta-imagery knowledge) and strategies (meta-imagery control). For example, knowledge of providing environmental cues (e.g., holding an implement) and the role of changing perspective dependant upon function are highlighted in both these models. What is required to understand meta-imagery is a model that has this key construct at its *centre* and explores the role of the commonly reported components of imagery (e.g., function, type, outcome) models in a meta-cognitive context. Furthermore, recently researchers have claimed that meta-cognition is a key component of expertise (Feltovich *et al.* 2006) and this, if proven, should be accounted for in any models that purport to explain imagery in sport.

The functional equivalent multi-modality account (FEMMAC)

An alternative theoretical model of how imagery may affect athletic performance can be sketched now, based on qualitative (Moran and MacIntyre 1998; MacIntyre and Moran 2007a,b) and experimental evidence (MacIntyre 2007). Central to this integrated model is a revised definition of imagery based on the findings that imagery and perception can occur simultaneously (in other words, athletes may be engaging in motor imagery during movement execution). Thus we subscribe to the idea that *imagery is an internal representation that gives rise to the experience of perception and action.* It is worth noting that a component of many previous definitions of both motor imagery and mental imagery is that it occurs in the absence of external input (see MacIntyre 2007). Meta-imagery processes are central to the model (see Figure 16.1) and relate directly to several of the models components.

As is evident from Figure 16.1, FEMMAC Proposes nine components of imagery, which are briefly outlined in Table 16.2. A second underlying assumption of this model is that imagery is posited to be functionally equivalent to perception; in other words they share common brain areas, have similar properties, and are similarly constrained. Furthermore, we propose that this equivalence includes *structural equivalence*, the idea that not just the content of an image is processed similarly in imagery and perception but that the representational format of perceptual experience is embodied in imagery. Evidence for the latter is accumulating and it enables stronger inferences to be made regarding the processes underlying imagery effects (e.g., Borst and Kosslyn 2008). Thus the FEMMAC model assumes functional and structural equivalence across the sense modalities. It is distinguishable from previous accounts which have attempted to encompass a functional equivalent account in that we are not proposing that functional equivalence can be increased or that 'the degree of equivalence between the imagery experience and the physical experience is a major determinant of imagery's effectiveness at modulating behaviour' (Ramsey *et al.* 2008, p. 209). Instead we postulate that functional equivalence occurs not at the level of application by the athlete (the phenomenological level) but that it occurs at a representational level. Instead we focus on the psychological processes that are accessible including meta-imagery.

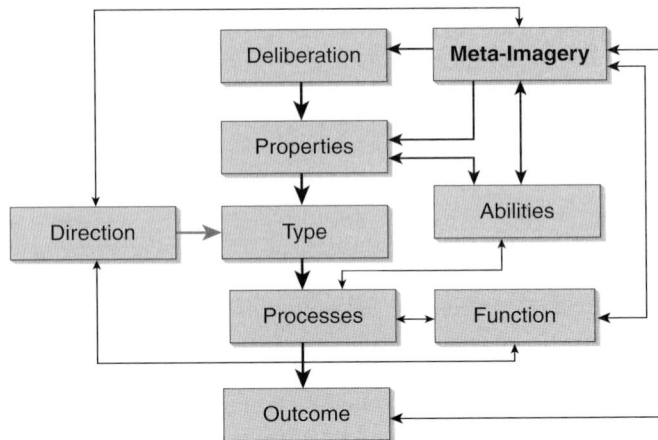

Fig.16.1 The functional equivalent multi-modality account (FEMMAC).

Table 16.2 Key components of the functional equivalent multi-modality account

Component	Definition	Sample of meta-imagery related issues
Deliberation	The level of conscious awareness during imagery (e.g., from mental practice setting to spontaneous or triggered imagery).	When should one use imagery? For instance, should an athlete block out imagery during specific times if it spontaneously occurs. What outcomes are they trying to achieve? Are they trying to employ it for a specific function, to achieve a desired outcome or are they aware of these?
Meta-imagery	Athletes' knowledge of, and control over, their *own* mental imagery skills and experiences, with three parts, knowledge, monitoring and control.	Meta-cognitive knowledge includes understanding of for instance, mental practice effect, mental travel phenomenon etc. Meta-cognitive monitoring refers to their awareness of their imagery and how, if they imagine an incorrect image (e.g., missed putt), they can re-wind their image and re-edit the image. Meta-cognitive control includes any strategy that enables the athlete to adapt their imagery, as in the above example, recalling a prior successful putt to help block out the image of a missed putt..
Properties	The sense modalities (and visual perspective) engaged in during imagery, including emotional and physiological concomitants and temporal characteristics.	Which of the senses are engaged in imaging? Are emotions engaged during imagery? Are any physiological concomitants present? What combination of imagery with movement occurs? Was the image time for the movement congruent with real time?
Abilities	The skill level on imagery abilities which can include specific modality imagery (e.g., visual, kinaesthetic), sub-components (e.g., mental rotation, imagery generation etc.) more general abilities (e.g., imagery use).	How skilled/accurate is the imager with regard to meta-imagery knowledge, meta-imagery monitoring, and meta-imagery control processes? How does their imagery ability determine the properties of their imagery? Which abilities are relevant for engaging different imagery processes and achieving desired outcomes
Type	This refers to the content of the athletes image, and encompasses the types described in the literature including CS, CG, etc.	Is the type of imagery they are employing relevant to both the processes and function of the image? Is the target of the image themselves or another athlete?

(Continued)

Table 16.2 (Continued) Key components of the functional equivalent multi-modality account

Component	Definition	Sample of meta-imagery related issues
Direction	Whether an image is facilitative or debilitative (e.g., recurring negative imagery).	How can one stop debilitative images when they occur? How can one use appropriate 'coping' imagery?
Processes	The cognitive systems employed to create, control and maintain an image including attention, working memory, and long-term memory.	Did the athlete generate an image from long-term memory or was it an entirely novel image? Were the processes fatiguing and did this influence negatively their performance?
Function	The purpose for which the athlete intended to employ imagery including for skill development, problem solving, changing arousal and affect and rehabilitation.	What is the purpose/goal of the imagery? Does the athlete have multiple functions in mind when they engage in the imagery? Did the athlete have a goal or was the image triggered by an external stimulus?
Outcome	The end result in terms of the change in performance, cognitions, or affective factors such as self-efficacy.	Was there a match between function and outcome? Was the outcome achieved and how did the athlete attribute their performance?

The FEMMAC approach attempts to explain imagery as a process from the generation of an image, either deliberately or spontaneously, to the outcome which can be a desired change in performance, self-efficacy, or arousal. While many of the aspects of the model overlap with those of other models (especially with regard to function, type and outcome), others appear to be unique. For instance, imagery deliberation and imagery direction are included on the basis of recent conceptualizations by Murphy *et al.* (2008). Although the inclusion of meta-imagery as a component in this models is a distinguishing characteristic of our model, so too is the 'imagery processes' item. This latter component encompasses the underlying processes that enable imagery to functionally exploit our perceptual and movement systems (see Jeannerod 2006).

New avenues for research

At least three avenues for further research may be identified in the field of meta-imagery processes in athletes. Firstly, additional qualitative studies (especially, those using diary research methodology; Bolger *et al.* 2003) are required to investigate elite athletes' insights into, and beliefs about the strategic control of their own imagery processes. Similar methods could also be applied fruitfully to elite coaches' experience of using imagery. Interestingly, several studies have shown that coaches play an important role in facilitating their athletes' imagery training (see White and Hardy 1998; Short *et al.* 2005) by either allocating time for mental practice or more directly engaging in imagery-based 'talk-throughs' with their athletes (see MacIntyre and Moran 2007a). What remains unexplored, however, is the constellation of beliefs about motor imagery that expert coaches have built up from their competitive experience. Such beliefs could play a vital role in mediating coach–athlete communication about the choice of mental skills training techniques to employ in a given sport. Secondly, based on the study of Denis and Carfantan (1985), research is required to develop and validate a psychometric instrument designed to measure the accuracy of elite athletes' meta-imagery beliefs. Such a study would be fascinating given the extensive database of empirical findings on imagery processes in athletes (e.g., see Weinberg 2008). Finally, the role of meta-imagery processes needs to be formally considered in models of imagery in sport psychology. In this regard, the putative components of the FEMMAC model should be further elaborated and tested.

References

Abma, C.L., Fry, M.D., Li, Y., and Relyea, G. (2002). Differences in imagery content and imagery ability between high and low confident track and field athletes. *Journal of Applied Sport Psychology*, **14**, 67–75.

Bolger, N., Davis, A., and Rafaeli, E. (2003). Diary methods: capturing life as it is lived. *Annual Review of Psychology*, **54**, 579–616.

Borst, G. and Kosslyn, S.M. (2008). Visual mental imagery and visual perception: structural equivalence revealed by scanning processes. *Memory and Cognition*, **36**, 849–62.

Calmels, C., D'Arripe-Longueville, F., Fournier, J.F., and Soulard, A. (2003). Competitive strategies among elute female gymnasts: an exploration of the relative influence of psychological skills training and natural learning experiences. *International Journal of Sport and Exercise Psychology*, **1**, 327–52.

Clarke, D. and Morris, K. (2005). *Golf: The Mind Factor*. London: Hodder and Stoughton.

Cleary, T.J. and Zimmerman, B.J. (2001). Self-regulation differences during athletic practice by experts, non-experts, and novices. *Journal of Applied Sport Psychology*, **13**, 185–206.

Cornoldi, C., DeBeni, R., and Giusberti, F. (1996). Meta-imagery: conceptualization of mental imagery and its relationship with cognitive behaviour. *Psychologische Beiträge*, **38**, 3/4, 484.

Cumming, J. and Hall, C. (2002). Deliberate imagery practice: the development of imagery skills in competitive athletes. *Journal of Sport Sciences*, **20**, 137–45.

Cumming, J., Nordin, S.M., Horton, R., and Reynolds, S. (2006). Examining the direction of imagery and self-talk on dart-throwing performance and self-efficacy. *The Sport Psychologist*, **20**, 257–74.

Denis, M. and Carfantan, M. (1985). People's knowledge about images. *Cognition*, **20**, 49–60.

Driediger, M., Hall, C., and Callow, N. (2006). Imagery use by injured athletes: a qualitative analysis. *Journal of Sport Sciences*, **24**, 261–72.

Driskell, J., Copper, C., and Moran, A. (1994). Does mental practice enhance performance? A meta-analysis. *Journal of Applied Psychology*, **79**, 481–92.

Dunlosky, J. and Metcalfe, J. (eds) (2008). *Metacognition: A Textbook for Cognitive, Educational, Lifespan and Applied Psychology*. New York: Sage.

Dunlosky, J., Serra, M.J., and Baker, J.M.C. (2007). Metamemory, in F.T. Durso (ed.), *Handbook of Applied Cognition I*. 2nd Edition. pp. 137–61. New York: John Wiley.

Durand-Bush, N., Salmla, J., and Green-Demers, I. (2001). The Ottawa Mental Skills Assessment Tool (OMSAT-3*). *The Sport Psychologist*, **15**, 1–19.

Evans, L., Hare, R. and Mullen, R. (2006). Imagery use during rehabilitation from injury. *Journal of Imagery Research in Sport and Physical Activity*, **1**, 1–21.

Feltovich, P.J., Prietula, M.J., and Ericsson, K.A. (2006). Studies of expertise from psychological perspectives, in K.A. Ericsson and N. Charness, R.R. Hoffman and P.J. Feltovich (eds), *The Cambridge Handbook of Expertise and Expert Performance*. pp. 41–68. Cambridge: Cambridge University Press.

Flavell, J.H. (1987). Speculations about the nature and development of metacognition, in F.E. Weinhert and R.H. Kluwe (eds), *Metacognition, Motivation and Understanding*. pp. 21–29. Hillsdale, NJ: Erlbaum.

Fournier, J.F., Deremaux, S., and Bernier, M. (2008). Content, characteristics and function of mental images. *Psychology of Sport and Exercise*, **9**, 734–48.

Guillot, A. and Collet, C. (2008). Construction of the motor imagery integrative model in sport: a review and theoretical investigation of motor imagery use. *International Review of Sport and Exercise Psychology*, **1**, 31–44.

Guillot, A., Collet, C., and Dittmar, A. (2005). Influence of environmental context on motor imagery quality. *Biology of Sport*, **22**, 215–26.

Hall, C.R. (2001). Imagery in sport and exercise, in R.N. Singer, H.N., Hausenblas, and C. Janelle (eds), *Handbook of Sport Psychology*. 2nd Edition. pp. 529–49. New York: Wiley.

Hall, C.R., Mack, D.E., Paivio, A., and Hausenblas, H.A. (1998). Imagery use by athletes: development of the sport imagery questionnaire. *International Journal of Sport Psychology*, **29**, 73–89.

Hall, C., Stevens, D., and Paivio, A. (2005). *The Sport Imagery Questionnaire: Test Manual.* West Virginia: Fitness Information Technology.

Halpern, D. F. (2003). *Thought and Knowledge: An Introduction to Critical Thinking.* 4th Edition. Mahwah, NJ: Lawrence Erlbaum.

Hanton, S., Fletcher, D., and Coughlan, G. (2005). Stress in elite sport performers: A comparative study of competitive and organizational stressors. *Journal of Sport Sciences,* **23**, 1129–41.

Hodges, N. J., Huys, R., and Starkes, J. L. (2007). Methodological review and evaluation of research in expert performance in sport, in, G. Tenebaum and R.C. Eklund (eds), *Handbook of Sport Psychology*. 3rd Edition. pp. 161–83. New York: John Wiley.

Holmes, P.S. and Collins, D.J. (2001). The PETTLEP approach to motor imagery: a functional equivalence model for sport psychologists. *Journal of Applied Sport Psychology*, **13**, 60–83.

Huber, J. (1997). Differences in problem representation and procedural knowledge between elite and nonelite springboard divers. *The Sport Psychologist*, **11**, 142–59.

Jackson, P.L. and Decety, J. (2004). Motor cognition: a new paradigm to study self–other interactions. *Current Opinion in Neurobiology*, **14**, 259–63.

Jeannerod, M. (2006). *Motor cognition: what actions tell to the self.* New York: Oxford University Press.

Kosslyn, S.M., Thompson, W.L., and Ganis, G. (2006). *The Case for Mental Imagery*. New York: Oxford University Press.

Kosslyn, S.M., Seger, C., Pani, J.R., and Hillger, L.A. (1990). When is imagery used in everyday life? A diary study. *Journal of Mental Imagery*, **14**, 131–52.

Levin, D.T. and Angelone, B.L. (2009). The visual metacognition questionnaire: a measure of intuitions about vision. *American Journal of Psychology*, **121**, 451–72.

MacIntyre, T. (2007). *Motor Cognition in Action: Exploring Kinaesthetic Imagery in sport*. Unpublished doctoral dissertation, School of Psychology, University College, Dublin, Ireland.

MacIntyre, T. and Moran, A. (2007a). A qualitative investigation of imagery use and meta-imagery processes among elite canoe-slalom competitors. *Journal of Imagery Research in Sport and Physical Activity*, **2(1)**, article 3, pp. 1–23.

MacIntyre, T. and Moran, A. (2007b). A qualitative investigation of meta-imagery processes and imagery direction among elite athletes. *Journal of Imagery Research in Sport and Physical Activity*, **2(1)**, article 4, pp. 1–20.

Mantle, H. (1996). Demonstration of dynamic imagery with international canoeist. Granstand, British Broadcasting Corporation. Cited in P. Holmes and D. Collins (2001), The PETTLEP approach to motor imagery: a functional equivalence model for sport psychologists. *Journal of Applied Sport Psychology*, **13**, 60–83.

Martin, K.A., Moritz, S.E., and Hall, C. (1999). Imagery use in sport: a literature review and applied model. *The Sport Psychologist,* **13**, 245–68.

Milton, J., Small, S.L., and Solodkin, A. (2008). Imagining motor imagery: Methodological issues related to expertise. *Methods*, **45**, 336–41.

McPherson, S.L. and Thomas, J.R. (1989). Relation of knowledge and performance in boys' tennis: age and expertise. *Journal of Experimental Child Psychology*, **48**, 190–211.

McPherson. S.L. (2000). Expert-novice differences in planning strategies during collegiate singles tennis competition. *Journal of Sport and Exercise Psychology*, **22**, 39–62.

Moran, A. and MacIntyre, T. (1998). 'There's more to an image than meets the eye:' A qualitative study of kinaesthetic imagery among canoe-slalomists. *The Irish Journal of Psychology*, **19**, 406–23.

Moran, A. and MacIntyre, T. (2008, 16 May). Motor cognition and mental imagery: new directions. Paper presented at conference on Functional, Algorithmic and Implementational Aspects of Motor Control and Learning, Liverpool Hope University.

Moran, A.P. (2002). In the mind's eye. *The Psychologist*, **15**, 14–15.

Moran, A.P. (2004). *Sport and Exercise Psychology: A Critical Introduction.* Hove, East Sussex: Routledge.

Moran, A.P. (2009). Cognitive psychology in sport: progress and prospects. *Psychology of Sport and Exercise.* **10**, 420–6.

Morris, T., Spittle, M., and Watt, A.P. (2005) *Imagery in Sport.* Champaign, Illinois: Human Kinetics.

Munroe-Chandler, K.J., Hall, C.R., Fishburne, G.J., and Shannon, V. (2005). Using cognitive general imagery to improve soccer strategies. *European Journal of Sport Science*, **5**, 41–9.

Munroe, K.J., Giacobbi, P.R., Hall, C., and Weinberg, R. (2000). The four Ws of imagery use: where, when, why, and what? *The Sport Psychologist*, **14**, 119–37.

Munzert, J. (2009). Cognitive motor processes: The role of motor imagery in the study of motor representations. *Brain Research Reviews*, **60**, 306–326.

Murphy, S.M. (1994). Imagery interventions in sport. *Medicine and Science in Sports and Exercise*, **26**, 486–94.

Murphy, S., Nordin, S.M., and Cumming, J. (2008). Imagery in sport, exercise and dance, in T.S. Horn (ed.), *Advances in Sport Psychology.* 3rd Edition. pp. 297–324. Champaign, IL: Human Kinetics

Nicklaus, J. and Boden, K. (1974). *Golf My Way.* New York: Simon and Schuster.

Nikulin, V.V., Hohlefeld, F.U., Jacobs A.M., and Curio, G. (2008). Quasi-movements: a novel motor-cognitive phenomenon. *Neuropsychologia*, **46**, 727–42.

Nordin, S. and Cumming, J. (2008). Types and functions of athletes' imagery: testing predictions from the applied model of imagery use by examining effectiveness. *International Journal of Sport and Exercise Psychology*, **6**, 189–206.

Nordin, S.M. and Cumming, J. (2005a). More than meets the eye: investigating imagery type, direction and outcome. *The Sport Psychologist*, **19**, 1–17.

Nordin, S.M. and Cumming, J. (2005b). Professional dancers describe their imagery: where, when, what, why and how. *The Sport Psychologist*, **19**, 395–416.

Orlick, T. and Partington, J. (1988). Mental links to excellence. *The Sport Psychologist*, **2**, 105–30.

Paivio, A. (1985). Cognitive and motivational functions of imagery in human performance. *Canadian Journal of Applied Sport Sciences*, **10**, 22S–28S.

Pitt, N. (1998). 'Out of the Woods'. *The Sunday Times*, 19 July, p. 5 (Sport).

Ramsay, R., Cumming, J., and Edwards, M.G. (2008). Exploring a modified conceptualization of imagery direction and golf putting performance. *International Journal of Sport and Exercise Psychology,* **6**, 207–23.

Rosenbaum, D.A. (2005). The Cinderella of psychology: The neglect of motor control in the science of mental life and behavior. *American Psychologist,* **60**, 308–17.

Shearer, D.A., Thomson, R., Mellalieu, S.D., and Shearer, C.R. (2007). The relationship between imagery type and collective efficacy in elite and non-elite athletes. *Journal of Sports Science and Medicine,* **6**, 180–7.

Short, S.E., Bruggeman, J.M., Engel, S.G., Marback, T.L, Wang, L.J., Willadsen, A., and Short, M.W. (2002). The effect of imagery function and imagery direction on self-efficacy and performance on a golf-putting task. *The Sport Psychologist*, **16**, 48–67.

Short, S.E., Ross-Stewart, L., and Monsma, E.V. (2006). Onwards with the evolution of imagery research in sport psychology. *Athletic Insight*, **8**, 3.

Short, S.E., Smiley, M. and Ross-Stewart, L. (2005). The relationship between efficacy beliefs and imagery use in coaches. *The Sport Psychologist,* **19**, 380–94.

Smith, D., Wright, C.J., Allsopp, A., and Westhead, H. (2007). It's all in the mind: PETTLEP-based imagery and sports performance. *Journal of Applied Sport Psychology*, **19**, 80–92.

Suinn, R.M. (1980). Psychology and sports performance: principles and applications, in R. Suinn and R.D. Clayton (eds), *Psychology in Sports: Methods and Applications*. Minneapolis, MN: Burgess.

Van Overschelde, J.P. (2008). Metacognition: knowing about knowing, in J. Dunlosky and R.A. Bjork (eds), *Handbook of Metamemory and Memory*. pp. 47–71. New York: Psychology Press.

Vanden Auweele, Y., Depreeuw, E., Rzewnicki, R. and Ballon, F. (1993). Elite performance and personality: from description and prediction to diagnosis and intervention, in R.N. Singer, M. Murphey, and L.K. Tennant (eds), *Handbook of Research on Sport Psychology*. pp. 257–89. New York: Macmillan.

Walsh, D. (2009). 'You get only one shot at this – you can't play the game again'. *The Sunday Times*, 29 March, p. 9. Sport.

Watt, A.P., Morris, T. and Andersen, M.B. (2004). Issues in the development of a measure of imagery ability in sport. *Journal of Mental Imagery*, **28**, 149–80.

Watt, A.P., Spittle, M., Jaakkola, T., and Morris, T. (2008). Adopting Paivio's general analytic framework to examine imagery use in sport. *Journal of Imagery Research in Sport and Physical Activity*, **3(1)**, article **4**, 1–15.

Weinberg, R. (2008). Does imagery work? Effects on performance and mental skills. *Journal of Imagery Research in Sport and Physical Activity*, **3(1)**, article 1, 1–21.

Weinberg, R., Butt, J., Knight, B., Burke, K.L. and Jackson, A. (2003). The relationship between the use and effectiveness of imagery: an exploratory investigation. *Journal of Applied Sport Psychology*, **15**, 26–40.

White, A. and Hardy, L. (1998). An in-depth analysis of the uses of imagery by high-level slalom canoeists and artistic gymnasts. *The Sport Psychologist*, **12**, 387–403.

Wilkinson, J. (2006). *My World*. London: Headline Book Publishing.

Williams, A.M. and Davids, K. (1995). Declarative knowledge in sport: a by-product of experience or a characteristic of expertise? *Journal of Sport and Exercise Psychology*, **17**, 269–75.

Woolfolk, R., Parrish, W., and Murphy, S.M. (1985). The effects of positive and negative imagery on motor skill performance. *Cognitive Therapy and Research,* **9**, 335–41.

Zimmerman-Schlattler, A., Schuster, C., Puhan, M.A., Siekierka, E., and Steurer, J. (2008). Efficacy of motor imagery in post-stroke rehabilitation: a systematic review. *Journal of Neuroengineering and Rehabilitation*, **5**, 8.

Chapter 17

The use of motor imagery in teaching surgical skills lessons from sports training

Robert E. Sapien and Rebecca G. Rogers

Surgical training and skills

Scant medical literature describes the use of mental imagery for medical training. One meta-analysis, conceptual report identifies potential applications for imaginary practice in surgery to include: learning a basic skill, diminishing the learning curve for new procedures, transferring skills from existing techniques, delaying the decay of skills, and preoperative preparation for a complex procedure (Hall 2002).

Four recent articles describe how mental imagery has been used to enhance medical instruction for medical students and physicians in training. Sanders *et al.* (2004) report the effect of imagery on training medical students to suture. Using a convenience sample of 65 second-year medical students, three randomized groups were generated. One group received three sessions actually practicing suturing on a pig foot. Group two received two sessions of suturing and one session of mental imagery rehearsal, and group three received one suturing session and two imagery sessions. The outcome measure was performance evaluation suturing on live rabbits (cognitive skill application). The authors report equivalent performance evaluations among all groups and concluded that motor imagery combined with physical practice was a cost-efficient alternative to repetitive practice of a surgical skill. Although not clearly stated in the article, this is presumably due to cost savings in faculty time and materials to physically practice compared with limited physical activity augmented with motor imagery practice.

Also, Bathalon *et al.* (2005) published a study in which 44 first-year medical students were instructed to perform a surgical cricothyrotomy (the entry into the upper trachea to ensure a patent airway) on a mannequin. The students were divided into three groups including a group which performed mental imagery combined with kinaesiology, a group that performed kinaesiology alone and a control group which used standard advanced trauma life support instruction prior to performing the cricothrotomy. Kinaesiology consisted of the physical demonstration of the cricothrotomy technique. The mental imagery was a five-minute session. Performance was evaluated one week later during cricothrotomy with an objective structured clinical exam (OSCE). The group with the best performance had used mental imagery combined with kinaesiology over either the kinaesiology alone or the advanced trauma life support instruction (Bathalon *et al.* 2005).

Two studies in 2008 further support the use of motor imagery in surgical skills training. In the first study, second-year medical students received standard instruction in suturing which included a didactic presentation, demonstrations by the instructor, physical practice by the medical student on pig's feet, and a live animal laboratory. They were then randomized to receive supplemental instruction/practice using either mental imagery or reading a textbook for equal amounts of time. The students who practiced using motor imagery outperformed those who supplemented their instruction with textbook reading (Sanders *et al.* 2008).

Finally, Komesu *et al.* (2009) conducted a multi-centre study on cystoscopy (insertion of a scope through the urethra to visualize inside the bladder) performance, in which gynaecology physicians in training (house officers) were randomized into one of two groups. All study participants were novice to the performance of cystoscopy and had performed fewer than three cystoscopies. One group received pre-operative mental imagery sessions administered by gynaecology faculty (intervention group) and the other group was instructed to prepare using standard of training at the participating institutions for the procedure, which was reading a chapter describing cystoscopy. Participants were assessed by a validated Global Scale of Operative Performance score and time taken to perform the cystoscopy. The imagery group demonstrated better performance as rated on the Global Scale of Operative Performance than the control group by 15.9%. Time to complete the procedure was not effected by motor imagery. The imagery group, however, rated their pre-operative preparation's usefulness higher than did the control group. Although limited in scope, all existing studies on the use of motor imagery in improving surgical skills have demonstrated either improved performance or equivalence with established training protocols. Since imagery is less expensive to perform than actual physical practice, imagery may provide a cost-efficient alternative to surgical training in a safe manner.

Sports training and skills

Sport training encompasses many facets including stage of training, purpose of training as well as the specific motor skill for which the individual is training. Stage of training refers to whether the individual is training as a novice or as an experienced, or even professional athlete. Training may be focused as follows: (1) to prepare for an impending competition or game; (2) for the acquisition of new or improvement of existing skills/technique; (3) motivation for an upcoming competition; or (4) simply to maximize training. Motor skills needed in sports training range from team versus individual sports, strength versus endurance skills, and gross motor versus fine motor skills.

Not only are motor skills and technique important in sports, but physical conditioning plays a major role in successful sport training. Physical conditioning may be building physical strength and endurance, or autogenic control of muscles, pulse, and blood pressure. It has been reported that biathletes trained in autogenic training to steady pulse and muscles, combined with mental imagery, increased their postural control and shooting stability (Paivio 1985; Groslamber *et al.* 1994). Mental state is equally important as physical performance and is the aspect of sports training which does not solely focus on the motor skill required in a particular sport. Mental state includes the motivation to perform, while maintaining the control to perform accurately and to the best of the individual's skill, strength, and talent (Short *et al.* 2005). Mental preparation varies with the individual. While some athletes perform well at high levels of anxiety prior and during competitions (i.e. 'psyche up') (Lee 1990) others desire lower levels of anxiety during competition (Hainin 1980). The ability to regulate anxiety level to improve performance is another aspect of mental imagery that can improve athletic performance.

While motor imagery has been used successfully to address all three aspects of sports training, less is known about using mental imagery to improve performance of other physical tasks requiring mental image manipulation such as architectural design or surgery. In this chapter, we will explore how mental imagery has been used in sports training, as well as how lessons learned from the sports literature may be used to improve performance of other physical tasks, such as surgical procedures.

Imagery has been referred to as mental rehearsal or practice, visualization, cognitive enactment, or motor imagery which mimics a real experience (Short *et al.* 2005, 2006; Guillot and Collet 2008). Imagery, however, need not be solely visual in guidance, and mental practice in only visual terms will not be equally effective for all individuals. As individuals differ in their ability to visualize, many may respond better to an auditory, kinaesthetic or olfactory 'visualization' (Callow *et al.* 2001). A mixture of these techniques may be best as one type of 'visualization' can enhance the experience of the others. Imagery can also be from an 'internal' or 'external' perspective, or both. Imagery from an internal perspective refers to the learner imaging doing a task, while external imagery refers to the learner seeing themselves as performing a task from a third-person perspective. In one study, 53.4% of athletes used internal imagery, 38.4% used external imagery, and 8.2% used both. First-person or third-person perspectives as well as individual ability to image may thus contribute to success of the visualization (Short *et al.* 2005).

Paivio and others have conceptualized that imagery ultimately effects behaviour generally by either cognitive or motivational mechanisms. Cognitive mechanisms are employed in the acquisition of skills and game plans (motor activities), whereas motivational mechanisms refer to the mental state, confidence, and level of anxiety in the sports contest (mental activities). Both cognitive and motivational approaches can be included in the same imagery activity.

There are five specific domains which have been described within these two general categories: (1) cognitive specific (CS); (2) cognitive general (CG); (3) motivational specific (MS); (4) motivational general-mastery (MG-M); and (5) motivational general-arousal (MG-A). CS imagery involves visualization of specific tasks or skills, such as a somersault or pitching a ball. It can be either fine motor such as finger placement on the baseball in preparing to throw a pitch, or gross motor such as the wind-up of the pitcher's entire body for the pitch. CS imagery is useful for skill and technique development. CG imagery ultimately collates CS skills into a general approach or plan. Reviewing strategic plays in a soccer game, for example, are the combination of the individual athlete's skills (CS) with those of their teammates to execute the strategic play (CG). The utility of CG has been demonstrated in gymnastics, canoe slalom races, and football (Fenker and Lambiotte 1987; Mace *et al.* 1987; MacIntyre *et al.* 2002). Athletes who practice CS have been shown to outperform athletes who practice CG only (Burhans *et al.* 1988). Performance of tasks with a high level of cognitive processing improves more by mental imagery practice than tasks which have lower cognitive demands.

Motivational domain pertains to the athlete's state of mind and their emotional state as they approach the sport in general, a specific game, and their performance and self-confidence (Martin *et al.* 1999). The MS domain involves attaining a specific goal, for example, seeing themselves cross the finish line in first place (visual) or feeling a competitor congratulating them by patting their back (kinaesthetic). This domain also affects effort and motivation in a sustained fashion. Golfers who practice goal setting with MS, ultimately practice more and set higher goals then those who used only CS (Martin *et al.* 1999). MG-M helps the athlete anticipate challenging situations which may arise during play by offering them coping mechanisms, hence achieving mastery of the situation. For example, an athlete may use motivational general mastery to quickly respond to a change in offensive strategy by the opposing team. The benefit to the athlete is composure so they can meet the challenge without it effecting their skill, technique, or performance. MG-A is the emotional state of the individual as they anticipate and ultimately participate in the sport. This varies with individuals, setting, and sport. While some athletes prefer a heightened state of arousal or anxiety for a competitive edge, others desire relaxation for control and focus, for example, being 'pumped up' as a swimmer or the calm focus of a golfer.

Beginners versus experienced athletes approach imagery differently. Novice athletes most often approach imagery with a focus on the CS domain. Novices must be familiar with the sport and task to be imaged for the imagery to be effective (Driskell *et al.* 1994). It would not be helpful for a diver to imagine a specific dive if they had not witnessed the dive, even if performed by another individual or still photos. Experienced athletes, however, advance to link specific tasks and personal performance through the CG domain. The emotional approach to performance is through motivational domains and tends to be greater in experienced athletes (MacIntyre *et al.* 2002). A study during motor imagery of novel and skilled hand movements demonstrated different areas of brain activation in novel compared with skilled movements. Novel movements tended to have increase activity in the cerebellum and increased striatal activation. Skilled movements of the same task showed more cortical (especially frontal and basal ganglion) activation (Lacourse *et al.* 2005). Recently, differences in brain area activity patterns using functional magnetic resonance imaging (fMRI) have been reported in novice versus expert and visual versus kinaesthetic imagery (Guillot, *et al.* 2008, 2009).

The use of motor imagery in surgical procedure preparation by the healthcare provider has some similarities to that of performance preparation by the athlete with regard to skill and accuracy. Preparation for a surgical procedure has both cognitive and motivational aspects, much like sports imagery. There is the cognitive element of the medical knowledge base, but there is also the cognitive aspect of the surgeon's skill set demonstrated through technical application, the actual surgical procedure. Learning and perfecting surgical skills involve fine and gross motor skills which are heavily cognitive (Rogers 2006). There is an association of surgical skills with visuospatial applications, psychomotor skills, and stress management which brings in the motivational aspects of procedure preparation. Therefore, the same five domains described for athletic motor imagery can be applied to mental imagery for surgical skill training – CS, CG, MS, MG-M, and MG-A. A CS application may be mentally practicing placing the aortic cross-clamp in a cardiac bypass, whereas the CG domain preparing for the operation may be the critically timed period the patient is on cardiac bypass, from aortic cross-clamping to cardiac re-perfusion. MS domain may include the mentally imagining the surgical team congratulating each other on the efficiency and limited time the patient was on bypass or even informing the patient's family of the successful procedure. An example of a surgical MG-M practiced with mental imagery may be the successful delivery of an infant with foetal distress via an expedient, crash cesarean section. Finally, a MG-A surgical example may be reinforcing mental focus for a prolonged neurosurgical spine procedure. One key difference between sports training and surgical training using mental imagery is that accomplishing all five domains in a single, 20-minute mental imagery may be challenging. Surgical procedures can be long and very complex technically. Dividing the procedure into smaller portions may be prudent in motor imagery training depending on the length and complexity of the impending procedure as well as the training stage of the participant.

State of mind-relaxation and hypnosis

Hypnosis has been defined as 'a natural, yet altered state of mind where selective thinking is maintained' (Simmerman 2007). Hypnosis induces a state of profound relaxation where the parasympathetic nervous system is activated and sympathetic nervous system activity is minimized. In this state of parasympathetic activation, safety and comfort are perceived, and suggestions (such as visual or kinaesthetic suggestions) are readily accepted. This is one condition for instruction and imagery to occur. In 2000, Liggett published that athletes using motor imagery with hypnosis reported more intense 'visualizations' visually, auditory, kinaesthetic, and affective. Additionally, due to the parasympathetic stimulation, control of autonomic function such as blood pressure and pulse is easier. Manipulating these autogenic parameters can be beneficial as reported in athletes participating in skiing/marksmanship biathlons where steadiness of rifle aim during intense physical activity is essential (Paivio 1985; Groslamber *et al.* 1994); similarly a surgeon's hands must be steady. The body–mind connection and its applicability to the athlete in healing and injury recovery are added benefits and may incorporate mental imagery to enhance healing (Newmark and Bogacki 2005).

A summary of motor imagery in sport (Guillot and Collet, 2008) indicates that relaxation may be useful before motor imagery, but may not be useful for the entire imagery session. Although not formally studied, hypnotic relaxation added to motor imagery in surgical skill training may be beneficial. Surgical procedures can be very complex and detailed, at times overwhelming the physician in training. Inducing a state of relaxation and perceived comfort and safety may help belay these feelings and enhance learning and preparation to perform the procedure. Unlike athletic competition, where a MG-A state of anxiety may be desirable for the competitive edge, anxiety is usually not desirable for the surgeon. As the surgeon's objective is not to outperform an opponent, but rather to optimize their performance to benefit the patient, mental focus and MG-M are more desirable for the surgeon. Using hypnosis to achieve a state of MG-A with low anxiety is both feasible and beneficial for the surgeon and the patient.

Proposed motor imagery session structure-preparing to perform a surgical procedure

♦ Schedule the session within 24 hours of the surgical procedure.

♦ Limit the session to 20 minutes.

♦ Know the outline of the mental imagery to be described before beginning the session.

♦ Identify challenges of participants to visualize and incorporate details using other 'visualizations' such as kinaesthetic, auditory, and olfactory.

♦ Instruct the participants to put themselves in a comfortable position.

♦ Instruct them to take a deep breath in and release the breath releasing, 'surface tension'.

♦ Instruct them to take another deep breath and release the breath releasing, 'any internal tension'.

♦ Give them the option of closing their eyes or keeping them open.

♦ Count backwards from 10 down to 1, instructing them to progressively relax their bodies from the head (10) to the toes (1).

♦ This should take less than 5 minutes, but do not rush the process.

♦ Begin CS guiding imagery, again using visual, kinaesthetic, and auditory details (e.g., not only describing visually imagining the surgical instrument, but also the sound of the surgical clamp opening or the weight of the laparoscope in the surgeon's hand may make the experience more vivid for the individual.) for 5 minutes.

♦ Progress to CG instruction, for example, an overview of the procedure from draping the patient to skin incision, through to closing the skin (5 minutes).

♦ Elaborate on the MS domain, for example, imagining the patient in stable condition throughout the procedure, greeting the family with the positive outcome of the procedure (1 minute).

♦ MG-M domain may be challenging because it is best to keep the visualization in a positive, successful image. Perhaps simple details such as 'any bleeding is easily controlled with well placed sutures', indicating mastery (1 minute).

- ♦ MG-A domain guides the participants to imagine themselves focused on the patient, calm and confident with their preparation (1 minute).
- ♦ Allow the participants' time to complete the imagery process (2–3 minutes).
- ♦ Indicate that you will count from 1 up to 5, and on the number 5 the participants will open their eyes, 'bringing with them the sense of a successful procedure'.

References

Bathalon, S., Dorion, D., Darveau, S., and Martin, M. (2005). Cognitive skills analysis, kinesiology and mental imagery in the acquisition of surgical skills. *The Journal of Otolaryngology*, **34**(5), 328–32.

Burhans, R.S., Richman, C.L., and Bergey, D.B. (1988). Mental imagery training: effects on running speed performance. *International Journal of Sport Psychology*, **19**, 26–37.

Callow, N., Hardy, L., and Hall, C. (2001). The effects of a motivational general-mastery imagery intervention on the sport confidence of high-level badminton players. *Research Quarterly for Exercise and Sport*, **72**(4), 389–400.

Driskell, J.E., Copper, C., and Moran, A. (1994). Does mental practice enhance performance? *The Journal of Applied Psychology*, **79**(4), 481–92.

Fenker, R.M. and Lambiotte, J.G. (1987). A performance enhancement program for a college football team: one incredible season. *The Sport Psychologist*, **1**, 224–36.

Groslamber, A., Candau, R., Grappe, F.B., and Rouillon, J.D. (1994). Effects of autogenic and imagery training on the shooting performance in the biathlon. *Research Quarterly for Exercise and Sport*, **74**(3), 337–41.

Guillot, A., and Collet, C. (2008). Construction of the motor imagery integrative model in sport: a review and theoretical investigation of motor imagery use. *International Review of Sport and Exercise Psychology*, **1**, 31–44.

Guillot, A., Collet, C., Nguyen, V.A, Malouin, F., Richards, C., and Doyon, J. (2008). Functional neuroanatomical networks associated with expertise in motor imagery. *NeuroImage*, **41**, 1471–83.

Guillot, A., Collet, C., Nguyen, V.A, Malouin, F., Richards, C., and Doyon, J. (2009). Brain activity during visual versus kinesthetic imagery: an fMRI study. *Human Brain Mapping*, **30**, 2157–72.

Hainin, Y.L. (1980). A study of anxiety in sports, in Stravb W.F. (ed.), *Sport Psychology: An Analysis of Athletic Behavior*. pp. 236–49. Ithaca, NY: Movement Press.

Hall, J.C. (2002). Imagery practice and the development of surgical skills. *American Journal of Surgery*, **184**, 465–70.

Komesu, Y., Urwitz, R., Begum, O., *et al.* (2009). Does mental imagery prior to cystoscopy make difference? A randomized controlled study. *American Journal of Obstetrics and Gynecology*, **201**(2), 218.e1–9.

Lacourse, M.G., Orr, E.L., Cramer, S.C., and Cohen, M.J. (2005). Brain activation during execution and motor imagery of novel and skilled sequential hand movements. *NeuroImage*, **27**, 505–19.

Lee, C. (1990). Psyching up for a muscular endurance task: effects of image content of performance and mood state. *Journal of Sport & Exercise Psychology*, **12**, 66–73.

Liggett, D.R. (2000). Enhancing imagery through hypnosis: a performance aid for athletes. *The American Journal of Clinical Hypnosis*, **43**(2), 149–57.

Mace, R.D., Eastman, C., and Carroll, D. (1987). The effects of stress inoculation training on gymnastics performance on the pommel horse: a case study. *Behavioral Psychotherapy*, **16**, 165–75.

MacIntyre, T., Moran, A., and Jennings, D.J. (2002). Is controllability of imagery related to canoe-slalom performance? *Perceptual and Motor Skills*, **94**, 1245–50.

Martin, K.A., Mortiz, S.E., and Hall, C.R. (1999). Imagery use in sport: a literature review and applied model. *The Sport Psychologist*, **13**, 245–68.

Newmark, T.S. and Bogacki, D.F. (2005). The use of relaxation, hypnosis and imagery in sport psychiatry. *Clinics in Sports Medicine*, **24**, 973–77.

Paivio, A. (1985). Cognitive and motivational functions of imagery in human performance. *Canadian Journal of Applied Sport Sciences,* **10**, 22–28.

Rogers, R.G. (2006). Mental Practice and acquisition of motor skills: examples from sports training and surgical education. *Obstetrics and Gynecology Clinics of North America*, **33**, 297–304.

Sanders, C.W., Sadoski, M., Bramson, R., Wiprud, R., and Van Walsum, K. (2004). Comparing the effects of physical practice and mental imagery rehearsal on learning basic surgical skills by medical students. *American Journal of Obstetrics and Gynecology,* **191**, 1811–4.

Sanders, C.W., Sadoski, M., Van Walsum, K., Bramson, R., Wiprud, R., and Fossum T.W. (2008). Learning basic surgical skills with mental imagery: using the simulation centre in the mind. *Medical Education*, **42**, 607–12.

Short, S.E., Tenute, A., and Feltz, D.L. (2005). Imagery use in sport: meditational effects for efficacy. *Journal of Sports Sciences*, **23**(9), 951–60.

Short, S.E., Ross-Stewart, L., and Monsma, E.V. (2006). Onwards with the evolution of imagery research in sport psychology. *Athletic Insight,* **8**(3), 951–60.

Simmerman, T. (2007). *Medical Hypnotherapy*. New Mexico: Peaceful Planet Press.

Chapter 18

Movement imagery, observation, and skill

Paul S. Holmes, Jennifer Cumming, and
Martin G. Edwards

Movement skill is essential to human development. Throughout our lives we not only learn, and acquire, new motor skills but also refine existing ones, allowing us to become more efficient in our movements. The necessity for physical practice in achieving skilled movement is well-established. In this regard, sport participants and musicians comprise a useful group to consider in that they are highly motivated and spend many hours physically practicing to improve specific movements that will determine a significant proportion of the outcome of their performance. Skilled individuals from these disciplines will have also experienced extensive practice over time and can, therefore, demonstrate relatively permanent patterns of skilled behaviour. Of particular interest to this chapter, however, is that many performers of sport and music regularly engage in additional, more covert, rehearsals of their chosen skill. There is emerging evidence that these rehearsal behaviours may also contribute to practice effects in acquiring motor skill.

Within the sport sciences, two of these more covert techniques, imagery and observational learning, have been extensively considered for skill acquisition, maintenance, and performance. It has been suggested that they can help learners acquire a 'mental blueprint or cognitive plan' (Morris *et al.* 2005 p. 216) of the action intended to be performed. The sport psychology and motor control literature provides strong support for the effectiveness of both applied techniques, with regard to movement skill, and it is generally assumed that these processes are able to contribute to the overall skill profile. However, despite their widespread use, there is a lack of a clear understanding of the efficacy of both approaches with regard to skill. As a result, procedures vary considerably, creating doubt about their contribution to movement abilities.

In this chapter, therefore, we will review literature demonstrating evidence that movement imagery and observation can modulate skill, the central tenet being the extent to which these two processes are able to contribute to some of the plastic adaptations normally associated with physical practice. The direct empirical literature in this area is new and somewhat sparse. Therefore, we will draw on indirect markers of plasticity and skill. We will also propose that consideration of the extent of similarity within brain activity processes between physical practice, imagery, and action observation can inform debate, and allow for predictions to be made, on the efficacy of imagery and observation intervention techniques purporting to develop skill.

In summary, we will consider how two covert processes, with no discernable movement, may contribute to relatively permanent change in brain structures and function similar to those seen following physical practice. We will consider briefly the neuroscientific processes thought to be involved in movement skill acquisition and modulation. We recognize that plastic changes can occur solely through physical practice, as has been shown clearly through research with rodents (e.g., Kleim *et al.* 2002). However, it is more probable that, in musicians and sports performers, change represents a combination of the contribution from physical and 'mental' practice behaviours. Therefore, in the following section, we do not disaggregate the two processes. As affect can been shown to influence skill, we will also consider this with movement imagery and observation interventions.

Neuronal plasticity and movement skill

A number of structural and functional neurophysiological markers have been proposed to identify the plastic changes associated with skill learning. In most cases these are thought to be brought about through a repetitive Hebbian modulation or efficiency of intracortical and subcortical excitatory mechanisms through synaptic and cortical plasticity (see Kolb and Whishaw 1998). Here we use the generic term 'plasticity' to encompass all of the possible mechanisms of neural reorganisation (e.g., synaptogenesis, sprouting of neurons, dendritic pruning, postsynaptic thickening and recruitment of functionally homologous pathways).

Short-term changes

Changes at the cortical level can occur over relatively short time periods. For example, training to perform synchronized thumb and foot movements has been shown to elicit a shift of the thumb motor map towards the map of the foot muscles and back within one hour (Liepert *et al.* 1999). Similarly, Classen *et al.* (1998) showed a shift in the transcranial magnetic stimulation (TMS) evoked thumb response, toward the trained direction, in less than half an hour. One of the mechanisms which may account for such rapid cortical plasticity is a modulation in the strength of cortico-cortical connections leading to measured change in the borders of the motor maps. This occurs through a process of long-term potentiation (LTP) and long-term depression (LTD) (see Shepherd 2004, for the full chemical process of LTP and LTD).

With regard to skill, however, it is the structurally and functionally efficient and relatively enduring changes in cortical properties that might be considered as most important. This concern will also be relevant for claims that plastic changes occur following periods of motor imagery or action observation if these techniques are to be recognised as significant in movement skill acquisition and maintenance.

Long-term changes

The mechanism underlying more long-term change in cortical organization seems to be synaptogenesis (i.e., the development and formation of synapses). Kliem *et al.* (2002) showed that cortical motor neurons of rats trained in reaching tasks had more synapses per cell than the neurons in untrained rat motor cortex. In addition, the size of dendritic trees of pyramidal cells in rat motor cortex correlated with the physical use of the contralateral limb (Jones and Schallert, 1994). Greater the dendritic absorption of pyramidal neurons was observed the more the limb was used. In contrast, decreased limb use was associated with pruning of dendritic trees. Further, skill learning-dependent synaptogenesis seems be cortex-specific. For example, Kleim *et al.* (1998) demonstrated that rats trained to perform reaching tasks showed size increases in the caudal forelimb motor map but not the rostral forelimb motor map. Kliem *et al.* (2002) extended this finding by showing an increase in the number of caudal forelimb synapses per neuron in layer V, the increase being specific to this area.

In a whole brain review, Doyon and Benali (2005) suggested that the learning of motor skills use cortico-striatal, cortico-cerebellar, and limbic (hippocampal) structures for consolidation and maintenance of spatio-temporal motor sequences in response to environmental manipulations. Similarly, Molina-Luna *et al.* (2008) demonstrated that the motor cortex representation for an action expands during skill learning and reverts to its original size once training is completed. Despite the changes in representation size, the skill is retained, rather than temporarily maintained, suggesting that motor cortex must be involved in encoding motor skill.

Possibly as a consequence of these more permanent structural changes, there is evidence that highly skilled behaviour shows a different profile of neural activity to that of the learner or the partially skilled. In this section we will consider some of these differences.

The parietal and motor regions have been shown to be active during skilled behaviour and it is considered that these areas particularly respond to familiar objects and skill related actions. Furthermore, skilled participants show greater activations of these areas when making skilled responses. Evidence for skill activating these brain regions comes primarily from data showing object skill deficits in apraxia. For example, Buxbaum et al. (2005) reported skilled gesture imitation deficits in patients with Ideomotor Apraxia following left-parietal lobe damage. They reported that patients were particularly impaired at gesturing object-based skilled actions such as hammering a nail or eating with a fork. In support of this data, Creem-Regehr and Lee (2005) used brain imaging and reported that imagined skilled object actions activated the same parietal regions of the brain (for reviews see also Johnson-Frey 2004; Lewis et al. 2006). In related studies, these areas of activation have been shown to be greater when made by skilled compared to non-skilled participants. For example, Calvo-Merino et al. (2006) reported great activations of the parietal and motor regions when professional dancers observed a video of a dance performance in which they were skilled compared to one for which they had limited skill. Furthermore, novices showed no such distinction, suggesting that the skill representations must be specific (see Fourkas et al. 2008 for similar effects).

In a novel study of motor experience in high-level shotgun shooters, Di Russo et al. (2005) identified significant changes in the electrical characteristics of shooting participants' movement-related cortical potentials: the bereitschaftpotentials and negative slope. These markers of motor preparation for voluntary movements were longer, and amplitudes were smaller for the finger triggering muscles when compared to non-shooting control participants. The authors interpreted these electrical changes as evidence of increased neural economy associated with skill learning. Of particular interest here, was that all the elite shooting participants in this study were members of national training squads working with sport psychologists and coaches. In all cases, the shooters were regularly using mental skills training and video-based coaching in addition to more traditional coaching (Dradi 2008). The measured changes in movement-related cortical potentials may reflect this wider training regime.

Similar claims for electrophysical efficiency have been made by Hatfield et al. (2006). They propose that skilled performers eliminate task-irrelevant cerebral cortical and subcortical connections and reduce the complexity in the organization of motor control processes. Their review provides numerous examples of superior psychomotor performance characterized by economy of cortical activity. As discussed above, it is likely that imagery and action observation comprise a significant role in the athletes' training programmes.

Most skill learning is goal-directed and so is influenced by our internal drives as well as by the task demands and environmental constraints. Emotional and motivational factors, therefore, might also modulate neural aspects of enduring skill learning. Whilst the research in this area is limited, there is some neurophysiological evidence for a link between the limbic system and pre-motor areas mediated by connections to the cingulate and prefrontal cortex (Schütz-Bosbach et al. 2007). Specifically, Oliveri et al. (2003) have shown a functional association between supplementary motor areas (SMA) and primary motor areas in the control of actions triggered by emotional visual stimuli. The authors concluded that SMA transforms motivations and emotional states into motor responses. Within the sport psychology literature, the motivational influence of imagery is well-known but whether it operates through the mechanisms discussed here remains to be tested.

In the literature presented so far, we have seen that physical practice is important for skill learning, presumably through a combined use of movement execution and feedback. In human learners of motor skill it is difficult to disaggregate the role that imagery and observation may have contributed to the longer term plastic changes, although anecdotal evidence would suggest its significance. However, a number of important questions remain concerning neuronal plasticity and the role of imagery and observation in motor skill learning and maintenance. What if physical practice is not possible due to environmental constraints, fatigue, or injury? What if physical practice is supplemented by more covert cognitive-based practices? What contributory (or, indeed, subductory) changes are brought about through the addition of movement imagery or observation to physical learning? Can these techniques lead to neural adaptation in the same way even when in isolation from physical practice?

Until fairly recently, researchers have typically addressed some of these questions through imagery and observational learning studies that have used motor performance and self-report measures as markers of change in brain mechanisms. As access to brain-imaging techniques increases, some of these studies can now be repeated to reveal the 'true' contribution of the psychological training. In many cases, researchers focus on the topographic match and temporal similarity in brain activity to support the theoretical justification for imagery and observation. The current evidence for this claim looks strong, albeit with some anomalies. Therefore we will review some of this literature and propose directions for applied work wishing to exploit this neural similarity.

Shared representation for movement imagery, observation, and execution: a mechanism for motor skill development?

Given that imagery and observation are assumed to have the potential to produce skill learning in a way similar to physical practice, then it seems likely that there are some shared neural substrates between motor imagery and action execution. For this proposition to hold true, these substrates should be active during action imagery, action observation, execution preparation, and anticipation, and, in some cases, actual motoric production. In the preceding chapters, support has been provided arguing for this 'shared' neural substrate between motor imagery and action execution. Whilst there is currently considerable debate as to the extent and exactness of the shared substrate (see Neuroimaging in the Sport Sciences, *Methods*, **45**; Vul *et al.* 2009), each process, logically, has the potential to influence the neuronal state of the individual, and, theoretically, could influence the other processes.

In this book, some authors have also demonstrated the similar peripheral effects of motor imagery on, for example, corticospinal facilitation (Chapter 4), electromyographic activity (Chapter 6), and autonomic nervous system activities (Chapter 7). These responses may reflect further similarity in the shared representation for motor preparation. During the covert behaviours, imagery or observation may activate forward loops in parietal cotex (see Wolpert *et al.* 1995; Wolpert and Kawato 1998). In addition, this activity in sensorimotor cortex may further enhance the development of the motor representation for skill learning.

Research associated with movement imagery and observation has generally shown that the techniques can also influence skill through the plastic mechanisms similar to those described in the section above (e.g. synaptopgenesis; dendritic pruning). Therefore, we will use the concept of shared motor representation to consider plastic change associated with imagery and observation strategies in the context of motor skill learning.

The authors of a number of neuroscientific experiments have interpreted their findings in support of this shared neuronal circuit idea (see meta-analysis by Grèzes and Decety 2001). The shared circuit concept is intuitively attractive,[1] and provides a strong theoretical model to support the inclusion of movement imagery and observation in skill learning. However, as stated earlier, the exactness of shared neural substrate is still under some discussion. For example, there is debate over whether primary motor cortex (M1) is active during movement imagery (see Chapter 3) and observation. Where activity has been recorded, there is further debate over its meaning. In the context of skilled behaviour, the concept of neural efficiency suggests reduced cortical functioning for advanced skill. This challenges whether M1 should be active at all during skilled behaviour. This issue is important. If shared neural substrates are argued to underpin the process by which imagery and observation support skill learning and maintenance, then controlling the variables that influence the extent and accuracy of the sharing must be considered. It is our belief that some of the variability found in studies comparing movement imagery, observation, and action execution can be attributed to the design of the procedure for the imagery and/or observation process. In addition, we have new evidence from our TMS studies which suggests that M1 activity, during action observation, may reflect inhibitory responses. This idea remains to be tested further.

Therefore, we suggest that research should attempt to address issues of neural sharing more fully and attempt to control for, and optimize, the 'functional equivalence' or shared substrates between the three processes through detailed consideration of the behaviours adopted during motor imagery and action observation. Some of the techniques that attempt to do this will be discussed later.

Shared representation: differences and similarities in neural substrates

Differences in neural substrates

Observation and imagery interventions are both mental practice techniques that are regularly used to contribute to the overall skill development profile. However, a key difference between them is that self-generated imagery tends to originate from an internal stimulus (i.e. recalled from long-term memory) whilst observation occurs by viewing an external model demonstrating the skill either live or from a video recording (McCullagh and Weiss 2001, 2002). Therefore, self-generated imagery, at a basic level, might be considered as a 'top-down', memory-driven process. In contrast, observation might be considered more 'bottom-up' and percept-driven (although we recognize the importance of top-down intentions in the observation process). Motor imagery techniques should, according to this consideration, show fewer neural similarities to motor execution as the perceptual information in contrast is more top-down.

It is surprising therefore that the vogue within the neurosciences has normally been to search for substrate *similarity* between motor imagery and execution (e.g. Grèzes and Decety 2001), and more recently, between movement observation and action execution (e.g. Filimon *et al.* 2007; Tkach *et al.* 2007). It is clearly of interest to consider aspects of convergence, and it is an attractive concept mechanistically for psychologist and others involved in skill development. However, given the differences that exist between the three processes, it may also be appropriate to consider

---

[1] For a detailed discussion of the shared circuit model, see Hurley (2008) which explains how control, mirroring, and simulation can enable imitation, deliberation, and mindreading. In the next section, we will discuss some of these issues in greater detail.

the substrates that are not shared, or are specific to only one process, in their ability to influence skill learning. Further, we propose that the concepts of neural 'functional equivalence' or 'sharedness' may have contributed to an oversimplification in the understanding of movement imagery and action observation. It may be that the amount of direct topographic mapping is less important than critical specific shared areas with shared temporal congruence. The advance of multi-technique approaches to research in this area (e.g. fMRI combined with EEG) may begin to address this concern. Accepting, and working within these limitations, we will use the broad concept of the shared circuit model to support our case in this chapter.

Similarities in neural substrates

The important issue for skill is that if the physical action, movement imagery, and observation share similar neural correlates then many of the procedures shown to be successful in physical practice should also be applied in these more covert mental practices.

The neuroscientific research supporting a shared memory representation has focused on central and peripheral function during the cognitive steps to action: the preparation phase of intending, planning and programming, and execution. A wealth of evidence has demonstrated that movement imagery and observation activate similar areas as those used to execute skilled action (see Fadiga et al. 1995, 1999; Gallese et al. 1996; Gerardin et al. 2000; Rizzolatti et al. 1996, 2001; Strafella and Paus 2000; Buccino et al. 2001, 2004; Ehrsson et al. 2003; Szameitat et al. 2007). For example, Buccino et al. (2001) reported functional magnetic resonance imaging (fMRI) brain activity when non-skilled individuals observed skilled actions made by the mouth, hand, or foot effectors. The data showed that observation of the skilled actions activated the premotor areas of the brain in a somatotopic organization, suggesting cohesion between observation and execution processes (see Szameitat et al. 2007 for similar effects from skilled action imagery).

These studies indicate that action observation, movement imagery, and execution, at one level, have a shared neural representation. Jeannerod's (1994) seminal paper suggested that the shared representation might also provide a motor skill learning mechanism through which observation and imagery simulate actions internally, allowing for skill development or practice independent of actual physical practice. More recent evidence, in support of this notion, comes from the findings of studies of simple movement where observation or imagery modulated subsequent action execution kinematics (e.g. Brass et al. 2000; 2001; Sturmer et al. 2000; Castiello et al. 2002; Edwards et al. 2003; Kilner et al. 2003; Heyes et al. 2005; Dijkerman and Smit 2007; Ramsey et al. 2008). Ramsey et al. (2008) used motion analysis tracking to measure movement responses following action imagery that was either congruent or incongruent to the execution task. Results showed that congruent imagery led to faster action initiation compared to the incongruent conditions. This suggests that action-planning processes seemed to be primed by the prior imagery (see Edwards et al. 2003 or Dijkerman and Smit 2007 for equivalent effects from observation). Similar effects have also been reported from brain-imaging studies. For example, Buccino et al. (2004) used an event-related fMRI design to measure relative changes in brain activity between observation and execution events of guitar chord action. Results showed that activations were largely similar in all observation and execution conditions. However, the period between observation and execution conditions showed strong activity where participants either had to imitate the observed chord, or freely play a chord of their own choice.

Neuroscientific research may also help to elaborate on the mechanism causing the beneficial effects of observation. Indeed, the similarity between the neural processes underlying imagery, observation, and action is now regularly used to explain observation's effectiveness (e.g. Hodges et al. 2007). Since the discovery of 'mirror' neurons in area F5 of macaque monkeys (Di Pellegrino et al. 1992), a wider network of mirror neurons, within the pre-motor, parietal, and temporal areas, seems to be active in humans during both action observation and action execution (for a review see Rizzolatti and Craighero 2004). Consequently, the term mirror neuron system (MNS) is now more commonly used and, despite some recent concerns (e.g. Hickok, 2009), is believed to contribute to the shared neural substrate.

Despite the potential for a testable explanation of the beneficial effects of imagery and observation, only rarely is there discussion of the impact of recent neuroscientific developments on skill learning within sport science research studies and reviews. Horn and Williams (2004) are one of few groups to have emphasized the importance of research that has considered motor imagery and shared neural substrates to advance observational learning. If the concept of shared representation underpins the potential for movement imagery and observation to modify skill, the two processes deserve further, more detailed, consideration.

Concerns with the shared representation model for imagery and observation: implications for skill

Our knowledge concerning any relatively permanent neural modulation from imagery and observation is limited and extends to just a few studies of simple movements 'learned' over a few hours or days (e.g. Lafleur *et al.* 2002; Nyberg *et al.* 2006). However, these studies do provide some evidence that these techniques can lead to distinct neuroplastic changes in the brain. Whether this is true for more complex motor skill, requiring months and years to acquire, remains to be shown.

Typically, imagery and observation conditions do not involve overt motor action. This lack of movement and subsequent lack of any significant direct proprioceptive feedback compromises the extent of LTP and LTD of synapses that is more readily available during physical practice. We accept that both imagery and observation might utilize forward models (e.g. Wolpert *et al.* 1995; Miall 2003), but the contribution to significant enduring plastic change is somewhat limited. In addition, we also suggest that there is evidence to support a distinction between the processes of imagery and observation in terms of their efficacy to access functional cortical and subcortical neural networks and thereby facilitate skill learning. For example, a motor image requires generation, maintenance and transformation which are not necessary in observation conditions. Further, the imagery procedure typically conflates visual perspective, movement agency and sensory modality. Again, these can be controlled easily within observation conditions (for a more comprehensive review of these issues, see Holmes and Calmels 2008). Since manipulation of these factors significantly alters the neural profile, it must also alter control over the potential for skill development.

There is evidence that some regional 'shared' areas, that are reported to be active during action execution and motor imagery, have very different functional roles during both processes. For example, regional cerebellar activity during motor imagery has been cited as evidence of 'shared neural substrate' or of a neural 'functional equivalence' between two or more processes (e.g. Montoya *et al.* 1998). This has been extended to validate imagery-based interventions (e.g. Holmes and Collins 2001; Murphy *et al.* 2008). Cerebellar activity during action execution typically reflects somatosensory feedback for precise, coordinated spatial and temporal control of movement. During traditional motor imagery, however, peripheral somatosensory feedback is significantly limited and, in learners, expected proprioceptive feedback is limited but cerebellar activity is still observed (e.g. Guillot *et al.* 2008). Closer inspection of the imagery-related activity reveals that the specific areas of cerebellum active during motor imagery are not the same as those active during movement execution. In the latter case, the active upper parts of posterior cerebellum are linked to the SMA and pre-motor cortex. Therefore, it is more probable that the activity recorded during imagery conditions reflects the *inhibition of movement* rather than any functionally equivalent activity related to the actual movement production. Indeed, Guillot *et al.* (2008) report that recruitment of the cortico-cerebellar system may be compensatory activity for poor imagers. The concept of neurological functional equivalence is appealing. However, when some areas are analyzed in greater detail, the matching seems less apparent.

It would seem inappropriate to report neural functional equivalence in cerebellum and other regions during imagery and execution conditions purely on the grounds of topography. We suggest that the *specificity* of the activity may be more appropriate to support a functional equivalence or shared circuit model and promote skill learning. Without the specific detail of spatial and temporal specificity, researchers should be cautious about suggesting activity is functionally related to the skilful physical activity. Neuroscience research that has considered skill in musicians supports this contention. Langheim *et al.* (2002) have shown that the contralateral primary motor cortex (cM1) was not active in skilled musicians during imagined performance, whilst activity was observed in functional cerebellar, superior parietal and frontal areas. This topographic profile was interpreted as reflecting spatial and temporal components of the skill, rather than any tacit motoric control. Therefore, it has been argued that, with increasing experience in the skill, the activation sites related to motor imagery may systematically change to reflect a more abstract, less motor-centred, internal representation of the behaviour (Lotze and Halsband 2006). Similarly, Sharma *et al.* (2008) have also suggested that, where M1 activity is observed during motor imagery, its role may be non-executive and perhaps related to spatial encoding. This new and interesting proposal remains to be tested further. If a shared neural circuit model is assumed to be the main mechanism to support imagery and observation's role in skill, it follows that the development of the process should focus on these abstract and less-motoric behaviours for skilled performers, and avoid direct motor activity comparisons.

The cM1 'shift' away from directly matched cortical motor sites is supported by further studies of amateur and professional musicians. Lotze *et al.* (2003) showed that the imagined musical performance of professionals was reflected in significantly lower cerebral activity compared to the amateurs' widely distributed activation maps. Again, the superior parietal and cerebellar shift from cM1 was interpreted as more efficient recruitment of sensoriomotor engrams and increased recruitment of temporal processes linked to the temporal information of the task. These interpretations would be consistent with skilled behaviour in sport. Lotze and Halsband (2006) have also offered two methodologically grounded explanations for the inconsistent finding of cM1 activity during motor imagery. First, cM1 activation during motor imagery conditions may be for a shorter time than activation during movement execution. Therefore, the temporal resolution of the technique used to provide the marker of cM1 activity may be significant. Given the importance of movement timing in skilled performance, this would seem important. Second, the imagined task could explain the different access to cM1. Simple finger flexions and extensions may access more neuronal assemblies of cM1 in comparison to more complex gross motor activities that can be inhibited. Lotze and Halsband concluded that, during motor imagery, M1 activity is intensity- and threshold-dependent.

Holmes and Calmels (2008) have offered two further considerations. First, as discussed above, there is sufficient doubt about the method and procedure to question the process and content of the imagery. Second, the influence of tacit knowledge in the imagery process has been questioned for some time (e.g. Jeannerod 1994) leading participants to make small movements through conscious instructional direction. Both these issues could also explain the variable activity seen in cM1. The M1 may be involved in motor imagery but its involvement is decreased and, in some studies (e.g. Sharma *et al.* 2008), spatially inexact in comparison with motor execution (those neurons that are involved are located more anterior to those active during execution).

Certainly, cM1 activity may be less of a required neuronal correlate during imagery conditions for elite performers. Therefore, M1 activity, during imagined behaviour, may reflect different processes to that during motor performance. Research that employs more consistent and clearly defined methods, where participant's imagery ability is evaluated through a wide range of procedures (see Guillot *et al.* 2008), would be welcome to resolve some of the issues identified here and develop the altered function debate.

In observation conditions, the findings are less clear as the process of observation may directly activate the MNS. For example, Orgs *et al.* (2008) considered electrophysiological markers in skilled dancers and non-dancers whilst the participants were watching dance and everyday movements. Power in the frequency bands 7.5–18Hz (alpha and beta) was significantly reduced (event-related desynchronization; ERD) but only for dancers in the dance observation condition. This phenomenon, it was proposed, reflected an indirect modulation of motor cortex, through a suppression of the central sensorimotor mu-rhythm, by the MNS. Further, it suggests ERD may be sensitive to both observation and execution conditions and a useful marker of expertise for skilled movements.

Physical practice versus movement imagery versus observation: what is the best combination?

Typically, researchers have compared the combination of physical practice and imagery against the separate conditions and a non-practicing control. A consistent finding is that a combined effect is most effective for skill learning (for a review see Jones and Stuth 1997). However, imagery alone can bring about significant and positive effects on performance (Driskell *et al.* 1984). Based on qualitative studies with athletes, imagery has also been proposed to have an effective role in skill practice, error detection and correction (e.g. Martin *et al.* 1999; Munroe *et al.* 2000).

In the case of observation, this strategy is more frequently termed observational learning, or modelling, and the process is widely used by coaches to convey information about a skill to be performed (for a review, see McCullagh and Weiss 2001, 2002). However, to clarify whether there is an advantage to using modelling in combination with physical practice over practice-only conditions, Ashford *et al.* (2006) carried out a meta-analysis on 68 investigations involving a range of motor skills. Consistent with the findings for imagery, the data revealed that additional benefits occur when participants use modelling *in combination* with physical practice compared to physical practice alone; the total amount of practice time being the same in both conditions. Observation strategies are also used by athletes for self-assessment, error detection and correction, and to make coaches' feedback more explicit (Hars and Calmels 2007). Within the sports science literature, the effects of observing a model on subsequent motor skill performance are well researched (for a review, see McCullagh and Weiss 2001, 2002). Indeed, modelling is considered to be one of the most important methods via which learning takes place (Bandura 1997).

Neuroscientific studies of a similar nature have also been carried out for imagery. For example, Pascual-Leone *et al.* (1995) used TMS and motor evoked potentials (MEPs) to map the size of the M1 given over to the muscles used in a piano skill execution task. They compared three groups of participants, with each either performing physical practice, imagery, or no practice for two hours a day over a five-day period. At baseline (i.e. before practice conditions), the size of the M1 associated with the muscles used in the piano skill execution task was standardized. After physical and imagery practice, participants showed increased areas of M1 associated with the skilled muscle execution, whereas no increases in activity size were found for the control group. Therefore, these data show that imagery and physical practice had the same effects on the motor homunculus. Although these findings have not been replicated in applied sport and performance research, the literature suggests that imagery is consistently more successful for skill learning than no practice control conditions, but not as effective as physical practice (Feltz and Landers 1983). This supports the idea that movement skill learning can occur without physical practice, as suggested in the imitation literature (see for example Meltzoff and Moore 1977; Prinz 1997), on the basis that both imagery and observation behaviours activate the same motor learning networks. This points to further commonalities between motor learning through imagery, observation (or imitation), and physical practice.

Stroke rehabilitation literature can also inform our understanding of observation and skill. Celnik *et al.* (2006) used TMS to test action observation memory encoding in adults who had experienced stroke. They tested conditions of motor training, action observation alone and a combination of both, for motor memory encoding, and measured motor cortex excitability. The data showed that the combination of observation and motor training particularly increased motor cortex excitability. The authors suggested that the two behaviours may have converged onto corticospinal action representation, encoding neurons in the M1 allowing for cross facilitation through Hebbian mechanisms, with the two processes strengthening the input to M1.

In a related paper, Stefan *et al.* (2008) explored the influence of action observation learning on evoked motor responses. Based on findings by Classen *et al.* (1998), they reported that TMS stimulation of the M1, associated with thumb activity, evoked a particular direction of thumb action. If participants physically, or through observation, learned a thumb action in the opposite direction to that that evoked at baseline, subsequent TMS stimulation would evoke the newly learned thumb action. Furthermore, Stefan *et al.* (2008) showed that the effects were dependent on the congruency between observed and physical practice learning. These findings are significant since they replicate, indirectly, those that have been found in the applied sport and performance literature in which the combination of physical practice with (motor) imagery has consistently been shown to be most efficacious for skill learning (for a review, see Nielson and Cohen 2008).

In an attempt to control some of the factors that influence the neural profile, coaches, psychologists and other practitioners using imagery and observation for skill learning and maintenance have been guided by various models purporting to address neural functional equivalence. For example, Guillot and Collet's (2008) motor imagery integrative model in sport (MIIMS) and Chapter 16 integrated multi-modality model of imagery (IMMMI) and Holmes and Collins' (2001) PETTLEP model. To date, only the PETTLEP model has been tested to any extent and will, therefore, be considered here.

Applied models of imagery and observation: practical considerations for skill development

In order to maximize the skill and performance benefits derived from imagery, Holmes and Collins (2001, 2002) proposed seven elements to consider when planning imagery interventions, represented in the acronym PETTLEP: Physical, Environment, Task, Timing, Learning, Emotion, and Perspective (for a recent review, see Cumming and Ramsey 2009). The model proposes that, in part, a shared representation is used for both motor imagery and action. The functional equivalence between the two behaviours is brought about through the manipulation of some, or all, of the seven elements. In contrast to traditional, relaxation-driven imagery techniques, the model supports motor imagery manipulations that interactively serve to closely approximate the real-life physical practice situation.

There is substantial evidence to indicate that adopting a PETTLEP approach to imagery practice will lead to more pronounced improvements in the performance of existing motor skills (e.g. Smith *et al.* 2001, Smith and Collins 2004; Callow *et al.* 2006; 2007; Wright and Smith 2007). For example, Smith *et al.* (2007) compared physical practice and two types of imagery practice (PETTLEP imagery versus traditional imagery) for the improvement of a turning jump on the balance beam for junior level gymnasts. The PETTLEP imagery group attempted to incorporate all seven elements in their imagery. For example, the gymnasts imaged a script while standing on the beam in the same gym in which the testing took place, and performed their imagery dressed in their normal gymnastics clothing (Physical, Task, Environment, and Emotion elements). The traditional imagery group received the same script, but performed their imagery at home dressed in their everyday clothes. After practicing three times per week for six weeks, both the physical practice and PETTLEP imagery groups demonstrated improvements in performance that did not significantly differ from each other. By comparison, the traditional imagery group showed no such improvement and was not significantly different from a control group who engaged in a placebo stretching task. Increasing the congruency between imagery and the conditions of physical practice would seem to be beneficial.

Also noteworthy within the PETTLEP model, and of relevance to this chapter, is the recommended use of self-observation (i.e. observing oneself perform at one's current skill level via videotaped recordings) for accessing the correct mental representations during imagery (Holmes and Collins 2001, 2002). To test this suggestion, Smith and Holmes (2004) examined whether the putting performance of skilled golfers could be further improved when an imagery intervention was supported with self-observation. Those who watched a videotape of themselves putting performed significantly better at post-test than a group receiving a written imagery script or a control group who read golf literature. Similarly, Caliari (2008), Li-Wei *et al.* (1992) and Ram *et al.* (2007) all found that a combined intervention of observing video clips and imaging the task led to greater improvements in performance than either modelling-only or imagery-only conditions. Alternatively, SooHoo *et al.* (2004) found similar improvements in the performance of a free-weight squat lift when modelling and imagery interventions were directly compared. In all of these studies, however, participants observed expert models perform the task. The disparity in performance level, between the observed model and that of the novice participant, may result in a less functionally equivalent observation. It is instead more likely that observing-self-as-the model would more closely activate the neural network overlapping between observation and physical practice, and lead to a corresponding stronger effect on performance. In one of the few studies to examine this proposal through electroencephalographic (EEG) neural markers, Holmes *et al.* (2006) attempted to manipulate the neural congruence of the observation and execution representation through manipulation of the physical and perspective elements of the PETTLEP model. EEG data were collected whilst international rifle shooters observed their worst shots in a competitive match on a life-size screen. Four incremental observation conditions were created, hypothesized to provide increasing functional equivalence with the physical shooting behaviour. The least and most 'functionally equivalent' conditions did show EEG profiles as predicted. However, the two middle conditions were less clear. The predicted linear relationship between behavioural functional equivalence and EEG profile was not found. This suggests that simply matching the physical characteristics in observation conditions does not guarantee access to a shared representation.

Overall, the evidence appears to favour the use of imagery and observation as complementary, rather than competing, interventions. As was noted by the elite gymnasts interviewed by Hars and Calmels (2007), prior-observation of a task may facilitate the generation of accurate and vivid images of that same task. On the other hand, imagery may enable performers to better encode and retain observed information (Bandura 1997). Rather than focusing research efforts on determining the separate effects of imagery and observation, more attention should be paid to maximizing the derived benefits for skill learning. For example, whilst it has been used in observation conditions, no model comparable to PETTLEP currently exists for creating more functionally equivalent observation interventions.

The importance of instructions in skill learning prior to the observation and imagery process

We have discussed the importance of clear instructions for moderation of the imagery process. For example, without clear guidance, visual perspective, visual angle, movement agency, and sensory modalities can be conflated and confused. Since the specific task demands to be imaged are essential to skill acquisition, the instructions relating to the imagery procedure have also been argued to be important (e.g. Holmes and Calmels 2008). If the imagery instructions are not clear, the content of the image may be very different to that prescribed both within and between individuals. This significantly compromises the similarity with the physical task and therefore the predicted development of the skill.

The observational neural profile is also sensitive to the instructions that are provided prior to the observation process, and may significantly influence skill acquisition mechanisms. Indeed, Engel *et al.* (2008) have gone so far as to question the bottom-up definition of observation. They report data that identify the important contribution of top-down movement intentions and goals irrespective of the biological movement being viewed.

Participants can be invited to observe movement with no specific goal, with the purpose of later imitation, or to merely recognize the movement. As for imagery, the nature of the instructions given to the participants is important since they can be differentiated by neural activity and, therefore, moderate the potential for skill development. This was reported by Decety *et al.* (1997) and Grèzes *et al.* (1998), which showed that cortical areas involved in the process of observation are dependent on the instructions given to the participants. For example, Decety *et al.* found that the dorsolateral prefrontal cortex and the pre-SMA were active when participants were provided with instructions to observe a movement, with the later requirement to imitate it. In contrast, the right parahippocampal gyrus was activated in situations where there was a requirement to just recognize the movement after its observation. There seems to be a requirement to 'hold' the observed actions within working memory, including motor areas, when the observer has to perform the action at some future time; this may include a form of imagery rehearsal. However, these essential areas are absent if the observer is not required or, possibly more significantly, is not told to observe for future performance. Clearly, the instructions provided to an individual may be as important as what they are being asked to image or the content of the observation condition.

Further practical consideration in the use of imagery and observation in skill learning

In the perceptual expertise literature (e.g. Starkes and Ericsson 2003), the development of optimal observational learning conditions has received some attention. Advances in computer-based technology mean that creating effective simulations for skill development is big business. Equipment is relatively inexpensive and accessible. Using video technology means that individuals can engage in the skill development environment at a self-regulated pace, in and out of season, when injured or fatigued (Williams and Ward 2003). We have already promoted the benefits of observation over imagery in terms of being able to manipulate and control visual content. However, are the benefits of video supported by neuroscience? Milner and Goodale (1995) proposed that different neural pathways are involved for perception and action. The ventral stream (from the striate cortex to the inferotemporal cortex) is considered important to perception and object recognition. In contrast, the dorsal stream (striate cortex to the posterior parietal areas) is linked to visual control of action. The two-dimensional quality of video, and the inferred analysis required during viewing may emphasize the ventral stream. Live demonstrations and physical practice for skill development will, intuitively, effectively train both the ventral and dorsal roots (Williams and Grant 1999). It may be that, as technology continues to improve, the virtual reality and 'total immersion' simulators that are now available will be able to address these neural incongruencies, leading to exciting possibilities for skill development.

Summary

This chapter has considered the role of motor imagery and action observation in movement skill development. The neuroscience literature provides strong support for the concept of some shared neural substrate between the behaviours. As a consequence, the physiological mechanisms proposed to be active during physical skill acquisition are also argued to be active during imagery and observation conditions. There remains some concern as to the full extent and meaning of the shared representation; suggesting limitations for this mechanism to explain fully the contribution of both imagery and observation to skill; although the evidence from studies in cognitive neuroscience and applied sport psychology that both imagery and observation can contribute significantly to plastic change during movement skill acquisition is strong. How these techniques might best be adopted by performers to facilitate long-term motor skill continues to challenging academics, coaches, and sport psychologists but there is no doubt that the input from cognitive neuroscience has made a major contribution to our understanding.

References

Ashford, D., Bennett, S., and Davids, K. (2006). Observational modelling effects for movement dynamics and movement outcome measures across differing task constraints: a meta-analysis. *Journal of Motor Behavior*, **38**, 185–205.

Bandura, A. (1997). *Self-Efficacy: The Exercise of Control.* New York: W. H. Freeman.

Brass, M., Bekkering, H., and Prinz, W. (2001). Movement observation affects movement execution in a simple response task. *Acta Psychologia*, **106**, 3–22.

Brass, M., Bekkering, H., Wohlschlager, A., and Prinz, W. (2000). Compatibility between observed and executed finger movements: comparing symbolic, spatial, and imitative cues. *Brain and Cognition*, **44**, 124–143.

Buccino, G., Binkofski, F., Fink, G.R., *et al.* (2001). Action observation activates premotor and parietal areas in a somatotopic manner: an fMRI study. *European Journal of Neuroscience*, **13**, 400–404.

Buccino, G., Vogt, S., Ritzl, A., *et al.* (2004). Neural circuits underlying imitation learning of hand actions: an event-related fMRI study. *Neuron*, **42**, 323–334.

Buxbaum, L.J., Kyle, K.M., and Menon, R. (2005). On beyond mirror neurons: internal representations subserving imitation and recognition of skilled object-related actions in humans. *Brain Research: Cognitive Brain Research*, **25**, 226–239.

Caliari, P. (2008). Enhancing forehand acquisition in table tennis: the role of mental practice. *Journal of Applied Sport Psychology*, **20**, 88–96.

Callow, N., Roberts, R., and Fawkes, J.Z. (2006). Effects of dynamic and static imagery on vividness of imagery, skiing performance, and confidence. *Journal of Imagery Research in Sport and Physical Activity*, **1**, Article 2.

Calvo-Merino, B., Glaser, D.E., Grezes, J., Passingham, R.E., and Haggard, P. (2006). Action observation and acquired motor skills: an FMRI study with expert dancers. *Cerebral Cortex*, **15**, 1243–1249.

Castiello, U., Lusher, D., Mari, M., Edwards, M.G., and Humphreys, G.W. (2002). Observing a human or a robotic hand grasping an object: differential motor priming effects, in W. Prinz and B. Hommel (eds), *Attention and Performance XIX*. Oxford: Oxford University Press.

Celnik, P., Stefan, K., Hummel, F., Duque, J., Classen, J., and Cohen, L.G. (2006). Encoding a motor memory in the older adult by action observation. *NeuroImage*, **29**, 677–684.

Classen, J., Liepert, J., Wise, S.P., Hallett, M., and Cohen, L.G. (1998). Rapid plasticity of human cortical movement representation induced by practice. *Journal of Neurophysiology*, **79**, 1117–1123.

Creem-Regehr, S.H. and Lee, J.N. (2005). Neural representations of graspable objects: are tools special? *Brain Research: Cognitive Brain Research*, **22**, 457–469.

Cumming, J. and Ramsey, R. (2009). Sport imagery interventions, in S. Mellalieu and S. Hanton (Eds), *Advances in Applied Sport Psychology: A Review*, pp. 5–36. London: Routledge

Decety, J., Grèzes, J., Costes, N. *et al.* (1997). Brain activity during observation of actions. Influence of action content and subject's strategy. *Brain*, **120**, 1763–1777.

Di Pellegrino, G., Fadiga, L., Fogassi, L., Gallese, V., and Rizzolatti, G. (1992). Understanding motor events: a neurophysiological study. *Experimental Brain Research*, **91**, 176–180.

Di Russo, F., Pitzalis, S., Aprile, T., and Spinelli, D. (2005). Effects of practice on brain activity: an investigation in top-level rifle shooters. *Medicine and Science in Sport and Exercise*, **37**, 1586–1593.

Dijkerman, H.C. and Smit, M.C. (2007). Interference of grasping observation during prehension, a behavioural study. *Experimental Brain Research*, **176**, 387–396.

Doyon, J. and Benali, H. (2005). Reorganization and plasticity in the adult brain during learning of motor skills. *Current Opinion in Neurobiology*, **15**, 161–167.

Driskell, J.E., Copper, C., and Moran, A. (1984). Does mental practice enhance performance? *Journal of Applied Psychology*, **79**, 4.481–492.

Edwards, M.G., Humphreys, G.W., and Castiello, U. (2003). Motor facilitation following action observation: a behavioural study in prehensile action. *Brain and Cognition*, **53**, 495–502.

Ehrsson, H.H., Geyer, S., and Naito, E. (2003). Imagery of voluntary movement of fingers, toes, and tongue activates corresponding body-part-specific motor representations. *Journal of Neurophysiology*, **90**, 3304–3316.

Engel, A., Burke, M., Fiehler, K., Bien, S., and Rösler, F. (2008). What activates the human mirror neuron system during observation of artificial movements: bottom-up visual features or top-down intentions? *Neuropsychologia*, **46**, 2033–2042.

Fadiga, L., Buccino, G., Craighero, L., Fogassi, L., Gallese, V., and Pavesi, G. (1999). Corticospinal excitability is specifically modulated by motor imagery: a magnetic stimulation study. *Neuropsychologia*, **37**, 147–158.

Fadiga, L., Fogassi, L., Pavesi, G., and Rizzolatti, G. (1995). Motor facilitation during action observation: a magnetic stimulation study. *Journal of Neurophysiology*, **73**, 2608–2611.

Feltz, D.L. and Landers, D.M. (1983). The effects of mental practice on motor skill learning and performance: a meta-analysis. *Journal of Sport Psychology*, **5**, 25–57.

Filimon, F., Nelson, J.D., Hagler, D.J., and Sereno, M.I. (2007). Human cortical representations for reaching: mirror neurons for execution, observation, and imagery. *NeuroImage*, **37**, 1315–1328.

Fourkas, A.D., Bonavolonta, V., Avenanti, A., and Aglioti, S.M. (2008). Kinesthetic imagery and tool-specific modulation of corticospinal representations in expert tennis players. *Cerebral Cortex*, doi:10.1093/cercor/bhn005.

Gallese, V., Fadiga, L., Fogassi, L., and Rizzolatti, G. (1996). Action recognition in the premotor cortex. *Brain*, **119**, 593–609.

Gerardin, E., Sirigu, A., Lehericy, S., *et al.* (2000). Partially overlapping neural networks for real and imagined hand movements. *Cerebral Cortex*, **10**, 1093–1104.

Grèzes, J. and Decety, J. (2001). Functional anatomy of execution, mental simulation, observation, and verb generation of actions: a meta-analysis. *Human Brain Mapping*, **12**, 1–19.

Grèzes, J., Costes, N., and Decety, J. (1998). Top-down effect of strategy on the perception of human biological motion: a PET investigation. *Cognitive Neuropsychology*, **15**, 553–582.

Guillot, A. and Collet, C. (2008). Construction of the motor imagery integrative model in sport: a review and theoretical investigation of motor imagery use. *International Review of Sport and Exercise Psychology*, **1**, 31–44.

Guillot, A., Collet, C., Nguyen, V.A., Malouin, F., Richards, C., and Doyon, J. (2008). Functional neuroanatomical networks associated with expertise in motor imagery. *NeuroImage*, **41**, 1471–1483.

Hars, M. and Calmels, C. (2007). Observation of elite gymnastic performance: processes and perceived functions of observation. *Psychology of Sport and Exercise*, **8**, 337–354.

Hatfield, B.D., Haufler, A.J., and Spalding, T.W. (2006). A cognitive neuroscience perspective on sport performance, in E.O. Acevedo and P. Ekkekakis (eds), *Psychobiology of Physical Activity*. pp. 221–241. Champaign, IL: Human Kinetics.

Heyes, C., Bird, G., Johnson, H., and Haggard, P. (2005). Experience modulates automatic imitation. *Brain Research: Cognitive Brain Research*, **22**, 233–240.

Hickok, G. (2009). Eight problems for the mirror neuron theory of action understanding in monkeys and humans. *Journal of Cognitive Neuroscience*, **21**, 1229–43.

Hodges, N.J. Williams, A.M. Hayes, S.J., and Breslin, G. (2007). What is modelled during observational learning? *Journal of Sports Sciences*, **25**, 531–545.

Holmes, P. S. and Calmels, C. (2008). A neuroscientific review of imagery and observation use in sport. *Journal of Motor Behavior*, **40**, 433–445.

Holmes, P.S. and Collins, D.J. (2001). The PETTLEP approach to motor imagery: a functional equivalence model for sport psychologists. *Journal of Applied Sport Psychology*, **13**, 60–83.

Holmes, P.S. and Collins, D.J. (2002). The problem of motor imagery: a functional equivalence solution, in I. Cockerill (ed.), *Solutions in Sport Psychology*. pp. 120–140. London, UK: Thomson Learning.

Holmes, P.S., Collins, D.J., and Calmels, C. (2006). Electroencephalographic functional equivalence during observation of action. *Journal of Sports Sciences*, **24**, 605–616.

Horn, R.R. and Williams, A.M. (2004). Observational learning: is it time we took another look? in A.M. Williams and N.J. Hodges (eds), *Skill Acquisition in Sport: Research, Theory and Practice*. pp. 175–207. London: Routledge.

Hurley, S. (2008). The shared circuit model (SCM): how control, mirroring, and simulation can enable imitation, deliberation, and mindreading. *Behavioral and Brain Sciences*, **31**, 1–58.

Jeannerod, M. (1994). The representing brain. Neural correlates of motor intention and imagery. *Behavioral and Brain Research*, **17**, 187–245.

Johnson-Frey, S.H. (2004). Stimulation through simulation? Motor imagery and functional reorganization in hemiplegic stroke patients. *Brain Cognition*, **55**, 328–331.

Jones, L. and Stuth, G. (1997). The uses of mental imagery in athletics: An overview. *Applied and Preventive Psychology*, **6**, 101–15.

Jones, T.A. and Schallert, T. (1994). Use-dependent growth of pyramidal neurons after neocortical damage. *The Journal of Neuroscience*, **14**, 2140–2152.

Kilner, J.M., Paulignan, Y. and Blakemore, S.J. (2003). An interference effect of observed biological movement on action. *Current Biology*, **13**, 522–525.

Kleim, J.A., Barbay, S., and Nudo, R.J. (1998). Functional reorganisation of the rat motor cortex following motor skill learning. *Journal of Neurophysiology*, **80**, 3321–3325.

Kleim, J.A., Barbay, S., Cooper, *et al.* (2002). Motor learning dependent synaptogenesis is localized to functionally reorganised motor cortex. *Neurobiology of Learning and Memory*, **77**, 63–77.

Kolb, B. and Whishaw, I.Q. (1998). Brain plasticity and behaviour. *Annual Reviews in Psychology*, **49**, 43–64.

Lafleur, M.F., Jackson, P.L., Malouin, F., Richards, C.L., Evans, A.C., and Doyon, J. (2002). Motor learning produces parallel dynamic functional changes during the execution and imagination of sequential foot movements. *NeuroImage*, **16**, 142–157.

Langheim, F.J.P., Callicott, J.H., Mattey, V.S., Duyn, J.H., and Weinberger, D.R. (2002). Cortical systems associated with covert musical rehearsal. *NeuroImage*, **16**, 901–908.

Li-Wei, Z., Qi-Wei, M., Orlick, T., and Zitzelsberger, L. (1992). The effect of mental-imagery training on performance enhancement with 7–10-year-old children. *The Sport Psychologist*, **6**, 230–241.

Lewis, J.W., Phinney, R.E., Brefczynski-Lewis, J.A., and DeYoe, E.A. (2006). Lefties get it 'right' when hearing tool sounds. *Journal of Cognitive Neuroscience,* **18**, 1314–1330.

Liepert, J., Terborg, C., and Weiller, C. (1999). Motor plasticity induced by synchronised thumb and foot movements. *Experimental Brain Research,* **125**, 435–439.

Lotze, M. and Halsband, U. (2006). Motor imagery. *Journal of Physiology*, **99**, 386–395.

Lotze, M., Scheler, G., Tan, H.R.M., Braun, C., and Birbaumer, N. (2003). The musician's brain: functional imaging of amateurs and professionals during performance and imagery. *NeuroImage*, **20**, 1817–1829.

Martin, K.A., Moritz, S.E., and Hall, C. (1999). Imagery use in sport: a literature review and applied model. *The Sport Psychologist*, **13**, 245–268.

McCullagh, P. and Weiss, M.R. (2002). Observational learning. The forgotten psychological method in sport psychology, in Van Raalte, J.L. and Brewer, B.W. (eds), *Exploring Sport and Exercise Psychology*. 2nd Edition. pp. 131–150. Washington, D.C.: American Psychologist Association.

McCullagh, P. and Weiss, M.R. (2001). Modeling: considerations for motor skill performance and psychological responses, in R.N. Singer, H.A. Hausenblas, and C.M. Janelle (eds), *Handbook of Sport Psychology*. 2nd Edition. pp. 205–238. New York: Wiley.

Meltzoff, A.N. and Moore, M.K. (1977). Imitation of facial and manual gestures by human neonates. *Science*, **198**, 75–78.

Miall, R.C. (2003). Connecting mirror neurons and forward models. *NeuroReport*, **14**, 2135–2137.

Milner, A.D. and Goodale, M.A. (1995). *The Visual Brain in Action*. Oxford: Oxford University Press.

Molina-Luna, K., Hertler, B., Buitrago, M.M., and Luft, A.R. (2008). Motor learning transiently changes cortical somatotopy. *NeuroImage*, **40**, 1748–1754.

Montoya, P., Lotze, M., Grodd, W., *et al.* (1998). *Brain activation during executed and imagined movements using fMRI*. Paper presented at the 3rd European Congress of Psychophysiology: Konstantz.

Morris, T., Spittle, M., and Watt, A.P. (2005). *Imagery in Sport*. Champaign, IL: Human Kinetics.

Munroe, K., Giacobbi, P.R., Hall, C., and Weinberg, R. (2000). The four Ws of imagery use: where, when, why, and what. *The Sport Psychologist*, **14**, 119–137.

Murphy, S., Nordin, S., and Cumming, J. (2008). Imagery in sport, exercise and dance, in T. Horn (ed.), *Advances in Sport Psychology*. Champaign, IL: Human Kinetics.

Nielsen, J.B. and Cohen, L.G. (2008). The Olympic brain. Does corticospinal plasticity play a role in acquisition of skills required for high-performance sports? *Journal of Physiology*, **586**, 65–70.

Nyberg, L. Eriksson, J., Larsson, A. and Marklund, P. (2006). Learning by doing versus learning by thinking: an fMRI study of motor and mental training. *Neuropsychologia*, **44**, 711–717.

Oliveri, M., Bablioni, C., Filippi, M.M. *et al.* (2003). Influence of the supplementary motor area on primary motor cortex excitability during movements triggered by neutral or emotionally unpleasant visual cues. *Experimental Brain Research*, **149**, 214–221.

Orgs, G., Dombrowski, J-H., Heil, M., and Jansen-Osmann, P. (2008). Expertise in dance modulates alpha/beta event related desynchronization during action observation. *European Journal of Neuroscience*, **27**, 3380–3384.

Pascual-Leone, A., Nguyet, D., Cohen, L.G., Brasil-Neto, J.P., Cammarota, A., and Hallett, M. (1995). Modulation of muscle responses evoked by transcranial magnetic stimulation during the acquisition of new fine motor skills. *Journal of Neurophysiology*, **74**, 1037–1045.

Prinz, W. (1997). Perception and action planning. *European Journal of Cognitive Psychology*, **9**, 129–154.

Ram, N., Riggs, S.M., Skaling, S., Landers, D.M., and McCullagh, P. (2007). A comparison of modelling and imagery in the acquisition and retention of motor skills. *Journal of Sports Sciences*, **25**, 587–597.

Ramsey, R., Edwards, M.G., and Cumming, J., (2008). Performance modulation following action imagery: a movement kinematic study of grasping. *Experimental Brain Research, 269*, 3–4.

Rizzolatti, G. and Craighero, L. (2004). The mirror-neuron system. *Annual Review of Neuroscience*, **27**,169–192.

Rizzolatti, G., Fadiga, L., Gallese, V., and Fogassi, L. (1996). Premotor cortex and the recognition of motor actions. *Brain Research: Cognitive Brain Research*, **3**, 131–141.

Rizzolatti, G., Fogassi, L., and Gallese, V. (2001). Neurophysiological mechanisms underlying the understanding and imitation of action. *Nature Review Neuroscience*, **2**, 661–670.

Schütz-Bosbach, S., Haggard, P., Fadiga, L., and Craighero, L. (2007). Motor cognition: TMS studies of action generation, in E.M. Wasserman (ed.), *Intentional Actions and the Serial Model of Action Generation*. pp. 463–478. Oxford: Oxford University Press.

Sharma, N., Jones, P.S., Carpenter, T.A., and Baron, J-C. (2008). Mapping the involvement of BA 4a and 4p during motor imagery. *NeuroImage*, **41**, 92–99.

Shepherd, G.M. (2004). *The Synaptic Organization of the Brain*. 5th Edition. New York, NY: Oxford University Press.

Smith, D., Wright, C., Allsopp, A., and Westhead, H. (2007). It's all in the mind: PETTLEP-based imagery and sports performance. *Journal of Applied Sport Psychology*, **19**, 80–92.

Smith, D. and Collins, D. (2004). Mental practice, motor performance and the late CNV. *Journal of Sport and Exercise Psychology*, **26**, 412–426.

Smith, D., Holmes, P., Whitemore, L., Collins, D., and Devonport, T. (2001). The effect of theoretically-based imagery scripts on field hockey performance. *Journal of Sport Behavior*, **24**, 408–419.

Smith, D. K. and Holmes, P. S. (2004).The effect of imagery modality on golf putting performance. *Journal of Sport and Exercise Psychology*, **26**, 385–395.

SooHoo, S., Takemoto, K.Y., and McCullagh, P. (2004). A comparison of modeling and imagery on the performance of a motor skill. *Journal of Sport Behavior*, **27**, 349–366.

Starkes, J.L. and Ericsson, K.A. (Eds.). (2003). *Expert performance in sports: Advances in research on sport expertise*. Champaign, IL: Human Kinetics.

Stefan, K., Classen, P., Celnik, P. and Cohen, L.G. (2008). Concurrent action observation modulates practice-induced motor memory formation. *European Journal of Neuroscience*, **27**, 730–738.

Strafella, A.P. and Paus, T. (2000). Modulation of cortical excitability during action observation: a transcranial magnetic stimulation study. *Neuroreport*, **11**, 2289–2292.

Sturmer, B., Aschersleben, G., and Prinz, W. (2000). Correspondence effects with manual gestures and postures: a study of imitation. *Journal of Experimental Psychology Human Perceptual Performance*, **26**, 1746–1759.

Szameitat, A.J., Shen, S., and Sterr, A. (2007). Effector-dependent activity in the left dorsal premotor cortex in motor imagery. *European Journal of Neuroscience*, **26**, 3303–3308.

Tkach, D., Reimer, J. and Hatsopoulos, N.G. (2007). Congruent activity during action and action observation in motor cortex. *The Journal of Neuroscience*, **28**, 13241–13250.

Vul, E., Harris, C., Winkielman, P., and Pashler, H. (2009). Voodoo correlations in social neuroscience. *Perspectives on Psychological Science, 4*, 274–90.

Williams, A.M. and Grant, A. (1999). Training perceptual skills in sport. *International Journal of Sport Psychology*, **30**, 194–220.

Williams, A.M. and Ward, P. (2003). Perceptual expertise: an integrated approach, in J.L. Starkes and K.A. Ericson (eds), *Expert Performance in Sport: Advances in Research on Sport Expertise*. pp 219–249. Champagne, IL: Human Kinetics.

Wolpert, D.M., Ghahramani, Z., and Jordan M.I. (1995). An internal model for sensorimotor integration. *Science, 269*, 1880–1882.

Wolpert, D.M. and Kawato, M. (1998). Multiple paired forward and inverse models for motor control. *Neural Networks*, **11**, 1317–1329.

Wright, C. and Smith, D. (2007). The effect of a short-term PETTLEP imagery intervention on a cognitive task. *Journal of Imagery Research in Sport and Physical Activity*, **2**, 1–16.

Chapter 19

From the mental representation of pain and emotions to empathy

Philip L. Jackson and Amélie M. Achim

In our daily interactions with other people, we rely on our senses to gather much information about the person from verbal and non-verbal exchanges as well as the context in which this interaction takes place. However, in order to reach beyond the observable, we must rely on our ability to remember, imagine, and infer the less obvious and for this we rely on mental representations. Compared to mental imagery, which involves the active maintenance or manipulation of a mental image, for example, of a movement in the case of motor imagery, mental representations can be more broadly defined as the implicit or explicit internalization of a behaviour wherein the behaviour can be a movement, a series of movements, a sensation, or even an emotion. The term action is proposed here to refer to these behaviours when they are linked to specific goals or intentions.

Mental representations of action can be recalled through external information, such as when we observe someone else, or completely from within, when we imagine an action. Recalling or evoking an action does not necessarily imply that one will produce the action. The mental representation of a specific movement triggered by motor imagery or observation does facilitate its future execution but does not automatically trigger an overt response. Similarly, the mental representation of an emotion does not imply the enactment of this emotion. One can think about sadness without becoming sad. Thus, the mental representations stemming from either a performed action, the observation of an action, or the imagination of an action are similar and share several properties including their cerebral basis. These representations, however, are not identical (Jeannerod 2001; Munzert et al. 2008) and the degree of similarity can depend on a number of factors, such as the target of the representation (e.g., self versus other; see Jackson et al. 2006a), the visual perspective from which the action is observed (Jackson et al. 2006b), as well as individual differences such as age (Leonard and Tremblay 2007) and imagery abilities (Guillot et al. 2008).

The sharing of a mental representation between an observer and another individual is thought to be one of the bases for social cognition and complex interaction like empathy. Understanding other people's sensory-motor state has clear adaptive advantages, and understanding emotional signals is especially important in the formation and maintenance of social relationships (Decety et al. 2007). Thus, the shared representations of an action are partly innate and dependant on the sensory characteristics of the target action, and partly adaptive and dependant on the individuals' experiences, including exposure to and practice with the action (Jackson et al. 2003; Cross et al. 2009).

Changes in the representation of motor actions have largely been discussed in previous chapters. This chapter will review the evidence for the Shared Representation Model beyond the motor literature, into the realm of sensations, notably pain and basic emotions. The last part of this chapter will discuss how shared representations are necessary to social learning but not sufficient to empathic understanding and healthy social interactions.

From nociception to the mental representation of pain

In parallel with the multitude of studies that have examined how motor imagery relates to actual movements, including shared cerebral representation between actions and action observation or imagination, a whole field of study has emerged that extended this paradigm to sensations such as touch (Keysers *et al.* 2004; Blakemore *et al.* 2005) and pain (de Vignemont and Singer 2006; Jackson *et al.* 2006c).

The particular case of pain is of special interest for a number of reasons. First, pain is conceived as a subjective experience triggered by the activation of a mental representation through actual or potential tissue damage. This representation can involve somatic sensory features, and affective-motivational reactions associated with the promotion of protective or recuperative visceromotor and behavioural responses, as well as different degrees of cognitive regulating mechanisms likely to involve mental imagery. Several imaging studies indicate that different parts of the network (sometimes referred to as the pain matrix) subserves more specifically, but not exclusively, distinct components such as the sensory (e.g., S1) and affective (e.g., anterior cingulate cortex [ACC]) aspects of this experience (Rainville 2002). Second, the response to the sight of a another person in pain can take at least two very different forms, either moving away from the target (fleeing the scene or preparing ourselves to receive the same pain) or getting closer to the target to provide help or support (prosocial attitude). Mental representations can therefore provide the primary referents from which a rich associative network can be established to evoke the notion of pain in the absence of a nociceptive stimulus (Jackson *et al.* 2006c). While pain perception involves both a sensation and its top-down interpretation, pain representation can be built through different routes, including pain observation (visual input) and pain imagination (no external input). The implication of imagery in the latter is obvious, but we will discuss in this chapter how observation can, in many circumstances involving pain and empathy, trigger mental (and often motor) imagery as well. Pain thus offers a unique sensory-affective state to investigate mental representations as well as the neural underpinning and foundation of human empathy.

Imaging the affective side of pain

Perhaps the first evidence of a shared mechanism between pain and pain observation or imagination stems from a single-neuron recording study of pain processing in psychiatric and neurological patients treated with psychosurgery. The objective of this initial study was to demonstrate that the ACC contains neurons that respond specifically to pain (but not to innocuous touch). The findings not only supported this hypothesis but also extended it by showing that at least one neuron responded to the observation of pain inflicted to another individual, in this case the neurosurgeon (Hutchison *et al.* 1999). It took five years to extend this intriguing (and mostly unnoticed) finding through a series of brain-imaging studies from different laboratories. Recently, a number of functional magnetic resonance imaging (fMRI) studies have shown that the observation of pain in others is mediated by several brain areas that are implicated in processing the affective and motivational aspects of one's own pain. One seminal experiment demonstrated that part of the ACC, the anterior insula, cerebellum, and brainstem were activated when subjects experienced a painful stimulus, as well as when they observed a signal indicating that their partner was receiving a similar stimulus (Singer *et al.* 2004). Because the participants could only see their partner's hand that received the painful stimulus and an arbitrary signal indicating the level of pain of the target (participant or partner), one could interpret such findings as evidence that an arbitrary visual cue can evoke, most likely through imagery, the mental representation of pain. Consistent results were found in an fMRI study with healthy volunteers showing that both feeling a moderately painful pinprick and seeing another person undergoing a similar stimulation were associated with activity in a common region of the right dorsal ACC (Morrison *et al.* 2004). Another fMRI study was conducted by our group to identify the extent of the neural network engaged in the perception of pain in other individuals, and the possible somatotopic organization of the representation of pain (Jackson *et al.* 2005). The participants in this experiment were shown still photographs depicting right hands and feet in painful or neutral everyday-life situations, and asked to assess the level of pain that these situations would produce. Significant activation was detected in regions involved in the affective aspects of the pain-processing network, notably the ACC and the anterior insula, but no significant change in activity was observed in the somatosensory cortex when comparing the activation from painful versus that of non-painful scenarios. In this last experiment, the task of the participants was both to observe a painful scenario and rate the level of pain. While the initial process of observing could evoke part of the pain representation, we think that the assessment process is what leads participants to use mental imagery. In order to provide an accurate rating the participant must hold the evoked representation within working memory, and we propose that mental imagery contributes to this process. In fact, 94% of participants answered 'yes' to the post-scanning question 'Did you imagine how much pain YOU would feel in these situations?'

In a follow-up fMRI study, again using pictures of hands and feet in painful scenarios, we instructed the participants to rate the level of pain perceived from two different perspectives. This time the imagery component was directly manipulated by asking them either to think about themselves (self) or to think about someone else (someone specific that they did not know; other) when assessing the level of pain (Jackson *et al.* 2006). The results indicated that both the self and the other cognitive perspectives were associated with activation in the neural network involved in the affective aspect of pain processing, comprising the ACC and the insula. Moreover, taking the self-perspective, which behaviourally yielded higher pain ratings than taking the perspective of others, involved the pain matrix more extensively, and was associated with activation of the secondary somatosensory cortex and the posterior part of the subcalosal cingulate cortex. Finally, distinct sub-regions were activated within the insular cortex for the two perspectives. The results of this study showed that the instruction was sufficient to modulate the cerebral response and further suggest that the differing instructions yielded different levels of imagery, which in the case of the self-perspective reached some level of somatosensory processing (S2, insula proper). Whether this somatosensory processing is somatotopically organized remains to be shown, as this study did not demonstrate any difference between the brain activation related to imagery of hand versus that of feet. These findings (see also Singer *et al.* 2006; Morrison *et al.* 2007; Zaki *et al.* 2007, for other consistent findings) highlighted both the similarities and self–other distinctiveness as important aspects of pain representation, and they are also coherent with the view that imagery can modulate this representation. In a meta-analysis of brain-imaging studies of pain empathy, we showed that cerebral activity in the ACC and insula related to the representation of pain was distributed in different sub-regions based not exclusively on the fact that painful stimulation was actually felt or not, but also based on how 'close' to the actual sensation the representation takes us (see Jackson *et al.* 2006, for a more extensive discussion of the self–other distinction). This 'closeness' can vary even in the absence of nociceptive stimulation for observed pain and pain imagery, as a function of the target (self or other) of the pain (see also Morrison and Downing 2007 for a discussion on the limits of the shared representation). Pain in others activates more anterior regions that project to the medial prefrontal cortex while pain in self is mediated by more posterior regions that have more extensive connections to regions involved in proprioception.

Beyond the affective representation

Earlier studies of pain and empathy all failed to show any activation in the somatosensory cortex during conditions of perception of pain in others, pointing out one possible limitation of the sharing mechanism for pain. However, subsequent studies, using different techniques such as transcranial magnetic stimulation (Avenanti *et al.* 2005, 2006), magnetoencephalography (Cheng *et al.* 2008), electroencephalography (EEG; Bufalari *et al.* 2007; Jackson *et al.* 2007; Fan and Han 2008) and even fMRI (Lamm *et al.* 2007) were able to demonstrate sensory-motor changes in relation with the mental representation of pain through observation and imagination of pain. The first study along this line showed that motor evoked potentials related to one specific muscle in the hand were inhibited when participants viewed a needle piercing the same muscle in another individual (Avenanti *et al.* 2005). A subsequent study further showed that viewing simple non-painful pricking of the hand was not sufficient to produce the motor inhibition, and that, contrary to our experiment (Jackson *et al.* 2006) specific instructions to change the cognitive perspective from which the stimuli were observed (from the self-perspective, from the other's), did not significantly change the magnitude of the motor evoked potential reduction (Avenanti *et al.* 2006). Using EEG and somatosensory evoked potential, the same team showed that viewing a needle piercing the hand of another person increased the P45 component of the somatosensory evoked potential induced by median nerve stimulation, while the P45 amplitude was reduced by the observation of non-painful tactile stimuli applied to the hand (Bufalari *et al.* 2007). The P45 component peaks early after stimuli onset (< 60 ms) and has been suggested to originate from S1 (possibly Brodmann area 1) contralateral to the stimulation (Allison *et al.* 1992). Using magneto-encephalography, Cheng *et al.* (2008) showed that the post-stimulus rebounds of the ~10-Hz somatosensory cortical oscillations was suppressed during the observation of limbs in painful and non-painful situations, and that the suppression was stronger in the former condition. Thus, seeing the pain in others spontaneously modulates somatosensory activity. This largely bottom-up response does not require imagery processes *per se*, but as discussed previously, imagery could potentially modulate the cerebral response related to somatosensory processing.

A more recent fMRI study capitalized on the possible difference between sensory and affective dimensions of pain and asked participants to focus either on one or the other in different conditions. The instructions changed between conditions from 'How much does it hurt?' (i.e., sensory aspect) to 'How unpleasant is it?' (i.e., affective aspect). As predicted, they found more activity in contralateral S1 when the focus was on the sensory dimension as opposed to the affective one (Lamm *et al.* 2007). Typically, the way to explain the difference between intensity and unpleasantness to participants in such experiments involves relating the former with the location where it hurts and the level as per a thermostat, and the latter with the way one feels, the emotion caused by the stimuli. Again, this argues that by using instructions that manipulate the imagery process taking place during observation and assessment of pain in others, either by changing the target person or the target dimension of the stimuli, it is possible to change the underlying functional cerebral organization.

A further demonstration of the specificity of the change in the somatosensory response during the observation and assessment of pain in others comes from recent results from our laboratory using EEG and non-painful tactile stimulation on the hand at a fixed frequency of 25 Hz (Jackson *et al.* 2007). By extracting specific time-frequency EEG components, we showed that the observation of hands and feet in potentially painful situations decreased the amplitude of the cerebral response in the contralateral parieto-occipital region, and that this diminution was greatest for the hand in pain condition compared to the hand in no pain, foot in pain, and foot in no pain conditions. This finding suggests that somatosensory cortical excitability can be modulated and, in this case, decreased, by the visual processing of pain stimuli during observation. This study did not allow us to determine whether the decreased somatosensory response was due to the automatic somatosensory resonance with the scenario, the assessment procedure that leads participants to use imagery to determine the level of pain shown, or both. Subsequent experiments by our group and others will try to better isolate these processes.

Altogether the more recent studies using mostly magneto-electric techniques support the notion that pain empathy taps not only the affective but also the sensory-discriminative component of pain processing. One explanation for the lack of sensory-discriminative activations in earlier studies may come from the fact that different components of the pain representation stemming from pain observation or pain imagination are triggered at different moments following the initial perception of the stimuli, as suggested by a recent report using EEG (Fan and Han 2008). One could propose that when imagery is involved in pain representation, it tends to be during the later stages.

One crucial difference in the types of stimuli used to trigger empathy for the pain of others in the different studies is also a source of potential disparity in the literature. While the bulk of studies have used stimuli of body parts receiving a painful stimulation, some have examined the cerebral response to the facial expression of pain in others (Botvinick *et al.* 2005; Simon *et al.* 2006; Saarela *et al.* 2007). These latter studies also report significant levels of activation within the ACC and insula in most conditions. The study by Simon *et al.* (2006) is particularly intriguing as it showed very different patterns of results between viewing male versus female models. In fact, the increased activation found in the amygdala, perigenual ACC, and somatosensory area during the viewing of male facial expressions of pain was shifted to a decrease in activation when participants of both sex looked at female facial expressions. One of the interpretation of the authors is that difference could be related to the fact that males generally express less pain than females and thus for similar levels of facial expression of pain, male expression are interpreted as being related to a more noxious stimuli. We would add that participants likely imagine that the males receive a more intense stimulus.

Factors contributing to the quality of pain representation

The latest studies on pain representation through observation and imagery have shifted their focus towards a number of factors that can modulate the level of representation one can establish through pain observation. One study by Gu and Han (2007) showed using fMRI that the typical regions of the cerebral pain matrix were activated (ACC/paracingulate, right insula/putamen, parietal, postcentral gyrus, occipitotemporal cortex) when participants assessed the pain of either real pictures of limbs or cartoon representations of same limbs, but the ACC activity associated with pain observation was stronger for the pictures than for the cartoons. Even more interesting was the finding that these pain-related activations were not found when participants observed the same stimuli but were asked to count the number of limbs instead of trying to assess the pain level. These results support the idea that the degree of reality of the stimuli, as well as top-down attention constraints, can modulate the level of involvement of the pain matrix during the observation of pain in others.

The level of experience with a specific situation can also change the cerebral response to the observation of a potentially painful situation. Cheng and colleagues (2007) demonstrated that physicians familiar with the practice of acupuncture responded differently than naïve participants to this practice. While the latter group showed the typical pain response including activation in the anterior insula, somatosensory cortices, and ACC, the former group did not. Moreover, the physicians showed additional activations in the medial and superior prefrontal cortices, as well as the temporoparietal junction, two regions known to be associated with emotion regulation and mentalizing (i.e., the ability to make inferences about mental states such as emotions, desires, and beliefs; Frith and Frith 2006) processes. This suggests that, with experience, people might be suppressing a typically automatic response to the pain of others. Note that changes in brain activity in these regulation-related regions were also reported in an fMRI study that compared a condition in which participants were told that the limb had been anaesthetised with another condition using the same scenarios without the pain control manipulation (Lamm *et al.* 2007). So the level of experience as well as specific knowledge about a situation can modulate the level of activity measured in the pain matrix and also involve additional regulating systems.

The gender of the observer has also been found in some circumstances to affect the cerebral response to the pain of others (e.g., Simon *et al.* 2006; Han *et al.* 2008). One might predict from the Shared Representation Model that the more we look at the target, the more the pain of others will resonate with our own system and the more pain we will attribute to others. But in fact, at the behavioural level, at least four of our recent studies on the observation of pain in others showed a significant gender difference with pain ratings of female being systematically higher than those of male, regardless of the gender of the target (Michon and Jackson 2008). Conversely, as suggested by the findings of Simon *et al.* described above (Simon *et al.* 2006), which used facial expressions of pain, the gender of the target being observed, regardless of the gender of the observer, can also play an important role in the attribution of pain to others. More studies need to explore the interaction between the gender of the model and the gender of the observer in order to get a better understanding of how this factor affects empathy for pain. It is clear, however, that both top-down learned processes which often rely on mental imagery (e.g., perspective-taking) and more automatic bottom-up processes (e.g., sensori-motor resonance) are involved in pain observation. The relationship between specific personality traits and the cerebral response to the pain of others is also likely to provide some answers along this line (e.g., Avenanti *et al.* 2008; Fecteau *et al.* 2008).

Interaction between pain and empathy

Based on the evidence that observing pain and the first-hand experience of pain share a number of neurophysiological processes, it is expected that experiencing both at the same time yields some additive or interactive mechanisms. In one experiment that we conducted, we showed that healthy participants generally overrated facial expressions of pain while they were themselves in pain (Ly *et al.* 2007). However, this pattern was not linear. Indeed, compared to non-painful warm stimulations, nociceptive stimulations increased the ratings of pain expression attributed to faces expressing low and moderate levels of pain but decreased the ratings of the high-pain expressions. Thus, the effects of pain in self and pain observation in others are not simply added to yield higher responses (in this case a rating). We propose that participants' ratings which are obtained in good part through imagery processes (for instance, perspective-taking) were influenced by their own state. The level of pain received by the participants was rated 'moderate' on average (5 out of 10), so it is possible that the perception of pain in others is affected not only by the level of pain observed but also by the congruency between self and other's pain.

A recent electroencephalography study using laser-evoked potentials supports the idea that pain empathy is influenced by one's own state. Valeriani *et al.* (2008) showed that observing pain in others reduced a cerebral component thought to be associated with the sensory component of the pain matrix (N1/P1). Further, they found that this somatic modulation of the signal was more important in individuals who rated the pain intensity as higher in themselves compared to what they attributed to others. These findings were interpreted as a demonstration that the pain-related empathic attitude towards another can be biased by one's own condition. Finally, the reverse relationship has also been tested. Loggia and colleagues (2008) examined whether observing an individual (an actor in this case) who draws an empathic response by telling a moving story can change the way people perceive nociceptive stimulations. They found that the subjects who were exposed to the condition in which the actor was drawing an empathic response rated on average the stimulations as more intense and more unpleasant than those for which the actor drew a negative attitude (i.e., telling a story in which the actor took advantage of a person with a disability). This effect was observed both when the actor was also receiving a painful stimulation and when the actor was not in pain, such that the hyperalgesic effect was not related to the state of the actor observed but rather to the attitude the participants held towards him.

Mental representation to reduce pain

The studies described so far had the objective of examining how much pain observation and pain assessment (which we propose triggers imagery) lead to a mental representation of pain and tap into its underlying cerebral mechanisms. Conversely, a number of studies have used imagery processes specifically to modulate the pain experience related to a number of conditions such as cancer, injury, and chronic pain. A complete review of this literature is beyond the scope of this chapter, but at least two different studies are worth mentioning. The first is a randomized controlled clinical trial that takes a holistic psychological approach to examine the use of imagery and relaxation to treat pain related to sports injury (Cupal and Brewer 2001). Thirty participants undergoing physical therapy after ligament reconstruction were randomly assigned to three groups: treatment (imagery + relaxation), placebo (encouragement, support), and control (no additional intervention). The imagery group showed more changes at 24 weeks after injury than the other two groups with regard to knee strength (increased), anxiety for possible reinjury (decreased), and pain (decreased). The second study conducted by our group proposed a more focused use of motor imagery to modulate phantom limb pain (Beaumont *et al.* 2009). A single-case multiple baseline design was conducted in six patients with chronic phantom limb pain. Patients' pain and imagery characteristics were assessed by questionnaires. After a randomly assigned baseline (3–5 weeks), participants followed a 4-week intervention, which combined observation and imagination of movements corresponding to their missing limb, both in the laboratory with a therapist and at home. The home-only intervention was then continued over four weeks. Four of the six patients decreased their reported pain levels by 32–43%. Time series analyses confirmed that three of these patients rated their pain gradually lower during the intervention. Although the idea to use alternate representations of the missing limb to reduce phantom limb pain is not new (e.g., Ramachandran and Rogers-Ramachandran 1996), the underlying mechanisms remain unclear. In our study, the effect of the imagery-based intervention was not related with the level of imagery self-reported by participants but there was preliminary evidence that participants did improve their capacity to produce movements with their phantom limb after the intervention.

Although most of the initial work on shared representations has involved motor actions (i.e., movements), there are now indications that other types of behaviour can show similar properties. Together, the findings from the cerebral basis of pain observation extend the Shared Representation Model of behaviour beyond the motor realm by introducing sensory and affective dimensions of actions that can also resonate with others and be used to modulate pain-related behaviour. This affective dimension opens the doors to another series of studies on basic emotions that are thought to be sufficiently universal to yield congruent representations in self and others, without necessarily having to experience them completely.

The mental representation of emotions

It is well-established that the experience of an emotion is associated with a characteristic pattern of autonomic responses (e.g., Lacey and Lacey 1958). About 25 years ago, Basch (1983) speculated that because there is a characteristic pattern of autonomic nervous systems responses associated with each emotion, a given affective expression, is likely to trigger a similar response in other members of that species. This idea is now supported by several lines of research suggesting that the perception of another person's emotion indeed activates the mental representation of that emotion in the observer. At the behavioural level, shared representation of emotions is supported by phenomenon such as facial mimicry and emotional contagion. The observation of emotional facial expressions in others has repeatedly been reported to produce spontaneous matching of facial gestures in the observer (e.g. Dimberg 1982; Dimberg *et al.* 2000; Moody *et al.* 2007). For instance, exposition to pictures of happy faces increases electromyographic (EMG) activity in the zygomatic major muscle, a muscle implicated in elevating the lips to form a smile, whereas pictures of angry faces increase EMG activity in the corrugators supercilii muscle, a muscle that knits the eyebrows during a frown (Dimberg 1982). Moreover, this pattern is observed even when the emotional stimuli are masked and the observer is not consciously aware of their presentation (Dimberg *et al.* 2000), suggesting that mimicry is an unconscious and automatic process.

The idea that mimicry represents not only a matching of the motor reaction, but instead an activation of the representation of the target emotion in the observer, is supported by studies showing that spontaneous facial reactions are triggered not only by facial expression of an emotion, but also by bodily expression and vocal prosody (Magnee *et al.* 2007). It was proposed that people may 'catch' the emotions of others as a result of feedback generated by elementary motor mimicry of others' expressive behaviour, producing a simultaneous matching emotional experience. It is also interesting to note that mimicry of a target also generates in the observer the autonomic response associated with the bodily state and facial expression being displayed (Basch 1983).

Interestingly, Levenson and Ruef (1992) found that a perceiver's accuracy in inferring a target's negative emotional states is related to the degree of physiological synchrony between the perceiver and the target. In other words, when the physiological state (e.g., heart rate, muscle activity) of two individuals is more closely matched, they are more accurate at perceiving each other's feelings. This was also suggested by our results on the interaction between pain and pain observation (Ly *et al.* 2007). Together, these results are consistent with the simulation theory of mind-reading (Gallese and Goldman 1998), a likely mechanism through which automatic activation of a mental representation by resonance mechanisms brings about higher order imagery processes that enables a deeper understanding of a person's mental state.

At the cerebral level, a few fMRI studies have revealed that common neural networks are activated during the observation of an emotion and during the imitation or the experience of that emotion. For example, Wicker *et al.* (2003) studied shared brain activations triggered by the observation and feeling of one of the basic emotions: disgust. In their study, they showed to participants short videos of people expressing disgust after smelling the content of a glass, and in separate runs presented the participants with disgusting odorants by means of a mask placed over their nose and mouth. Their results revealed that both observing expressions of disgust and feeling disgusted activated the insula, including an overlapping region. These results are consistent with the idea that part of the mechanism for the internal representation of an emotion and for the representation of that same emotion in others is similar. Likewise, Carr *et al.* (2003) asked participants to either simply observe or to actively imitate and internally generate the target emotion depicted by facial expressions. In line with their hypothesis, observation and imitation generated similar patterns of brain activation. These brain regions showing shared activation included the premotor cortex, the inferior prefrontal cortex, the posterior parietal cortex, the insula, and the amygdala. Except for the posterior parietal cortex, these regions showed greater activation during imitation than during observation of emotional facial expressions, but showed significant activation relative to a low-level baseline during both conditions.

The insula and the amygdala are two brain regions typically involved in emotional processing. Activation of these brain regions during the observation of an emotion, and the increased activation in these regions during imitation of emotional expressions suggest that imitating other's facial expression could help to increase/improve the internal representation of the emotion. We suggest that in such a paradigm, in order to imitate correctly, we imagine the mental state of the other person to reproduce accurately the expression. This suggestion is in line with Damasio's description of secondary emotions, which can be initiated either by top-down or bottom-up processes, but in any case involve a rich internal representation, akin to mental imagery, that is added to and interacts with the automatic, pre-organized response (Damasio 1994).

The premotor cortex, the inferior prefrontal cortex, and the posterior parietal cortex are part of a fronto-parietal mirror neuron system involved in shared representation of a variety of body movements. In line with Carr *et al.*'s study (2003), Leslie *et al.* (2004) also observed common patterns of brain activation in this brain network for the observation and active imitation of short movies of people either smiling or frowning. In addition, their study included a condition in which the subjects were asked to imitate hand movements (moving fingers), and they observed common activation of the premotor cortex and inferior frontal cortex for the imitation of hand movement and the imitation of facial expressions. The authors concluded that there is a common imitation circuit for multiple body parts. However, the areas generally involved in emotional processing such as the insula and the amygdala were not significantly recruited in their study, even during the imitation of emotional facial expressions. One explanation for this lack of emotion-related activation is that subjects were instructed to imitate the 'facial movement' rather than to focus on the associated emotional expression, thereby not requiring any imagination of the emotional state of the other. As discussed in the previous section on pain, the focus of one's attention during the observation of another's emotion will likely modulate the level of imagery involved and the ensuing level of representation.

Emotions are complex phenomenon that can be mentally represented both in terms of their associated body expressions (i.e., facial expressions, body posture, etc.) and in terms of the internal feeling and associated autonomic manifestations. These different components are intimately linked, but one can take precedence over the other depending on the context or the specificity of the task. Based on current evidence, it can be hypothesized that the representation of the sensori-motor aspect of an emotion activates the fronto-parietal 'mirror neuron system' whereas the representation of the affective aspect of an emotion activates brain regions associated with emotional processing. According to Carr *et al.* (2003) and Iacoboni and Lenzi (2002), the insula could act as a relay between the emotional limbic system and the 'cold' fronto-parietal network that supports action representations. It is through this combined emotional/non-emotional pathway that imitation (including both conscious imitation and unconscious mimicry) of emotional facial expression would lead to a representation of both the motor and the affective aspects of the emotion. Because this system is not only activated during imitation, but also during the observation of emotional facial expressions (Carr *et al.* 2003), it is thought to play a role in identifying the emotion of others. Moreover, activation of this system is not limited to the imitation or observation of emotions. In their study, Kim *et al.* (2007) presented participants with neutral facial expressions and asked them to imagine the person in the picture showing a happy facial expression or an angry facial expression. When compared to neutral facial expression, imagining emotional (both happy and angry) facial expressions showed significant activation in several brain regions including the amygdala and premotor cortex. These results support the idea that these brain regions (limbic system and fronto-parietal 'mirror neuron system') represents a neural correlate of the representation of emotions whether this representation is triggered by the observation, imagination, or expression of the actual emotion.

The association between the motor aspect of an emotion and the activation of the limbic system (generally associated with the experience of an emotion) is well illustrated by Hennenlotter *et al.*'s study (2009). This group examined the effect of botulinum toxin induced denervation of frown muscle on the brain response elicited during intentional imitation of angry facial expressions. They observed an attenuation of the activation of the left amygdala during the imitation of angry faces in subject previously injected with the botulinum toxin as compared to a control group. The functional coupling between amygdala activation and part of the dorsal pons (possibly the peri-aqueductal grey matter) implicated in the autonomic manifestations of emotional stress was also attenuated in the injected group. Moreover, in the control group, there was a significant correlation between the activation of the left amygdala and the individual intensity of brow movements. In line with Damasio's model of the interrelationship between stimulus driven and cognitive processing of emotions (1994), these results show that feedback from the face can influence the experiential aspect of an emotion, and the opposite (expression of felt emotions) is also known to be true. This also implies that imagery of one aspect of an emotion (expression or feeling) will likely activate the representation of the other aspect of the emotion, and thus facilitates imagery of that other aspect.

The studies mentioned here have all focused on basic emotions, and it is unclear at this point whether this pattern of shared brain activations would also support the shared representation of more complex mental states. These more complex mental states, which include social emotions (e.g., shame), intentions, motivations, beliefs, etc., are not only expressed by facial and/or body expressions, but also require the observer to draw some inferences based on other sources of perceived information, including information about the context, and on their personal knowledge and experience with similar situations. We argue that processing of such complex emotions is unlikely without some level of mental imagery.

Combining subjective measures and cerebral evidence

The evidence for shared representations based on the activation of similar cerebral networks for the observation of a behaviour and the actual behaviour is growing, but would probably not be as compelling without some behavioural and subjective measures to corroborate the self–other correspondence. Yet the evidence from these sources is not as consistent as the patterns of cerebral activations. In our early study, we not only demonstrated that a good part of the pain matrix was involved in the perception and assessment of pain in others, but we also showed that people who attributed more pain to the scenarios showed more activity within the ACC (Jackson *et al.* 2005). In that study, we did not, however, find any relationship with the self-rated level of empathy people reported from Davis' Interpersonal Reactivity Index (IRI; Davis 1983). In their initial transcranial magnetic stimulation study (Avenanti *et al.* 2005) and a subsequent EEG study (Valeriani *et al.* 2008), Aglioti's group also failed to find any relationship between the motor evoked potential amplitude and laser evoked potential, and measures of trait empathy. They did however find an association between the neural response and subjective measures of pain intensity taken with visual analogue scales.

Other studies did find some link between changes in brain activity and subjective measures of trait empathy. Singer and colleagues reported that the higher participants scored on this type of questionnaire, the higher was their activation in anterior insula and ACC during a task where they received a signal that another person was receiving pain (Singer *et al.* 2004, 2006). Jabbi *et al.* (2007) also observed a positive correlation between self-rated empathy and activation of a brain region of interest encompassing the insula and adjacent frontal operculum (IFO). In their study, participants were presented with short videos of people tasting a liquid and reacting with a facial expression of pleasure, disgust or a neutral expression, or were exposed to pleasant, unpleasant or neutral substances. Significant correlations were observed between scores on the IRI and bilateral activation of the IFO during observation of emotional expression of disgust and pleasure, but not during the experience of those emotions. When considering separately the different IRI subscales, Jabbi *et al.* (2007) observed that both the Personal Distress and the Fantasy subscales correlated significantly with IFO activation during emotion observation (both disgust and pleasure). It is interesting to note that both of these subscales measure the tendency to share the affective states of others, be it with someone being directly observed (Personal Distress subscale) or with fictional characters (Fantasy subscale). Another study has addressed the relationship between self-rated empathy and brain activation during observation and imitation of facial expression, but this time in a group of children (Pfeifer *et al.* 2008). Similarly to the results reported in adults (Jabbi *et al.* 2007), this study observed a significant correlation between scores on the IRI and activation triggered by observation of emotional expressions in the bilateral inferior frontal gyri and adjacent premotor cortex (likely including the frontal operculum), right insula, left amygdala, and left fusiform gyrus (Pfeifer *et al.* 2008). In the same study, brain activation in the bilateral insula, right inferior frontal gyrus and left amygdala also showed significant correlations with parental reports of the child's interpersonal skills as indexed by the Interpersonal Competence Scale (Cairns *et al.* 1995).

Overall, even though the relationship between the cerebral response attesting to the shared representation and the self-rated subjective measures is not always consistent, this type of report remains an important source of information for mostly internal processes (i.e., mental representations). It is interesting to note that the studies that did observe a relationship between self-rated empathy and brain activation all used stimuli involving affective representations, rather than somatosensory representations.

Although this idea would need to be directly tested, it is consistent with the fact that the items used in the empathy scales evaluate a person's tendency to assess and/or react to another person's mental states, rather than to another person's sensations.

Moreover, these questionnaires do not distinguish between voluntary/explicit perspective-taking, which certainly involves mental imagery, and the more automatic reaction to another person's expressed feelings, which could lead to mental imagery but does not necessarily involve this process. Perhaps the development of new questionnaires is required; and to achieve this, we need comprehensive models on which to base the structure of the different subscales.

Shared representations as the foundation of human empathy

Altogether, there is increasing evidence for shared representations between self and other for action understanding, the perception of pain in others, and emotion recognition. However, the fast pace with which this literature has grown in recent years has led to a fair degree of generalizations and over-interpretations, in particular when it comes to clarifying the role of this mechanism in social interactions. We have elaborated a model of human empathy that relies on these shared representations as one building block for a more complex framework. Other models have also taken this perception-action mechanism as subserving more than motor acts. This kind of model is important to draw the extent as well as the limits of this sharing mechanism. For instance,

Preston and DeWaal agree with our view that such a system automatically prompts the observer to resonate with the emotional state of another individual, with the observer emulating the motor representations and associated autonomic and somatic responses of the observed target (Preston and DeWaal 2002). Others have proposed that the perception-action coupling mechanism offers an interesting foundation for intersubjectivity because it provides a functional bridge between first-person (self) information and third-person (other) information, an implicit connection between the self and the other (Decety and Sommerville 2003). In order to use this representation within a social context after the initial resonance mechanisms, however, other processes are required. For instance, we need to track the source (agent) of a representation if that of the self and that of the other are fairly similar and we need to be able to switch voluntarily between them. We also need to modulate the initial resonance so we are not immersed by other people's emotions. Recent models of empathy do take into account these interacting processes, and we argue that these secondary processes rely in great part on mental imagery.

Despite the various definitions of empathy, there is broad agreement on three components that we have identified as: (1) an affective response to another person, which is based on the shared representation mechanisms; (2) a cognitive capacity to deliberately take the perspective of the other person (which also presupposes self-awareness and likely involves imagery); and (3) some form of emotion regulation (Decety and Jackson 2004, 2006; Decety and Lamm 2006; Decety et al. 2007). Some scholars favour a particular aspect over the others in their definitions. For instance, Hoffman (1981) views empathy as a largely involuntary vicarious response to affective cues from another person, while Batson (1997) emphasize people's intentional role-taking ability, which taps mainly into cognitive resources (and prosocial attitude). These two aspects represent different routes by which empathy can be triggered and in which the automatic tendency to mimic the expressions of others (bottom-up processing) and the capacity for the imaginative and wilful transposition of oneself into the feelings and thinking of another (top-down processing) are differentially involved. Moreover, both aspects tap, to some extent, similar neural mechanisms that underpin emotion processing. As discussed previously, it is unlikely, however, that the overlap between self- and other representations is absolute. Such a complete overlap between self and other could lead to personal distress (i.e., a self-focused, aversive response to another's emotional state). This would consequently hamper the ability to switch between self- and other perspectives and would not constitute an adaptive behaviour. Therefore, regulatory processes are at play to prevent confusion between self- and other feelings. Contrary to the first two components, these regulating processes likely stem from both automatic and controlled mechanisms. The importance to distinguish between automatic versus controlled processes comes from the rehabilitation framework in which we operate. If we are to develop means to intervene and improve (or in some case reduce) people's shared representation processes and ultimately empathy in neurological and psychiatric populations, we need to identify which part can be modified through deliberate and conscious acts, and which ones need more implicit types of learning. Evolutionary speaking, the end product of the three distinct components of empathy can then lead to a defensive, aggressive, or prosocial stance towards the other person. Our work on empathy focuses on the latter, as we believe that we can imagine the actions and emotions of others to help us understand and eventually care about them. The form of the behavioural response that follows empathy is proposed in some models (Goubert et al. 2005) but has been largely neglected thus far.

Conclusion

The same processes that allow us to evoke motor information either through simple observation or even in the absence of external stimulation during motor imagery, are also at play when sensory and affective information is evoked. This initial representation can then be regulated through higher level cognitive abilities and yield social skills. Altogether, the findings from the pain and emotion observation literature illustrate how shared representations are not fixed perception-action matching mechanisms but can be modified over years of experience, through changes in the individual as well as changes within the environment. The study of the development of this mechanism in children promises some novel and fascinating lines of research, and the debate rages on as to whether and, if so, to what level non-human primates (Call and Tomasello 2008) also share this ability to represent mentally the actions of others.

Acknowledgements

This work was made possible thanks to grants awarded to P.L.J. from the National Sciences and Engineering Research Council of Canada (NSERC), NARSAD – The World's Leading Charity Dedicated to Mental Health Research, and salary grants from the Fonds de la Recherche en Santé du Québec (FRSQ) and the Canadian Institutes of Health Research (CIHR). A.M.A. is supported by a fellowship from the CIHR.

References

Allison, T., McCarthy, G., and Wood, C.C. (1992). The relationship between human long-latency somatosensory evoked potentials recorded from the cortical surface and from the scalp. *Electroencephalography and Clinical Neurophysiology*, **84**, 301–14.

Avenanti, A., Bueti, D., Galati, G., and Aglioti, S.M. (2005). Transcranial magnetic stimulation highlights the sensorimotor side of empathy for pain. *Nature Neuroscience*, **8**, 955–60.

Avenanti, A., Minio Paluello, I., Bufalari, I., and Aglioti, S.M. (2006). Stimulus-driven modulation of motor-evoked potentials during observation of others' pain. *Neuroimage*, **32**, 316–24.

Avenanti, A., Minio-Paluello, I., Bufalari, I., and Aglioti, S.M. (2008). The pain of a model in the personality of an onlooker: influence of state-reactivity and personality traits on embodied empathy for pain. *Neuroimage*, **44**, 275–83.

Basch, M.F. (1983). Empathic understanding: a review of the concept and some theoretical considerations. *Journal of the American Psychoanalytic Association*, **31**, 101–26.

Batson, C.D. (1997). Self–Other merging and empathy-altruism hypothesis: reply to Neuberg *et al.* (1997). *Journal of Personality and Social Psychology*, **73**, 517–22.

Beaumont, G., Carrier, J.N., Fortin, M., *et al.* (2009), Improving the mental representation of action to decrease phantom limb pain. *Pain Research and Management*, **14**, 127.

Blakemore, S.J., Bristow, D., Bird, G., Frith, C., and Ward, J. (2005). Somatosensory activations during the observation of touch and a case of vision-touch synaesthesia. *Brain*, **128**, 1571–83.

Botvinick, M., Jha, A.P., Bylsma, L.M., Fabian, S.A., Solomon, P.E., and Prkachin, K.M. (2005). Viewing facial expressions of pain engages cortical areas involved in the direct experience of pain. *Neuroimage*, **25**, 312–9.

Bufalari, I., Aprile, T., Avenanti, A., Di Russo, F., and Aglioti, S.M. (2007). Empathy for pain and touch in the human somatosensory cortex, *Cerebral Cortex*. **17**, 2553–61.

Cairns, R.B., Leung, M.C., Gest, S.D., and Cairns, B.D. (1995). A brief method for assessing social development: structure, reliability, stability, and developmental validity of the Interpersonal Competence Scale. *Behavioural Research Therapy*, **33**, 725–36.

Call, J. and Tomasello, M. (2008). Does the chimpanzee have a theory of mind? 30 years later. *Trends in Cognitive Sciences*, **12**, 187–92.

Carr, L., Iacoboni, M., Dubeau, M.C., Mazziotta, J.C., and Lenzi, G.L. (2003). Neural mechanisms of empathy in humans: a relay from neural systems for imitation to limbic areas. *Proceedings of the National Academy of Sciences U.S.A.*, **100**, 5497–502.

Cheng, Y., Lin, C.P., Liu, H.L., *et al.* (2007). Expertise modulates the perception of pain in others, *Current Biology*. **17**, 1708–13.

Cheng, Y., Yang, C.Y., Lin, C.P., Lee, P.L., and Decety, J. (2008). The perception of pain in others suppresses somatosensory oscillations: a magnetoencephalography study. *Neuroimage*, **40**, 1833–40.

Cross, E.S., Kraemer, D.J., Hamilton, A.F., Kelley, W.M., and Grafton, S.T. (2009). Sensitivity of the action observation network to physical and observational learning. *Cerebral Cortex*, **19**, 315–326.

Cupal, D. and Brewer, B. (2001). Effects of relaxation and guided imagery on knee strength, reinjury anxiety, and pain following anterior cruciate ligament reconstruction. *Rehabilitation Psychology*, **46**, 28–43.

Damasio, A.R. (1994). *Descartes Error: Emotion, Reason and the Human Brain*. New York: G.P. Putnam's Sons.

Davis, M.H. (1983). Measuring individual differences in empathy: evidence for a multidimensional approach. *Journal of Personality and Social Psychology*, **44**, 113–26.

de Vignemont, F. and Singer, T. (2006). The empathic brain: how, when and why? *Trends in Cognitive Sciences*, **10**, 435–41.

Decety, J. and Jackson, P.L. (2004). The functional architecture of human empathy. *Behavioural Cognitive Neurosciences Reviews*, **3**, 71–100.

Decety, J. and Jackson, P.L. (2006). A social neuroscience perspective of empathy. *Current Direction in Psychological Sciences*, **15**, 54–8.

Decety, J., Jackson, P.L., and Brunet, E. (2007), The cognitive neuropsychology of empathy, in T.F. Farrow and P.W. Woodruff (eds), *Empathy in Mental Illness and Health*. New York: Cambridge University Press.

Decety, J. and Lamm, C. (2006). Human empathy through the lens of social neuroscience. *Scientific World Journal*, **6**, 1146–63.

Decety, J. and Sommerville, J.A. (2003). Shared representations between self and other: a social cognitive neuroscience view. *Trends in Cognitive Sciences*, **7**, 527–33.

Dimberg, U. (1982). Facial reactions to facial expressions. *Psychophysiology*, **19**, 643–7.

Dimberg, U., Thunberg, M., and Elmehed, K. (2000). Unconscious facial reactions to emotional facial expressions. *Psychological Science*, **11**, 86–9.

Fan, Y. and Han, S. (2008). Temporal dynamic of neural mechanisms involved in empathy for pain: an event-related brain potential study. *Neuropsychologia*, **46**, 160–73.

Fecteau, S., Pascual-Leone, A., and Théoret, H. (2008). Psychopathy and the mirror neuron system: Preliminary findings from a non-psychiatric sample. *Psychiatry Research*, **160**, 137–44.

Frith, C.D. and Frith, U. (2006). The neural basis of mentalizing. *Neuron*, **50**, 531–4.

Gallese, V. and Goldman, A. (1998). Mirror neurons and the simulation theory of mind-reading. *Trends in Cognitive Sciences*, **2**, 493–501.

Goubert, L., Craig, K.D., Vervoort, T. *et al.* (2005). Facing others in pain: the effects of empathy. *Pain*, **118**, 285–8.

Gu, X. and Han, S. (2007). Attention and reality constraints on the neural processes of empathy for pain. *Neuroimage*, **36**, 256–67.

Guillot, A., Collet, C., Nguyen, V.A., Malouin, F., Richards, C., and Doyon, J. (2008). Functional neuroanatomical networks associated with expertise in motor imagery. *Neuroimage*, **41**, 1471–83.

Han, S., Fan, Y. and Mao, L. (2008). Gender difference in empathy for pain: an electrophysiological investigation. *Brain Research*, **1196**, 85–93.

Hennenlotter, A., Dresel, C., Castrop, F., Ceballos Baumann, A.O., Wohlschlager, A.M., and Haslinger, B. (2009). The link between facial feedback and neural activity within central circuitries of emotion – new insights from botulinum toxin-induced denervation of frown muscles. *Cerebral Cortex*, **19**, 537–42.

Hoffman, M.L. (1981). Is altruism part of human nature? *Journal of Personality and Social Psychology*, **40**, 121–37.

Hutchison, W.D., Davis, K.D., Lozano, A.M., Tasker, R.R., and Dostrovsky, J.O. (1999). Pain-related neurons in the human cingulate cortex. *Nature Neuroscience*, **2**, 403–5.

Iacoboni, M. and Lenzi, G.L. (2002). Mirror neurons, the insula, and empathy. *Behavioral and Brain Sciences*, **25**, 39–40.

Jabbi, M., Swart, M., and Keysers, C. (2007). Empathy for positive and negative emotions in the gustatory cortex. *Neuroimage*, **34**, 1744–53.

Jackson, P.L., Brunet, E., Meltzoff, A.N., and Decety, J. (2006a). Empathy examined through the neural mechanisms involved in imagining how I feel versus how you feel pain. *Neuropsychologia*, **44**, 752–61.

Jackson, P.L., Lafleur, M.F., Malouin, F., Richards, C., and Doyon, J. (2003). Functional reorganization associated with motor sequence learning using mental practice with motor imagery. *Neuroimage*, **20**, 1171–80.

Jackson, P.L., Meltzoff, A.N., and Decety, J. (2005). How do we perceive the pain of others? A window into the neural processes involved in empathy. *Neuroimage*, **24**, 771–9.

Jackson, P.L., Meltzoff, A.N., and Decety, J. (2006b). Neural circuits involved in imitation and perspective-taking. *Neuroimage*, **31**, 429–39.

Jackson, P.L., Rainville, P., and Decety, J. (2006c). To what extent do we share the pain of others? Insight from the neural bases of pain empathy. *Pain*, **125**, 5–9.

Jackson, P.L., Voisin, J., Mercier, C., Canizales, D.L., Marcoux, L.A., and Lauzon, P.O. (June 2007). Pain observation modulates the cerebral response to a vibrotactile stimulation. *Human Brain Mapping Organization Conference*, Chicago.

Jeannerod, M. (2001). Neural simulation of action: a unifying mechanism for motor cognition. *Neuroimage*, **14**, s103–9.

Keysers, C., Wicker, B., Gazzola, V., Anton, J.L., Fogassi, L., and Gallese, V. (2004). A touching sight: SII/PV activation during the observation and experience of touch. *Neuron*, **42**, 335–46.

Kim, S.E., Kim, J.W., Kim, J.J. *et al.* (2007). The neural mechanism of imagining facial affective expression. *Brain Research*, **1145**, 128–37.

Lacey, J. and Lacey, B. (1958). Verification and extension of the principle of autonomic response-stereotypy. *American Journal of Psychology*, **71**, 50–73.

Lamm, C., Nusbaum, H.C., Meltzoff, A.N., and Decety, J. (2007). What are you feeling? Using functional magnetic resonance imaging to assess the modulation of sensory and affective responses during empathy for pain. *PLoS ONE*, **2**, e1292.

Leonard, G. and Tremblay, F. (2007). Corticomotor facilitation associated with observation, imagery and imitation of hand actions: a comparative study in young and old adults. *Experimental Brain Research*, **177**, 167–75.

Leslie, K.R., Johnson-Frey, S.H., and Grafton, S.T. (2004). Functional imaging of face and hand imitation: towards a motor theory of empathy. *Neuroimage*, **21**, 601–7.

Levenson, R.W. and Ruef, A.M. (1992). Empathy: a physiological substrate. *Journal of Personality and Social Psychology*, **63**, 234–46.

Loggia, M.L., Mogil, J.S., and Bushnell, M.C. (2008). Empathy hurts: compassion for another increases both sensory and affective components of pain perception. *Pain*, **136**, 168–76.

Ly, T.N., Jackson, P.L., Jakmakjian, E., and Rainville, P. (2007) The interaction between the experience of pain and the perception of pain in others, *Canadian Pain Society Meeting*, Ottawa.

Magnee, M.J., Stekelenburg, J.J., Kemner, C., and de Gelder, B. (2007). Similar facial electromyographic responses to faces, voices, and body expressions. *Neuroreport*, **18**, 369–72.

Michon, P.E. and Jackson, P.L. (March 2008). Différences dans l'interprétation de la douleur d'autrui selon le genre. *30e congrès annuel de la SQRP*, Trois-Rivières.

Moody, E.J., McIntosh, D.N., Mann, L.J., and Weisser, K.R. (2007). More than mere mimicry? The influence of emotion on rapid facial reactions to faces. *Emotion*, **7**, 447–57.

Morrison, I. and Downing, P.E. (2007). Organization of felt and seen pain responses in anterior cingulate cortex. *Neuroimage*, **37**, 642–51.

Morrison, I., Lloyd, D., di Pellegrino, G., and Robets, N. (2004). How do we perceive the pain of others? A window into the processes involved in empathy. *Neuroimage*, **24**, 771–9.

Morrison, I., Peelen, M.V., and Downing, P.E. (2007). The sight of others' pain modulates motor processing in human cingulate cortex. *Cerebral Cortex*, **17**, 2214–22.

Munzert, J., Zentgraf, K., Stark, R., and Vaitl, D. (2008). Neural activation in cognitive motor processes: comparing motor imagery and observation of gymnastic movements. *Experimental Brain Research*, **188**, 437–44.

Pfeifer, J.H., Iacoboni, M., Mazziotta, J.C., and Dapretto, M. (2008). Mirroring others' emotions relates to empathy and interpersonal competence in children. *Neuroimage*, **39**, 2076–85.

Preston, S.D. and de Waal, F.B.M. (2002). Empathy: Its ultimate and proximate bases. *Behavioral and Brain Sciences*, **25**, 1–71.

Rainville, P. (2002). Brain mechanisms of pain affect and pain modulation. *Current Opinion in Neurobiology*, **12**, 195–204.

Ramachandran, V.S. and Rogers-Ramachandran, D. (1996). Synaesthesia in phantom limbs induced with mirrors. *Proceedings in Biological Science*, **263**, 377–86.

Saarela, M., Hlushchuk, Y., Williams, A., Schürmann, M., Kalso, E., and Hari, R. (2007). The compassionate brain: humans detect intensity of pain from another's face. *Cerebral Cortex*, **17**, 230–7.

Simon, D., Craig, K.D., Miltner, W.H., and Rainville, P. (2006). Brain responses to dynamic facial expressions of pain. *Pain*, **126**, 309–18.

Singer, T., Seymour, B., O'Doherty, J., Kaube, H., Dolan, R.J., and Frith, C.D. (2004). Empathy for pain involves the affective but not sensory components of pain. *Science*, **303**, 1157–62.

Singer, T., Seymour, B., O'Doherty, J.P., Stephan, K.E., Dolan, R.J., and Frith, C.D. (2006). Empathic neural responses are modulated by the perceived fairness of others. *Nature*, **439**, 466–9.

Valeriani, M., Betti, V., Le Pera, D. *et al.* (2008). Seeing the pain of others while being in pain: a laser-evoked potentials study. *Neuroimage*, **40**, 1419–28.

Wicker, B., Keysers, C., Plailly, J., Royet, J.P., Gallese, V., and Rizzolatti, G. (2003). Both of us disgusted in my insula: the common neural basis of seeing and feeling disgust. *Neuron*, **40**, 655–64.

Zaki, J., Ochsner, K.N., Hanelin, J., Wager, T.D., and Mackey, S.C. (2007). Different circuits for different pain: patterns of functional connectivity reveal distinct networks for processing pain in self and others. *Social Neuroscience*, **2**, 276–91.

Index